MW01488985

© 2022 Sharon Rush – Growise Ltd

The Low-FODMAP Cookbook: 400 Quick & Easy Gut-Friendly Recipes to Relieve the Symptoms of IBS and Other Digestive Disorders | 30-Day Organized Meal Plan to Beat Bloat and Soothe Your Gut Effortlessly

ISBN 9798832563589

10 9 8 7 6 5 4 3 2 1

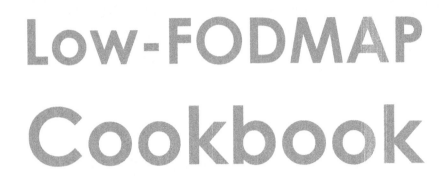

Low-FODMAP Cookbook

400 Quick & Easy Gut-Friendly Recipes to Relieve the Symptoms of IBS and Other Digestive Disorders. 30-Day Organized Meal Plan to Beat Bloat and Soothe Your Gut Effortlessly

Sharon Rush

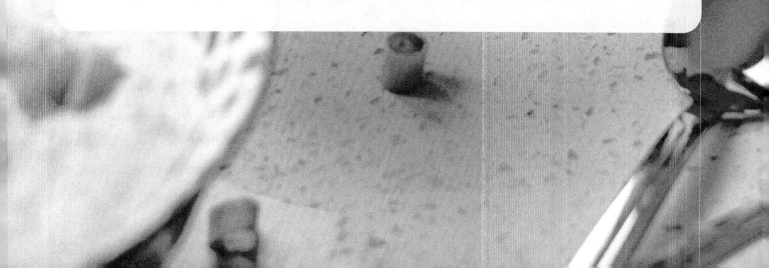

Table of Contents

Introduction

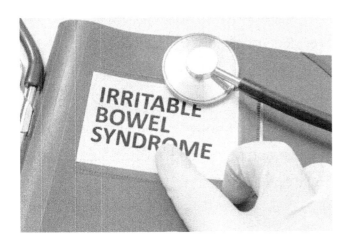

Irritable bowel syndrome (IBS) affects one out of every ten individuals worldwide, and it's a chronic disorder characterized by stomach discomfort and bloating, excessive gas, diarrhea or constipation, or both on a regular basis. While doctors are adept at recognizing the problem, they have a poor track record at resolving it. If you have IBS, one or more food intolerances, or other chronic digestive problems, this is the book for you and are tired of feeling ill. The low-FODMAP diet was the first to be scientifically demonstrated to treat IBS symptoms. It can also assist with Cohn's disease, ulcerative colitis, and celiac disease (alongside a fully gluten-free diet). The program has changed many people's lives, and it might work for you as well.

FODMAP stands for fermentable, poorly absorbed short-chain carbohydrates that offer quick food for intestinal bacteria and may induce digestive pain. Fermentable Oligosaccharides, Disaccharides, Monosaccharides, and Polyols (FODMAP) is an acronym for fermentable oligosaccharides, disaccharides, monosaccharides, and polyols. If this all seems a little too complicated, keep in mind that saccharide is only another term for sugar. Polyols are sugar alcohols, sugar molecules with an alcohol side chain, whereas oligosaccharides, disaccharides, and monosaccharides are carbohydrates made up of sugar molecules.

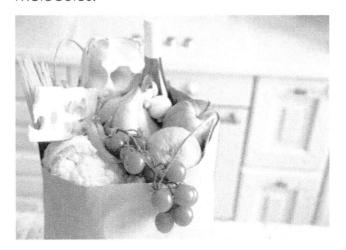

Chapter 1: What is Low-FODMAP Diet and IBS- An Overview

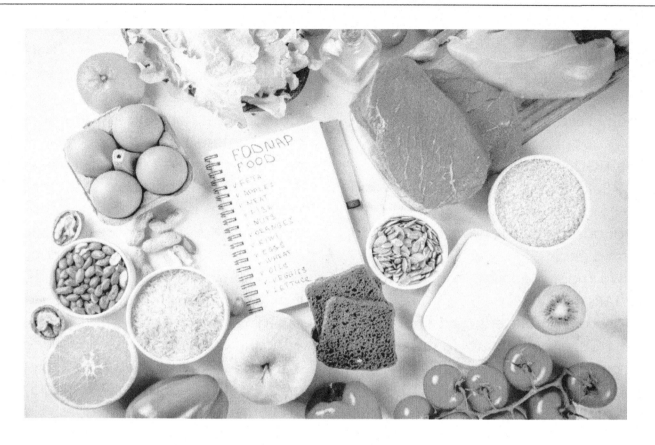

The low-FODMAP diet was created by researchers in 1999, and it has been proved to treat at least three out of four persons with IBS, a condition that has previously been difficult to control. It also shows promise in treating celiac disease, Cohn's disease, and ulcerative colitis symptoms that remain. FODMAPs are a type of naturally occurring sugar that is not absorbed in the small intestine and instead travels through the rest of the digestive system to the large intestine, where bacteria live (which is normal and healthy). Unabsorbed sugars (FODMAPs) provide a food supply for these bacteria. When bacteria digest FODMAPs, they ferment them, resulting in the production of gas, which can cause excessive flatulence, gassiness, bloating, abdominal distension, and discomfort. FODMAPs can also slow down the movement of the intestines, causing constipation or diarrhea (or a mix of both) in those who are sensitive to them. As a result, it's extremely evident how FODMAPs cause IBS symptoms.

1.1. FODMAP

FODMAP is an acronym that stands for:

FERMENTABLE
Bacteria in the large intestine ferment these poorly absorbed carbohydrates (bowel).

OLIGOSACCHARIDES
Saccharide means sugar, and oligo means little. So they are individual sugars that have been linked to form a chain.
The two main oligosaccharides that are FODMAPs are:
Fructans are fructose sugars that have been linked together to form a chain (with glucose at the very end).
Galactooligosaccharides (GOS) are oligosaccharides made up of galactose sugars bonded together at the end with fructose and glucose.

DISACCHARIDES
Saccharide means sugar, and di means two. So they are two separate sugars that have been combined to form a double sugar.
Lactose, a FODMAP disaccharide composed of an individual glucose sugar connected to an individual galactose sugar, is the most significant FODMAP disaccharide.

MONOSACCHARIDES
Saccharide means sugar, and mono signifies one. So they are sugars in their own right.

Excess fructose is a key FODMAP monosaccharide. Fructose does not have to be avoided entirely. On the low fodmap diet, only foods that contain more fructose than glucose (also known as "excess fructose") should be avoided.
An item is acceptable for the low fodmap diet if it contains more glucose than fructose or if glucose and fructose are present in equal ("balanced") proportions.
If a food (for example, a piece of fruit) contains more glucose than fructose or equal amounts of fructose and glucose, it is suitable to eat; however, only one piece of suitable fruit should be consumed at a time. This doesn't mean you can only have one piece of fruit per day! You can have several but spread them out so that you only have one per sitting.

AND **P**OLYOLS

A polyol is a sugar molecule with an alcohol side chain attached. Polyols are also known as sugar alcohols but don't worry; they won't get you drunk!
Sorbitol and mannitol are the two polyols found most frequently in foods.

1.2. Irritable Bowel Syndrome

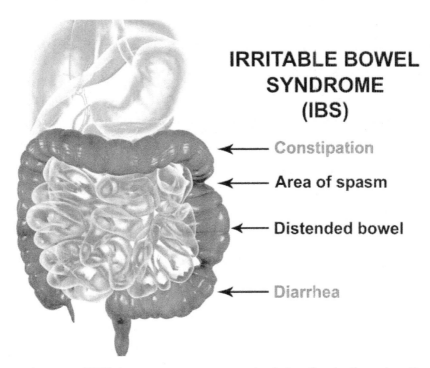

Irritable bowel syndrome (IBS) is a common gastrointestinal disorder that affects around 15% of the population. Males and ladies of various ages are affected. Excess flatulence, stomach bloating, distension, pain, or discomfort, and changed bowel habits are all symptoms (diarrhea, constipation, or a combination of both). The intensity of these symptoms varies from day to day and week to week. Because IBS is diagnosed based on the pattern of symptoms, it's critical to rule out other disorders with similar symptoms, such as celiac disease and inflammatory bowel disease (IBD), which can potentially be mistaken for IBS. Before starting a low-FODMAP or gluten-free diet, everyone with IBS symptoms should be evaluated for these illnesses, so if you haven't already, talk to your doctor about getting tested. However, keep in mind that IBS and other digestive diseases can coexist.

FODMAPs cause IBS

FODMAPs all have the same characteristics:

1. They have a low absorption rate in the small intestine. This implies that many of these molecules skip past the small intestine without being absorbed instead of traveling straight to the colon. This is due to their inability to be broken down or their delayed absorption. Our capacity to digest and absorb various FODMAPs varies from person to person: Fructose absorption varies from person to person; some people do not produce enough lactase (the enzyme needed to break down lactose), and the capacity to absorb polyols (which are the wrong shape to pass easily through the small intestinal

15

lining) also varies. Fructans and galactooligosaccharides (GOS) are poorly absorbed in everyone since none of us can digest them.

2. They are little molecules that are eaten in high doses. The body tries to "dilute" tiny, concentrated molecules by pumping water into the gastrointestinal system when they are poorly absorbed. Extra fluid in the gastrointestinal system can produce diarrhea and interfere with the gut's muscular activity.

3. They're "quick food" for the bacteria that exist in the big intestine naturally. Billions of bacteria live in the large intestine (and the bottom section of the small intestine). If chemicals aren't absorbed in the small intestine, they make their way to the large intestine. These food molecules are seen as rapid food by the bacteria that reside there, and they are swiftly broken down, releasing hydrogen, carbon dioxide, and methane gases. The length of the chain determines how rapidly the molecules are fermented: In comparison to fiber, which comprises considerably longer chain molecules known as polysaccharides, oligosaccharides, and simple sugars ferment relatively quickly. In most meals, many forms of FODMAPs are present. Their effects are cumulative since they all produce distension in the same way until they reach the lower small intestine and colon. This indicates that the degree of intestinal distension can be determined by the overall quantity of FODMAPs taken rather than the amount of anyone FODMAP. Suppose someone who has trouble digesting lactose and absorbing fructose consumes a meal with some lactose. In that case, fructans, polyols, GOS, and fructose, the effect on the intestine will be $1 + 1 + 1 + 1 + 1 = 5$ times larger than if they ate the same quantity of simply one of that FODMAPs. As a result, we must take all FODMAPs into account while changing our diet.

1.3. Symptoms of IBS

Common IBS Symptoms

Constipation

Diarrhea

Mixed bowel habits

Mucus in bowel movements

Feeling of incomplete bowel movements

Looser and/or more frequent stools

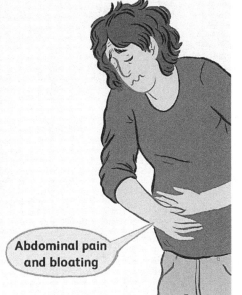

Abdominal pain and bloating

1.4. Moderate and Low-FODMAP Foods and Grocery List

Vegetables:
- ☐ green beans
- ☐ bell peppers
- ☐ carrots
- ☐ lettuce
- ☐ tomatoes
- ☐ zucchini
- ☐ bok choy
- ☐ alfalfa
- ☐ bean sprouts

Proteins:
- ☐ beef
- ☐ chicken
- ☐ pork
- ☐ lamb
- ☐ fish
- ☐ eggs
- ☐ tofu
- ☐ tempeh
- ☐ shellfish

Fruits:
- ☐ bananas
- ☐ oranges
- ☐ grapes
- ☐ raspberries
- ☐ strawberries
- ☐ blueberries
- ☐ cranberries
- ☐ grapefruit
- ☐ lemons, limes

Grains:
- ☐ GF breads
- ☐ GF cereals
- ☐ oats
- ☐ rice
- ☐ polenta
- ☐ quinoa
- ☐ popcorn

Dairy:
- ☐ lactose-free milk
- ☐ lactose-free yogurt
- ☐ soy milk
- ☐ oat milk
- ☐ rice milk
- ☐ hard cheeses
- ☐ brie
- ☐ camembert

Sweeteners:
- ☐ sugar
- ☐ brown sugar
- ☐ stevia
- ☐ pure maple syrup

Nuts:
- ☐ almonds
- ☐ pumpkin seeds

Fruits	pomegranate (seeds from ½ small), rambutan (3 whole)
Vegetables	asparagus (3 spears), beet (½ medium), broccoli (½ cup), Brussels sprouts (½ cup), butternut squash (¼ cup), savoy cabbage (1 cup), fennel (½ cup), green peas (⅓ cup), snow peas (10 pods), sweet corn (½ cob)
Legumes	well-rinsed canned chickpeas (up to ¼ cup),* well-rinsed canned red or brown lentils (up to ¼ cup)*
Nuts	almonds (up to 10), hazelnuts (up to 10), one handful of all other nuts and all seeds; 2 tablespoons of nut and seed butters

Fruits	all others not mentioned above
Vegetables	alfalfa sprouts, avocados, bamboo shoots, bean shoots, bell peppers, bok choy, broccoli, carrots, cauliflower, celery, Chinese cabbage, chives, cucumber, eggplant, endive, ginger, green beans, lettuce, mushrooms, olives, parsnips, potatoes, pumpkin, Swiss chard, spinach, scallions (green part only), squash (all summer and winter varieties except for butternut squash), rutabaga, sweet potatoes, taro, tomatoes, turnips, watercress, yams, zucchini
Cereals, grains, and starches	arrowroot, buckwheat, cornmeal, cornstarch, millet, oats, popcorn, potatoes, quinoa, rice, sorghum, tapioca
Legumes	tempeh, tofu
Drinks	regular tea and coffee, many herbal teas and infusions
Fiber supplements	chia seeds, flaxseeds, oat bran, psyllium, rice bran

1.5. Implementing Low-FODMAP Diet

If you've been diagnosed with IBS, or if you've had bloating and abdominal discomfort without a change in bowel habits, or if you and/or your doctor believe you should follow the low fodmap diet for another reason, your first step should be to contact a registered dietitian who specializes in gastrointestinal nutrition. That isn't to argue that following a low fodmap diet is impossible, but it will necessitate major dietary and lifestyle modifications. You'll need to understand your illness, which foods are appropriate, and what will happen if you don't stick to the diet. To keep your symptoms under control, we recommend sticking to the low fodmap diet for at least two months and avoiding any FODMAPs. Whether your symptoms have improved after this period, slowly reintroduce one FODMAP group at a time to determine if you can handle it. This is easiest to accomplish with the assistance of a qualified dietitian, who will examine your symptoms and recommend the best course of action, but for additional information on how to do it yourself and meal plans, go here.

At first, you may find certain components of the low fodmap diet to be overwhelming. Each morning, you'll have to ask yourself the following questions: What will I be doing today? Is it necessary for me to bring food? Should I eat something before I leave? Will there be something I can eat there? If you have to follow a specific diet, it can begin to control your thinking, and some individuals are better at dealing with this than others. Seek therapy or other assistance if you're having problems adapting. Here are some more considerations to keep in mind while creating a low fodmap diet to your specific needs:

Consider all the FODMAP groups. They all have the potential to cause bowel distension and other IBS symptoms.

No one can absorb fructans, GOS, or polyols well. This means you should always avoid them when first implementing the low fodmap diet.

Only some people have lactose or fructose malabsorption. A breath hydrogen test will tell you whether or not you need to limit lactose or excess fructose in your diet.

Some FODMAPs cause more trouble in some people than others. This depends on the proportions of each FODMAP in their diet, how well or poorly they absorb fructose and lactose, and how sensitive they are to each FODMAP, which could be related to which bacteria they have in their bowel. You'll learn which FODMAPs give you the most trouble through a combination of clinical tests and trials in your diet.

1.6. Alternatives on a Low-FODMAP Diet

SUGGESTED ALTERNATIVES TO WHEAT-BASED FOODS		
	Wheat-based varieties	Suggested alternatives
Bread	white, whole wheat, multigrain, and sourdough breads, pita bread, many "rye breads"	corn tortillas, gluten-free bread,* gluten-free flatbread,* 100% spelt bread (for some people)
Pasta, noodles, and grains	regular pasta, spelt pasta, most instant noodles, egg noodles, udon, gnocchi, bulgur, farro	gluten-free pasta,* glass (mungbean) noodles, rice noodles (vermicelli), wheat-free soba (buckwheat) noodles
Breakfast cereals	most are made from wheat and may also contain excess dried fruit or be sweetened with fruit juice	many gluten-free breakfast cereals, cornflakes, wheat-free fruit-free muesli, oatmeal, quinoa flakes, rice flakes, rice puffs
Crackers	wheat-based varieties, water crackers	corn thins, gluten-free crackers, gluten-free crispbread (such as buckwheat), rice cakes or crackers (but check for onion powder)
Cakes and baked goods	most are made from wheat	flourless cakes, gluten-free cakes,* gluten-free baking mixes*
Cookies	wheat-based varieties	almond macaroons, gluten-free cookies*
Pastry and bread crumbs	made with wheat flour	gluten-free pastry mixes,* cornflake crumbs, gluten-free bread crumbs* (although wheat-based crumbs can usually be tolerated in small amounts)
Other cereal products	semolina, couscous, bulgur	buckwheat, chestnut, chia seeds, corn, millet, polenta, potatoes, quinoa, rice, sago, sorghum, tapioca, and their flours

	High-FODMAP varieties	LowFODMAP alternatives
Flours and grains (including legume products)	barley, bulgur, chickpea flour (besan),* couscous, durum, Kamut®, lentil flour,* multigrain flour, pea flour,* rye, semolina, soy flour,* triticale, wheat bran, wheat flour, wheat germ	arrowroot, buckwheat flour, cornmeal, cornstarch, gluten-free flour blends,** glutinous rice, ground rice, malt, millet, oat bran, oatmeal, polenta, popcorn, potato flour, quinoa, rice (brown, white), rice bran, rice flour, sago, sorghum, tapioca, wild rice
Cereals	wheat-based and mixed-grain breakfast cereals, muesli	baby rice cereal, cream of buckwheat, rice-or corn-based breakfast cereals, oatmeal, wheat-free, fruit-free muesli
Pasta and noodles	noodles, pasta, spaetzle, gnocchi	glass (mungbean) noodles, rice noodles, rice vermicelli, 100% buckwheat soba noodles, gluten-free pasta
Breads, cookies, and cakes	breads (including sourdough), bread crumbs, cookies, cakes, croissants, muffins, and pastries containing wheat and rye	gluten-free breads,** corn tortillas and taco shells, plain rice cakes and crackers, gluten-free cookies,** gluten-free cakes and pastries**
Dairy foods and alternatives	regular milk, ice cream, soft cheeses (in amounts greater than ½ cup), yogurt	lactose-free milk; most lactose-free yogurts and kefir; lactose-free ice cream; calcium-fortified soy,† rice, oat, and quinoa milks, yogurts, and ice creams; butter and margarine; hard and ripened cheeses, including Brie and Camembert; gelato and sorbets made from suitable fruits and sweeteners; moderate servings of cream (less than ½ cup)
Meat and vegetarian protein sources	certain sausages (check for onion and dehydrated vegetable powders)	bacon, eggs, fish, poultry, plain red meat, tempeh, tofu
Nuts and seeds	pistachios and cashews	all other nuts and seeds; nut and seed butters not made from pistachios or cashews (no more than a handful of nuts and seeds or 2 tablespoons of nut or seed butters in a meal)
Vegetables	artichokes (globe and Jerusalem), asparagus, cauliflower, garlic, leeks, mushrooms, onions (yellow, red, white, onion powder), scallions (white part), shallots, snow peas, sugar snap peas	alfalfa sprouts, bamboo shoots, bean sprouts, bok choy, bell pepper, carrot, chayote, Chinese cabbage, cucumber, eggplant, green beans, lettuce (butter, iceberg, romaine), olives, parsnip, potatoes, pumpkin, rutabagas, Swiss chard, spinach, scallion (green part only), squash (all tested varieties except butternut squash—note that not all have been tested), taro, turnips, watercress, yams, zucchini

Fruits	apples, apricots, Asian pears, blackberries, boysenberries, cherries, figs, mangoes, nectarines, peaches, pears, persimmon, plums, prunes, tamarillo, watermelon, white peaches	bananas, blueberries, cantaloupe, cranberries, durian, grapefruit, grapes, honeydew melon, kiwi, lemons, limes, mandarin oranges, oranges, passion fruit, papaya, raspberries, star fruit, strawberries, tangelos, tangerines, tomatoes
Spreads and condiments	most commercial relishes, chutneys, onion-containing gravies, stock and bouillon cubes, dressings, and sauces	jam, marmalade, mayonnaise, mustard, soy sauce, garlic-free sweet chili sauce or hot sauce, tamari, vinegar
Sweeteners	agave nectar, honey, high-fructose corn syrup, corn syrup solids, fructose, fruit juice concentrate; sorbitol, mannitol, maltitol, xylitol	sucrose (table sugar, cane sugar), including superfine sugar, confectioners' sugar, brown sugar, raw sugar; glucose; maple syrup, molasses, rice syrup; artificial sweeteners not ending in "ol" (e.g., aspartame, saccharine, and stevia)
Fats and oils	applesauce as oil replacer in low-fat baked goods	vegetable oils, butter, ghee, lard, drippings, margarine, garlic-infused oil as an onion and garlic substitute
Others		baking powder, baking soda, cocoa, coconut, gelatin, salt, xanthan gum, fresh and dried herbs and spices

Chapter 2: Elimination Diet and 7-day Meal Plan

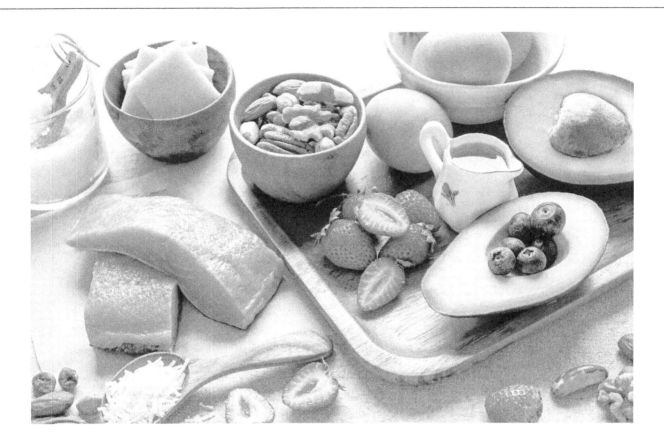

2.1. Elimination Diet

The following points will help you learn as much as possible about your IBS triggers while on the FODMAP elimination phase of this program.

1. This is a temporary learning diet. It's not a long-term diet.

2. Begin at a reasonable hour. Start at the beginning of a two-week period, when you have some additional time to plan meals, go grocery shopping, and prepare food. Start shortly after you've emptied your bowels and before the next episode of constipation starts in if you have IBS with constipation or a mixed-bowel pattern.

3. Take a vacation from your vitamin and mineral supplements if you can. Set your supplements aside for the time being unless you're taking a recommended vitamin or mineral to correct a confirmed nutrient deficit. Some vitamin supplements have a detrimental influence on IBS symptoms, and they might be contributing to your condition. Large amounts of vitamin C or magnesium, for example, might produce diarrhea.

Some calcium and iron supplements might induce bloating and constipation. Fructose and other FODMAPs are included in several chewable or powdered vitamins and minerals.

4. Maintain as much consistency as possible in the remainder of your regimen. Any changes in your symptoms can then be linked to your food adjustment. In collaboration with your prescribing physician, continue to take the majority of your recommended drugs. Some drugs are only given "as required," which means you shouldn't take them if you don't need them. As a general rule, start no additional therapies for your IBS during the first several weeks of the program. There are exceptions to this rule, and you should follow your healthcare provider's advice.

5. Make every effort to keep to the diet. The fewer exceptions you make, the better; after following it for at least two weeks, you'll have learned a lot about your IBS. However, if you make a mistake or consume any FODMAPs out of need, the project will not be damaged, so don't go hungry. Just keep going. Plan ahead of time, carry food if necessary, and make as few exceptions as possible.

6. Don't make snap judgments. You may believe that one kind of FODMAP is not a concern because you consume it on a regular basis. You could believe that ordinary bread and yogurt, for example, aren't a concern because you consume them frequently and don't have any symptoms. Eliminate them nevertheless; eating these items during the elimination period will prevent you from adopting a truly low-FODMAP diet.

7. Concentrate solely on this program. If you try to mix several dietary techniques for IBS management, you can end up with an over-restricted diet. Let go of preconceived conceptions, assumptions, and fear-based dietary limitations. Yes, your gym trainer recommended a paleo diet, and your acupuncturist recommended "GAPS," but you've always avoided nightshade plants after seeing them on TV induce inflammation, and you've heard that individuals with IBS should avoid red meat and caffeine. Allow these notions to fade away for a few weeks as you experiment with this new method.

2.2 Steps of Elimination Diet

Day of the week	Food Program
1	Elimination of suspect foods
Da 2 a 14	Annotation of worsening or improvement of symptoms
15	Reintroduction of a food
Da 16 a 17	Stop the food and note any symptoms
18	Reintroduction of another food
Da 19 a 20	Stop the food and note any symptoms
21	Reintroduction of a third food
Da 22 a 23	Stop the food and note any symptoms
The same process until all suspect foods have been tested	

Basic elimination diet

Food group	Allowed foods	Foods to eliminate
Animal protein	chicken, turkey, pork	eggs, dairy products
Cereals	corn, barley, rice, oats, millet, potatoes, sweet, quinoa, tapioca	wheat
Fats	non-hydrogenated vegetable oils	butter, margarine, cream
Foods always allowed		
Fruits, vegetables, spices, sweeteners, legumes, and nuts		

Level II Elimination Diet

Food group	Allowed foods	Eliminated foods
Animal Protein	Lamb	eggs, dairy products, meat
Vegetable Protein	Anyone	legumes and dried fruit
Cereals	Corn, rice, potato, sweet, tapioca	Wheat, millet, barley, spelled, oats
Vegetables	All others	Peas, tomato
Fruits	All others	Citrus fruits, strawberries
Sweeteners	Whole cane sugar, maple syrup	All others, including aspartame
Fats	Coconut, Olive, Sunflower, Sesame	Butter, lard, margarine, corn oil, soybean oil, peanut oil
Other foods	Salt, pepper, spices, vanilla, lemon extract	Chocolate, coffee, tea, cola, alcohol, sugary drinks

A ONE WEEK FOOD DIARY CHART

(LOG IN ALL FOODS, SUPPLEMENTS, ALCOHOL USE, AND MEDICATIONS TAKEN AND TIMES. NOTE THE SYMPTOMS YOU HAVE AND WHAT TIMES AS WELL)

	DAY 1	DAY 2	DAY 3	DAY 4	DAY 5	DAY 6	DAY 7
MORNING FOODS							
MORNING SYMPTOMS							
AFTERNOON FOODS							
AFTERNOON SYMPTOMS							
EVENING FOODS							
EVENING SYMPTOMS							

2.4 12 Minutes Exercises for IBS

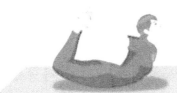

2 miuntes
(Bow Pose)

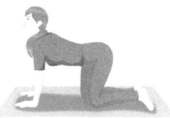

2 miuntes
(Cat Stretch)

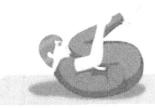

2 miuntes
(Wind-relieving Pose)

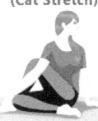

2 miuntes
(Sitting Half Spinal Twist)

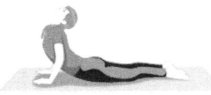

2 miuntes
(Cobra Pose)

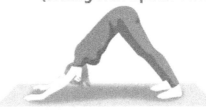

2 miuntes
(Downward-facing Dog Pose)

Chapter 3: Basic Recipes

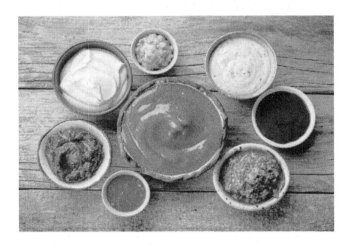

1. Balsamic Vinaigrette

Prep time: 5 min | Serves: 10 | Difficulty: Moderate |
Nutrition: Calories: 82kcal | Fat: 0.1 g | Protein: 0.2g
| Carbohydrates: 3.8 g.

Ingredients
- ¼ cup garlic-infused extra-virgin olive oil
- ¼ cup balsamic vinegar
- 1 teaspoon sugar
- ½ teaspoon salt
- ¼ teaspoon freshly ground black pepper

Instructions
- Whisk together the oil, vinegar, sugar, salt, and pepper in a small mixing bowl until the sugar and salt have dissolved. Serve right away, or cover and chill for up to 4 days.

2. Blue Cheese Dressing

Prep time: 5 min | Serves: 12 | Difficulty: Moderate |
Nutrition: Calories: 64kcal | Fat 1.8g | Protein 0.4g |
Carbohydrate 1g

Ingredients
- ⅓ cup crumbled Gorgonzola cheese
- ⅓ cup mayonnaise
- ⅓ cup lactose-free sour cream
- 1 tablespoon fresh lemon juice

Instructions
- Combine the cheese, mayonnaise, sour cream, and lemon juice in a small bowl.
- Cover securely with plastic wrap and refrigerate until ready to serve.

3. Smoky Ranch Dressing

Prep time: 5 min | Serves: 10-18 | Difficulty: Moderate |

Nutrition: Calories: 71kcal | Fat 2g | Protein 0.5g |
Carbohydrate 2g

Ingredients
- ¼ cup mayonnaise
- ¼ cup lactose-free sour cream
- 1 tablespoon garlic-infused olive oil
- 2 tablespoons fresh lime juice
- 1 teaspoon sugar
- ½ teaspoon salt
- ¼ teaspoon sweet smoked paprika
- 1 teaspoon chia seeds (optional)

Instructions
- Stir together the mayonnaise, sour cream, oil, lime juice, sugar, salt, paprika, and seeds, if using, in a small mixing bowl until well blended. Before serving, carefully cover and refrigerate for 30 minutes.

4. Lemon French Dressing

Prep time: 5 min | Serves: 12 | Difficulty: Moderate |
Nutrition: Calories: 82kcal | Fat 1g | Protein
0g | Carbohydrates 7.2g

Ingredients
- ¼ cup fresh lemon juice
- 3 tablespoons olive oil
- 1 tablespoon garlic-infused olive oil
- ½ teaspoon salt
- ½ teaspoon dry mustard
- ½ teaspoon sweet paprika
- 1½ teaspoons sugar

Instructions
- Combine the lemon juice, oils, salt, mustard, paprika, and sugar in a blender or small bowl and mix until smooth. Serve right away.

5. Basil Pesto

Prep time: 5 min | Serves: 12 | Difficulty: Moderate |
Nutrition: Calories: 78kcal | Fat 1.5g | Protein 0.3g |
Carbohydrate 1.2g

Ingredients
- ¼ cup water
- ½ cup pine nuts
- 1 cup garlic-infused olive oil
- 4 cups tightly packed fresh basil
- 1 cup grated Parmesan cheese
- 1½ teaspoons salt

Instructions

- Grind the pine nuts and water in a blender or food processor until the nuts are split up into small bits. Add the oil and basil alternately, in thirds, while the blades are rotating on medium-high, and process until the mixture is homogeneous and the texture of sand. If your blender comes with a tamper, use it to press the basil leaves closer to the blades as needed. Stir in the Parmesan cheese and salt on low speed until barely blended.
- Refrigerate the pesto securely covered or freeze small portions for later enjoyment; ice cube trays or 12-pint canning jars work nicely for this.

6. Cilantro-Chile-Mint Pesto

Prep time: 5 min | Serves: 5 | Difficulty: Moderate | Nutrition: Calories: 86kcal | Fat:5g | Carbohydrate:2g | Protein: 1.2g

Ingredients

- 1 small fresh green or red chile, chopped
- 1 tablespoon minced fresh ginger
- 2 tablespoons water
- 3 tablespoons fresh lime juice (from I large lime)
- 2 tablespoons walnut pieces
- ¼ cup olive oil
- 1 teaspoon sugar
- 1 teaspoon salt
- 2 cups tightly packed fresh cilantro leaves
- 1 cup tightly packed fresh mint leaves

Instructions

- Combine the chile, ginger, water, lime juice, walnuts, oil, sugar, and salt in a food processor or blender and purée until smooth. Open the lid's hole, and jam handfuls of cilantro and mint leave into the blender while the machine is running; you may need to cover the hole in the lid with your hand in between additions of leaves to prevent spattering.
- Continue to process until you have a coarse paste. If preferred, chill until ready to serve or freeze in little pieces.

7. Beef Stock

Prep time: 50 min | Serves: 12 | Difficulty: Moderate | Nutrition: Calories: 152kcal | Fat 7g | Protein 12g | Carbohydrates 2.9g

Ingredients

- 1 small onion, quartered
- 1 garlic clove
- 2 tablespoons olive oil
- 10 cups water and/or pan drippings
- 2 carrots, coarsely chopped
- 1 bay leaf
- 10 whole peppercorns
- 1 teaspoon salt
- 1 tablespoon reduced-sodium soy sauce

Instructions

- Preheat the oven to 400 degrees Fahrenheit. In a baking pan, roast the beef bones for 1 hour.
- Sauté the onion and garlic in the olive oil in a large stockpot over medium heat. Remove the onion and garlic from the pot when they are translucent and set aside for another use, leaving the flavored oil in the pot.
- Add the beef bones, drippings or water, carrots, water, bay leaf, peppercorns, salt, and soy sauce, as well as the bay leaf, peppercorns, salt, and soy sauce. Bring to a boil over high heat, then lower to a low level and cover and simmer for 112 to 2 hours, or until the stock has reduced by approximately 20%. As required, skim any froth from the surface.
- Cool the stock until it's safe to handle, then strain it to remove the bones and other particles with a slotted spoon or a sieve. Remove the solids and throw them away. Use right away, or cover and store in the refrigerator for up to 3 days, or freeze for up to 3 months. If desired, the firm fat on top of the stock can be readily removed once it has chilled.

8 Chicken Stock

Prep time: 5 min | Serves: 12 | Difficulty: Moderate | Nutrition: Calories: 123kcal | Fat 2g | Protein 8g | Carbohydrate 6g

Ingredients

- 1 small onion, quartered
- 1 garlic clove
- 2 tablespoons olive oil
- 1 carcass from a roasted chicken, including bones and skin
- 2 large carrots, coarsely chopped
- 10 cups water and/or pan drippings
- 1 bay leaf
- 10 whole peppercorns
- 1 teaspoon salt
- 1 tablespoon reduced-sodium soy sauce

Instructions

- Sauté the onion and garlic in the olive oil in a large stockpot over medium heat. Remove the onion and garlic from the pot when they are transparent and set aside, leaving the flavored oil in the pot.
- Add the chicken carcass, carrots, water and drippings, bay leaf, peppercorns, salt, and soy sauce to the pot. Bring to a boil over high heat, then lower to a low level and cover and simmer for 112 to 2 hours, or until the stock has reduced by approximately 20%.
- Allow the stock to cool completely before removing the particles with a slotted spoon or straining through a sieve. Remove the solids and throw them away. Use right away, or cover and store in the refrigerator for up to 3 days, or freeze

for up to 3 months. The solidified fat can be readily removed once the stock has cooled if desired.

9. Seasoned Salt

Prep time: 5 min | Serves: 30 | Difficulty: Moderate |
Nutrition: Calories: 12kcal | Fat 0g | Proteins 0g | Carbohydrates 0.5g

Ingredients
- 1 tablespoon medium salt crystals
- 1 tablespoon black peppercorns
- 1 tablespoon coriander seeds
- 1 tablespoon mustard seeds
- 1 teaspoon red pepper flakes

Instructions
- Combine the salt, peppercorns, seeds, and red pepper flakes in a small bowl.
- Fill a pepper mill or grinder halfway with the mixture. Serve at the table, with fresh seasoned salt sprinkled on top of your favorite foods if preferred.

10. Taco Seasoning Mix

Prep time: 5 min | Serves: 32 | Difficulty: Moderate |
Nutrition: Calories: 16kcal | Fat 0.2g | Protein 0g | Carbohydrate 3g

Ingredients
- ¼ cup cornstarch
- ¼ cup ground ancho chile
- ¼ cup ground ancho chile
- 2 tablespoons ground cumin
- 1 teaspoon sweet smoked paprika
- 2 teaspoons salt

Instructions
- In an airtight container, combine the cornstarch, ground chile, cumin, paprika, and salt. Though Taco Seasoning Mix may be stored forever, for the best flavor, use it within six months.

11. Garlic -Infused Olive Oil

Prep time: 20 min | Serves: 12 | Difficulty: Moderate |
Nutrition: Calories: 98kcal | Fat 2g | Protein 0g | Carbohydrate 2g

Ingredients
- 1 cup plus 1 teaspoon extra-virgin olive oil
- 8 garlic cloves

Instructions
- Heat the oil and garlic in a small, heavy saucepan over medium heat until the garlic starts to crackle and little bubbles rise continuously to the surface. Reduce the heat to low and cook for 10 minutes, or until the garlic is soft.
- Allow it cool for a few minutes before removing the garlic and storing the oil in the refrigerator for up to 4 days, carefully sealed.

12. Zippy Ketchup

Prep time: 5 min | Serves: 12 | Difficulty: Moderate |
Nutrition: Calories: 97kcal | Fat 2g | Protein 1.2g | Carbohydrate 8g

Ingredients
- 1 14.5-ounce can diced tomatoes
- 1 tablespoon garlic-infused olive oil
- 1 small red chile, fresh or dried, minced
- ⅓ cup sugar
- ⅓ cup apple cider vinegar
- ¼ teaspoon sweet smoked paprika
- ¼ teaspoon ground allspice
- ⅛ teaspoon ground cloves
- ½ teaspoon salt, or more as needed

Instructions
- Combine the tomatoes, juices, oil, chile, sugar, vinegar, spices, and salt in a 3-quart pot. Bring the mixture to a boil over medium-high heat, then lower to low heat and cook, uncovered, for 1 hour.
- Remove the saucepan from the heat and set it aside to cool for 30 minutes or until the ketchup is safe to handle. Puree the ketchup in a blender until it is completely smooth.
- Refrigerate the ketchup in a firmly closed glass jar for up to 4 days, or freeze for 2 to 3 months.

13. Marinara Sauce

Prep time: 35 min | Serves: 10 | Difficulty: Moderate |
Nutrition: Calories: 79kcal | Fat 0g | Protein 1.8g | Carbohydrate 10.9g

Ingredients
- 4 tablespoons olive oil or garlic-infused olive oil
- 4 tablespoons olive oil or garlic-infused olive oil
- 1 bunch scallions (green parts only), thinly sliced
- 1 28-ounce can be crushed or finely chopped tomatoes
- 1 14.5-ounce can crush or finely chopped tomatoes
- ½ teaspoon salt, or more as needed
- 1 tablespoon dried basil
- 1 tablespoon dried oregano
- 1 tablespoon sugar

Instructions
- For three minutes over medium heat, sauté the scallion greens in the oil in a 4-quart pot. Toss in the tomatoes, along with their juices, as well as the salt, basil, oregano, and sugar. Bring the sauce to a boil, covered, over medium-high heat; decrease the heat to low and cook for about 30 minutes.
- Serve immediately or cover tightly and refrigerate for up to 4 days.

14. Spicy Peanut Sauce

Prep time: 5 min | Serves: 7 | Difficulty: Moderate |
Nutrition: Calories: 85 kcal | Carbohydrate 6g | Fat 2.5g | Protein 1g

Ingredients
- 6 tablespoons natural peanut butter
- 2 tablespoons reduced-sodium soy sauce
- ½ cup canned coconut milk
- 1 tablespoon minced fresh ginger
- 2 teaspoons sugar
- 1 teaspoon toasted or spicy sesame oil

Instructions
- Whisk together the peanut butter, soy sauce, coconut milk, ginger, sugar, and sesame oil in a medium bowl until smooth. Serve as soon as possible.
- Refrigerate any leftovers for up to 4 days in an airtight jar; bring to room temperature before serving.

15. Pineapple -Teriyaki Sauce

Prep time: 5 min | Serves: 7 | Difficulty: Moderate |
Nutrition: Calories: 55kcal | Fat 1.8g | Protein 1g | Carbohydrate 6g

Ingredients
- ¼ cup reduced-sodium soy sauce
- ½ cup crushed pineapple, with juice
- 1 tablespoon toasted or spicy sesame oil
- 1 tablespoon garlic-infused olive oil
- 1 tablespoon rice vinegar
- 1 tablespoon minced fresh ginger
- 2 tablespoons light brown sugar
- ¼ teaspoon red pepper flakes (optional)

Instructions
- Whisk together the soy sauce, pineapple and juice, oils, vinegar, ginger, brown sugar, and red pepper flakes in a large glass or ceramic bowl. Place the steak, fish, or chicken in the marinade and marinate for up to 10 hours in the refrigerator; alternatively, pour the marinade into a zipped bag and marinate in it.
- Remove the meat, fish, or poultry from the marinade and prepare the grill. Transfer the marinade to a small saucepan, bring to a boil, and cook for 2 to 3 minutes until it has reduced and thickened somewhat. During grilling, brush the marinade on the meat, fish, or poultry several times. Any remaining marinade should be discarded.

16. Sourdough Bread Croutons

Prep time: 45 min | Serves: 12 | Difficulty: Moderate |
Nutrition: Calories: 164kcal | Fat 1.8g | Protein 2g | Carbohydrate 17g

Ingredients
- 2 tablespoons melted butter
- 2 tablespoons extra-virgin olive oil
- 5 cups stale sourdough bread, cut into ½-inch cubes
- ¼ teaspoon salt
- ¼ teaspoon freshly ground black pepper
- ¼ teaspoon poultry seasoning

Instructions
- Preheat the oven to 250 degrees Fahrenheit.
- Drizzle the melted butter and oil over the bread cubes in a large mixing basin. Season the bread cubes evenly with salt, pepper, and poultry seasoning, and mix well.
- Place the bread cubes on two baking pans that haven't been oiled and bake for 20 minutes. Return the pans to the oven for another 20 minutes after stirring. Allow the bread cubes to cool to room temperature after turning off the oven and opening the door slightly.
- Transfer the cubes to a firmly closed container after they have cooled. To avoid mold, make sure the cooled croutons are totally dry before storing them.

17. Toasted Bread Crumbs

Prep time: 25 min | Serves: 22 | Difficulty: Moderate |
Nutrition: Calories: 78kcal | Fat 0.8g | Protein 0.2g | Carbohydrate 18g

Ingredients
- 1 Bread loaf

Instructions
- Preheat the oven to 250 degrees Fahrenheit.
- Place the bread pieces on a wire rack on top of an ungreased cookie sheet in a single layer. The bread should be baked until it is dry, about 20 minutes; it does not need to brown. Allow the bread to cool to room temperature after turning off the oven and propping the door open. Break the bread slices into 2-inch pieces with your hands.
- In a blender or food processor, grind the bread in tiny batches until it has the texture of gritty sand.
- To avoid mold, cool the bread crumbs fully before storing them in an airtight container for up to a month.

18. Salsa Verde

Prep time: 15 min | Serves: 1 | Difficulty: Moderate |
Nutrition: Calories: 53kcal | Fat 1g | Protein 0.2g | Carbohydrates 1.9g

Ingredients
- 2 handfuls of flat-leaf parsley, rinsed and dried
- 3 anchovy fillets in oil, drained (optional)
- 2 teaspoons capers, rinsed and drained
- 1 tablespoon garlic-infused olive oil
- 2 tablespoons olive oil
- 2 tablespoons fresh lemon juice, or to taste
- Salt and freshly ground black pepper

Instructions

- In a food processor or blender, add the parsley, anchovy fillets (if using), and capers and pulse until smooth.
- Gradually drizzle in the garlic-infused oil and olive oil, mixing thoroughly after each addition.
- Toss in the lemon juice and season to taste with salt and pepper. Place in a dish or jar, cover, and keep refrigerated for up to 5 days.

19. Basil Pesto

Prep time: 45 min | Serves: 1 | Difficulty: Moderate | Nutrition: Calories: 102 kcal | Fat 2.6g | Protein 1.3g | Carbohydrate 7g

Ingredients

- 2 handfuls of basil leaves, rinsed and dried
- 2 tablespoons garlic-infused olive oil
- 2 tablespoons olive oil, plus more as needed
- 1/3 cup pine nuts
- 1/3 cup grated Parmesan
- Salt and freshly ground black pepper

Instructions

- In a food processor or blender, mix the basil, garlic-infused oil, olive oil, pine nuts, and Parmesan until well incorporated.
- Season with salt and pepper to taste.
- If you want a more liquid pesto for drizzling, add extra oil. Cover with a thin coating of olive oil and spoon into a dish or jar.
- Refrigerate for up to 5 days or freeze for up to 2 months after covering.

20. Sun-Dried Tomato Spread

Prep time: 20 min | Serves: 1 | Difficulty: Moderate | Nutrition: Calories: 134kcal | Carbohydrate 3g | Fat 5.5g | Protein 2g

Ingredients

- 1 cup sun-dried tomatoes in oil, drained, and roughly chopped (oil reserved)
- 1/4 cup roughly chopped flat-leaf parsley
- 2 heaping tablespoons reduced-fat cream cheese, at room temperature
- 1 tablespoon garlic-infused olive oil
- 3 tablespoons olive oil
- Salt and freshly ground black pepper

Instructions

- In a food processor or blender, mix the sun-dried tomatoes, saved oil, parsley, and cream cheese until thoroughly incorporated.
- Add the garlic-infused oil and olive oil in small increments until the mixture is virtually smooth.
- Season with salt and pepper to taste.
- Place in a dish or jar, cover, and keep refrigerated for up to 3 days.

21. Olive Tapenade

Prep time: 20 min | Serves: 1 | Difficulty: Moderate | Nutrition: Calories: 83kcal | Fat 4.8g | Protein 0.1g | Carbohydrate 0.7g

Ingredients

- 1 cup pitted black olives
- 1 1/2 ounces anchovy fillets in oil, drained
- 2 heaping tablespoons gluten-free mayonnaise
- 2 teaspoons garlic-infused olive oil
- 2 teaspoons olive oil
- 2 teaspoons fresh lemon juice
- Pepper to taste (optional)

Instructions

- In a food processor or blender, combine all of the Ingredients and process until smooth. The
- tapenade should still have some texture to it. Place in a dish or jar, cover, and keep refrigerated for up to 5 days.

22. Mango Salsa

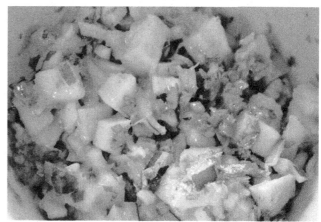

Prep time: 10min | Serves: 6 | Difficulty: Moderate | Nutrition: Calories: 64kcal | Fat 0g | Protein 0g | Carbohydrate 16g

Ingredients:

- 2 ripe mangoes, peeled and diced
- 1 serrano chili, finely chopped (optional)
- 2 green onions, finely chopped
- 1/2 red pepper, finely chopped
- 1/2 yellow pepper, finely chopped
- 1 cup fresh cilantro, finely chopped Juice of 1 lime (about 2 tablespoons), or to taste

Instructions:

- In a bowl, combine the mango chunks with the chopped chiles, green onions, red and yellow bell peppers, cilantro, and lime juice to make a dip or guacamole complement.

23. Celery Root Tahini Dip

Prep time: 10min | Serves: 6 | Difficulty: Moderate
Nutrition: Calories: 149kcal | Fat 2.9g | Protein 0.7g | Carbohydrate 23g

Ingredients:
- 1 medium celery root, skinned and chopped (about 2 cups)
- 2 tablespoons of olive oil or coconut oil
- 1/2 an onion
- 1 to 2 cloves garlic
- 1 teaspoon turmeric
- 1/2 to 1 teaspoon sea salt
- 1 1/2 teaspoons of Herbs de Provence mixture or rosemary
- 2 tablespoons tahini Juice of 1/2 a lemon (about 1/8 cup)
- 1/8 teaspoon each sea salt and pepper, or to taste

Instructions:
- Drain the celery root and throw it in a bowl after boiling it for about 5 minutes or until soft.
- In the same oil, fry the onions and garlic, then add the celery root, turmeric, sea salt, and herbs. Cook, constantly stirring, until the celery root is gently caramelized.
- Combine the tahini and lemon juice in a mixing bowl. At this stage, you can eat the combination as is, mash it with a potato masher, or blend it.
- To taste, season with salt and pepper.

24. Basic Nut or Seed Pâté

Prep time: 5min | Serves: 8 | Difficulty: Moderate
Nutrition: Calories: 68kcal | Fat 2g | Protein 0.2g | Carbohydrate 7g

Ingredients:
- 2 cups of seeds or nuts (such as sunflower seeds, pumpkin seeds, almonds, macadamia nuts, or cashews)
- Juice of 3 lemons (about 3/4 cup)
- 1/4 cup of water
- 1 heaping teaspoon of sea salt
- 4 cloves garlic

Instructions:
- In a coffee grinder or high-powered blender, grind the nuts or seeds. We recommend grinding a quarter cup at a time. If you use a coffee grinder in a basin, set aside the powdered mixture.
- In a blender or food processor, combine the lemon juice, water, salt, and garlic.
- Blend in the powdered mixture with the lemon juice mixture. You may need to add a few more tablespoons of water and lemon juice to achieve the required consistency.

25. Lemon Gone Wild Dressing

Prep time: 5min | Serves: 6 | Difficulty: Moderate
Nutrition: Calories: 69kcal | Fat 1g | Protein 0.2g | Carbohydrate 19g

Ingredients:
- 1/4 cup extra-virgin olive oil
- 2 tablespoons fresh lemon juice
- 3/4 teaspoon minced fresh garlic
- 3/4 teaspoon salt
- 1/8 teaspoon freshly cracked black pepper
- 3/4 teaspoon fresh thyme leaves

Instructions
- Gently whisk together all of the ingredients in a mixing bowl to properly combine, but keep the vinaigrette clear (not emulsified) for a better presentation.

26. Asian Dressing

Prep time: 5min | Serves: 2 | Difficulty: Moderate
Nutrition: Calories: 140kcal | Fat 4.2g | Protein 1g | Carbohydrate 21g

Ingredients:
- 1/4 cup sesame oil
- 4 tablespoons vegetable oil
- 1/4 cup soy sauce
- 1/4 cup rice wine vinegar
- 2 tablespoons maple syrup
- 1 tablespoon light miso paste (optional)

Instructions
- Combine all ingredients in a large mixing bowl and whisk vigorously to combine.

27. Shannon's Spicy Caesar Dressing

Prep time: 5min | Serves: 15 | Difficulty: Moderate
Nutrition: Calories: 165kcal | Fat 3.2g | Protein 3.4g | Carbohydrate 15g

Ingredients:
- 1 cup flaxseed, olive, or hemp oil
- Juice of 1 to 2 lemons (about 1/2 cup)
- 1/3 cup raw tahini
- 1 to 2 cloves garlic
- Nama Shoyu, or 1/2 teaspoon sea salt

Instructions
- Combine all of the ingredients in a blender and process until smooth.

28. Angela's Happy Mayo

Prep time: 10min | Serves: 2 | Difficulty: Moderate
Nutrition: Calories: 94kcal | Fat 2.5g | Protein 0.9g | Carbohydrate 26g

Ingredients:
- 1/2 cup raw tahini
- 1 to 2 tablespoons fresh lemon juice
- 2 tablespoons yacon syrup, or 6 soaked honey dates, pitted
- 1 teaspoon sea salt

- Juice of 1 orange (about 1/4 cup)
- 2 tablespoons fresh dill
- 1 cup water

Instructions
- Combine all ingredients in a mixing bowl and toss with your favorite salad or spread over a favorite sandwich.

---

29. Home-style Mayonnaise

Prep time: 5min | Serves: 2 | Difficulty: Moderate

Nutrition: Calories: 182kcal | Fat 2.9g | Protein 3.4g | Carbohydrate 24g

Ingredients:
- 1 egg
- 1 teaspoon dry mustard
- 1/2 teaspoon each white pepper and sea salt
- Pinch of cayenne pepper
- 3 tablespoons lemon juice
- 1 cup olive oil or safflower oil
- 1 tablespoon hot water

Instructions
- Blend the egg, mustard, white pepper, salt, cayenne pepper, and lemon juice together in a blender until smooth.
- While the mixer is still running, slowly drizzle in the oil.

Chapter 4: Breakfast, Brunch, and Muffins

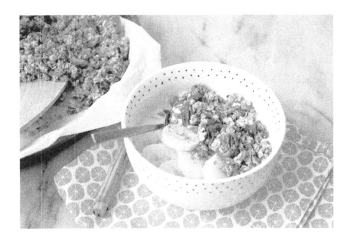

1. Bacon and Zucchini Crustless Quiche

Prep time: 50 min | Serves: 8 | Difficulty: Moderate
Nutrition: Calories: 258kcal | Fat 5.6g | Protein 4g | Carbohydrate 25g

Ingredients
- 2 large zucchinis, grated
- 1 1/2 cups (6 ounces/180 g) grated cheddar
- 2 tablespoons canola oil
- 6 large eggs, lightly beaten
- Salt and freshly ground black pepper
- Green salad, for serving (optional)

Instructions
- Preheat the oven to 350 degrees Fahrenheit (170 degrees Celsius). Line a 9-inch quiche dish or pie pan with parchment paper and grease it.
- Using paper towels, cover a plate. Turn the heat to medium and add the bacon to an unheated skillet. Cook for approximately 10 minutes, or until crispy, flipping periodically.
- Drain on the platter that has been prepared. Break the bacon into little pieces after it has cooled enough to handle.
- In a large mixing bowl, combine the bacon, zucchini, cheese, oil, and eggs.
- Salt & pepper to taste. Bake for 20 to 25 minutes, until firm and golden brown, in the baking dish.
- Before slicing, remove from the oven and set aside for 5 minutes. Serve it warm or chilled, with a green salad on the side, if preferred.

2. Scrambled Eggs

Prep time: 20 min | Serves: 4 | Difficulty: Moderate
Nutrition: Calories: 282kcal | Fat 0.7g | Protein 6.5g | Carbohydrate 21g

Ingredients
- 10 large eggs
- 3/4 cup lactose-free milk
- Salt and freshly ground black pepper

- 3 tablespoons salted butter
- Toasted gluten-free, soy-free bread, for serving

Instructions
- In a large mixing bowl, crack the eggs and whisk in the milk until well blended.
- Salt & pepper to taste.
- In a medium frying pan, melt the butter over low heat.
- Pour the egg mixture into the pan. To avoid sticking, carefully push the egg mixture from the pan's perimeter into the center using a wooden spoon.
- Cook for another 4 to 5 minutes, gently stirring occasionally, until the eggs are almost done—the yolks should still be creamy and a little runny.
- Serve with toasted gluten-free bread right away.

3. Omelet Wraps

Prep time: 20 min | Serves: 6 | Difficulty: Moderate
Nutrition: Calories: 159kcal | Fat 2.2g | Protein 7.5g | Carbohydrate 19g

Ingredients
- Nonstick cooking spray
- 6 large eggs
- 6 thin slices cooked turkey breast
- 1 heaping tablespoon cranberry sauce
- 1 avocado, pitted, peeled, and sliced (optional)
- 1 tomato, sliced
- 2 handfuls of baby spinach leaves, rinsed and dried
- 1/2 cup (60 g) grated carrot (1 medium)

Instructions
- Spray a medium nonstick frying pan with cooking spray and place it over medium heat.
- In a small bowl, crack one egg and whisk it with a fork. Pour the egg into the heated pan and tilt it to coat the bottom; the omelet should be about 5 inches (12 cm) across.
- Cook for 30 to 60 seconds before flipping the omelet using a spatula or pancake-turner, being careful not to damage it. Cook for another 30 to 60 seconds, then remove from the pan and place on a platter. To create 6 omelets, repeat with the remaining eggs.
- Allow cooling before serving. Place an omelet on a flat surface to assemble.
- Place a piece of turkey breast in the center of the omelet, followed with 1/2 teaspoon cranberry sauce, a few slices of avocado and tomato, baby spinach leaves, and a dusting of carrot.
- To encapsulate the filling, fold the bottom third of the omelet toward the center, then fold in the

left and right sides (almost as if you were rolling a burrito).

- Using the leftover omelets and filling, repeat the process. Serve right away, or cover and keep refrigerated until ready to eat.

4. Light Omelet with Chicken and Spinach

Prep time: 20 min | Serves: 2 | Difficulty: Moderate
Nutrition: Calories: 343kcal | Fat 5.2g | Protein 9.5g | Carbohydrate 29g

Ingredients
- 4 large eggs
- 1/4 cup roughly chopped basil
- 1/4 cup roughly chopped flat-leaf parsley
- Salt and freshly ground black pepper
- 1 tablespoon canola oil
- 1/2 cup shredded cooked chicken
- A small handful of baby spinach leaves, rinsed, dried, and chopped
- 1/2 red bell pepper, diced
- 1/4 cup grated cheddar

Instructions
- In a medium mixing bowl, whisk together the eggs, basil, and parsley.
- Salt & pepper to taste.
- In a medium frying pan, heat the oil over medium heat.
- Pour in the egg mixture and tilt the pan to coat the bottom.
- Cook until the top is almost set. Carefully raise the edges of the omelet with a spatula or pancake turner and shake it loose.
- On one half of the omelet, scatter the chicken, spinach, bell pepper, and cheese. To cover the filling, fold the other half over the top.
- Cook for a few minutes until the mixture is hot and the cheese is beginning to melt. Remove the omelet from the pan and slice it in half (or serve it whole with two forks!).
- Split the Ingredients in half and create two smaller omelets if desired.

5. Roasted Sweet Potato and Bell Pepper Frittata

Prep time: 45 min | Serves: 6-8 | Difficulty: Moderate
Nutrition: Calories: 191kcal | Fat 5.2g | Proteins 10 mg | Carbohydrate 29g

Ingredients
- 1 large sweet potato, peeled (if desired) and chopped
- 2 red bell peppers, seeded and cut into quarters
- Olive oil for drizzling and greasing the pan
- 1 large handful of baby spinach leaves, rinsed and dried
- 10 large eggs
- Salt and freshly ground black pepper

Instructions
- Preheat the oven to 350 degrees Fahrenheit (180 degrees Celsius). In a glass baking dish, combine the sweet potato and bell peppers, sprinkle with olive oil, and bake for 10 to 15 minutes, until golden brown and soft.
- Remove the pan from the oven, cover it in foil, and set it aside to cool. Turn on the oven. Remove the skins off the cooled peppers and discard them. Using a large knife, cut the peppers into big pieces.
- A 9-inch (23-cm) ovenproof frying pan should be greased. A layer of sweet potato goes on the bottom, followed by a layer of bell peppers on top. Add a few spinach leaves as a finishing touch.
- Finish with a layer of bell peppers before continuing with the other veggies.
- In a bowl, lightly beat the eggs and season with salt and pepper. Pour the eggs over the veggies, tilting the dish slightly to ensure that they are equally distributed and cover any gaps.
- Bake for 20 to 30 minutes, or until firm in the center when touched. Remove the pan from the oven and set it aside to cool for 5 minutes before slicing.

6. Cheese and Herb Scones

Prep time: 20 min | Serves: 10-12 | Difficulty: Moderate
Nutrition: Calories: 179kcal | Fat 6g | Protein 7.9g | Carbohydrate 18g

Ingredients
- 3/4 cup low-fat milk, lactose-free milk, or suitable plant-based milk, plus more for brushing
- 1 large egg
- 1/2 cup grated Parmesan
- 1/2 cup grated cheddar
- 3 to 4 heaping tablespoons chopped herbs (such as oregano, thyme, and flat-leaf parsley)
- 1 cup cornstarch, plus more for kneading
- 1 cup tapioca flour
- 1/2 cup soy flour
- 1 teaspoon xanthan gum or guar gum
- 2 teaspoons gluten-free baking powder
- 5 tablespoons unsalted butter, cut into cubes, at room temperature

Instructions
- Preheat the oven to 400 degrees Fahrenheit (200 degrees Celsius). Using parchment paper, line a baking sheet.
- In a mixing dish, combine the milk and the egg. Combine the Parmesan, cheddar, and herbs in a mixing bowl.
- In a medium mixing bowl, sift the cornstarch, tapioca flour, soy flour, xanthan gum, and baking powder three times (or whisk in the bowl until well combined).

- With your fingertips, rub in the butter until the mixture resembles fine bread crumbs. With a big metal spoon, stir in the milk mixture all at once until the dough begins to hold together.
- Using cornstarch, lightly dust your work surface. With your hands, gently pull the dough together and turn it out onto a floured surface. Knead the dough lightly by pushing and rotating it until it is just smooth (use a light touch, or the scones will be tough).
- Roll out the dough to a thickness of 1-inch (2.5 cm) with a lightly floured rolling pin and cut out 10 to 12 scones using a 2-inch (5 cm) biscuit or cookie cutter.
- To achieve this, use a straight-down motion (if you twist the cutter, the scones will rise unevenly during baking).
- To keep the cutter from sticking, coat it with cornstarch before each cut. Brush the tops of the scones with milk and place them about 13 inches (1 cm) apart on the baking sheet.
- Bake for 10 to 12 minutes, or until golden brown and well done. Take the scones out of the oven and cover them in a clean dish towel right away (this will help give them a soft crust). Warm the dish before serving.

7. Chocolate Scones

Prep time: 30 min | Serves: 10-12 | Difficulty: Moderate
Nutrition: Calories: 188kcal | Fat 7.8g | Protein 8.4g | Carbohydrate 49g
Ingredients
- 2⁄3 cup low-fat milk, lactose-free milk, or suitable plant-based milk, plus more for kneading
- 1 large egg
- 1 cup cornstarch, plus more for dusting
- 1 cup tapioca flour
- 1⁄2 cup soy flour
- 2 heaping tablespoons cocoa
- 1 teaspoon xanthan gum or guar gum
- 13⁄4 teaspoons gluten-free baking powder
- 1⁄4 cup superfine sugar
- 5 tablespoons unsalted butter, cut into cubes, at room temperature
- 1⁄2 cup chocolate chips*
- Jam or butter, for serving

Instructions
- Preheat the oven to 400 degrees Fahrenheit (200 degrees Celsius). Using parchment paper, line a baking sheet.
- In a mixing dish, combine the milk and the egg. In a medium mixing bowl, sift the cornstarch, tapioca flour, soy flour, cocoa, xanthan gum, baking powder, and sugar three times (or whisk in the bowl until well combined).
- With your fingertips, rub in the butter until the mixture resembles fine bread crumbs. Combine the chocolate chips with the rest of the

Ingredients and stir to combine. With a big metal spoon, stir in the milk and egg combination all at once until the dough begins to hold together.
- Using cornstarch, lightly dust your work surface. With your hands, gently pull the dough together and turn it out onto a floured surface.
- Knead the dough lightly by pushing and rotating it until it is just smooth (use a light touch, or the scones will be tough). Roll out the dough to a thickness of 1-inch (2.5 cm) with a lightly floured rolling pin and cut out 10 to 12 scones using a 2-inch (5 cm) biscuit or cookie cutter.
- To achieve this, use a straight-down motion (if you twist the cutter, the scones will rise unevenly during baking).
- To keep the cutter from sticking, coat it with cornstarch before each cut. Brush the tops of the scones with milk and place them about 13 inches (1 cm) apart on the baking sheet. Bake for 10 to 12 minutes, or until golden brown and well done.
- Take the scones out of the oven and cover them in a clean dish towel right away (this will help give them a soft crust). Serve warm with butter and jam.

8. Blueberry Pancakes

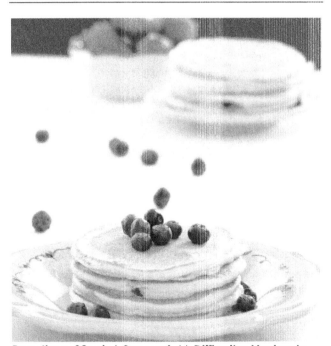

Prep time: 30 min | Serves: 4-6 | Difficulty: Moderate
Nutrition: Calories: 235kcal | Fat 9.2g | Protein 9.2g | Carbohydrate 21g
Ingredients
- 2 large eggs
- 11⁄2 cups low-fat milk, lactose-free milk, or suitable plant-based milk
- 1 cup superfine white rice flour
- 1⁄2 cup (cornstarch

- 1/2 cup soy flour
- 2/3 cup packed light brown sugar
- 1 tablespoon plus 1 teaspoon gluten-free baking powder
- 1 teaspoon xanthan gum or guar gum
- 4 tablespoons salted butter, melted
- Nonstick cooking spray
- 1 cup fresh or frozen blueberries
- Maple syrup and/or whipped cream, for serving (optional)

Instructions

- In a small dish or liquid measuring cup, whisk together the eggs and milk.
- In a large mixing bowl, sift the rice flour, cornstarch, soy flour, brown sugar, baking powder, and xanthan gum three times (or whisk in the bowl until well combined).
- Make a well in the center and slowly pour in the milk mixture, stirring well to combine. Cover and leave aside for 15 minutes after adding the melted butter.
- Spray a large nonstick frying pan or griddle with cooking spray and heat over medium heat. Working in batches, pour enough batter to make four 4-inch (10-cm) pancakes (approximately 1/2 cup/125 ml each) and cook for one minute, or until they begin to firm.
- Cook for another 2 minutes after adding 8 blueberries to each pancake. Cook for another 2 minutes, or until well cooked.
- To keep warm, transfer to a platter and cover loosely with foil. To create a total of 12 pancakes, repeat with the remaining batter and berries. Serve immediately with the leftover blueberries and maple syrup (if wanted) and/or whipped cream for an extra delectable treat.

9. Pumpkin Muffins

Prep time: 40 min | Serves: 12 | Difficulty: Moderate
Nutrition: Calories: 209kcal | Fat 8g | Protein 11g | Carbohydrate 34g
Ingredients
- 1 cup superfine white rice flour
- 1/2 cup cornstarch
- 1/2 cup potato flour
- 2 teaspoons gluten-free baking powder
- 1 teaspoon baking soda
- 1 teaspoon xanthan gum or guar gum
- 2 teaspoons pumpkin pie spice
- 1 heaping tablespoon ground cinnamon
- 3 tablespoons unsalted butter, melted
- 3/4 cup (200 g) gluten-free, low-fat vanilla yogurt
- 2 large eggs
- 1 1/2 cups mashed cooked pumpkin, kabocha, or other suitable winter squash (from about 18 500 g peeled and seeded raw squash)
- 1 cup superfine sugar

Instructions

- Preheat oven to 325 degrees Fahrenheit (170 degrees Celsius) and line a 12-cup muffin tin with paper liners.
- In a large mixing bowl, sift together the rice flour, cornstarch, potato flour, baking powder, baking soda, xanthan gum, pumpkin pie spice, and cinnamon three times (or whisk in the bowl until well combined). In a medium mixing dish, combine the melted butter, yogurt, and eggs.
- Combine the squash and sugar in a mixing bowl. Add to the flour mixture and whisk until just mixed with a heavy metal spoon (do not overmix).
- Fill the muffin cups two-thirds full with the batter. Bake for 15–20 minutes, or until golden brown and a toothpick inserted in the center comes out clean. Cool for 5 minutes in the pan before turning out onto a wire rack to cool fully.

10. Banana–Chocolate Chip Muffins

Prep time: 40 min | Serves: 12 | Difficulty: Moderate
Nutrition: Calories: 220kcal | Fat 8.5g | Protein 9g | Carbohydrate 26g
Ingredients
- 1 cup superfine white rice flour
- 1/2 cup cornstarch
- 1/2 cup soy flour
- 2 teaspoons gluten-free baking powder
- 1 teaspoon baking soda
- 1 teaspoon xanthan gum or guar gum
- 2 large eggs
- 1 cup superfine sugar
- 3 tablespoons unsalted butter, melted
- 1 teaspoon vanilla extract
- 2 bananas, peeled and mashed
- 1/3 cup low-fat milk, lactose-free milk, or suitable plant-based milk
- 3/4 cup gluten-free, low-fat vanilla yogurt
- 1 cup chocolate chips*
Instructions
- Preheat oven to 325 degrees Fahrenheit (170 degrees Celsius) and line a 12-cup muffin tin with paper liners.
- In a large mixing bowl, sift the rice flour, cornstarch, soy flour, baking powder, baking soda, and xanthan gum three times (or whisk in the bowl until well combined).
- In a medium mixing bowl, whisk together the eggs and sugar until thick and frothy. In a large mixing bowl, add the melted butter, vanilla, mashed bananas, milk, and yogurt (do not overmix).
- Add to the flour mixture and whisk until just mixed with a heavy metal spoon. Fold in the chocolate chunks gently. Fill the muffin cups two-thirds full with the batter. Bake for 15 to 20

minutes, or until a toothpick inserted in the center comes out clean.

11. Vanilla-Rhubarb Muffins

Prep time: 40 min | Serves: 12 | Difficulty: Moderate
Nutrition: Calories: 221kcal | Fat 7.8g | Protein 8.4g | Carbohydrate 29g

Ingredients
- 1 1/4 cup finely chopped rhubarb
- 1 1/2 cups superfine sugar
- 1 cup superfine white rice flour
- 1/2 cup tapioca flour
- 1/2 cup cornstarch
- 2 teaspoons gluten-free baking powder
- 1 teaspoon baking soda
- 1 teaspoon xanthan gum or guar gum
- 3 tablespoons unsalted butter, melted
- 1/2 teaspoon vanilla extract
- 3/4 cup gluten-free, low-fat vanilla yogurt
- 2 large eggs

Instructions
- In a small saucepan, combine the rhubarb and 1⁄4 cups (55 g) sugar and cover with water. Bring to a boil over high heat, then lower to medium and simmer for 10 minutes, or until vegetables are soft.
- Drain the water and set it aside to cool. Preheat oven to 325 degrees Fahrenheit (170 degrees Celsius) and line a 12-cup muffin tin with paper liners. In a large mixing bowl, sift together the rice flour, tapioca flour, cornstarch, baking powder, baking soda, and xanthan gum three times (or whisk in the bowl until well combined).
- In a medium mixing basin, combine the melted butter, vanilla, yogurt, eggs, and the remaining 1⁄4 cups (275 g) sugar.
- With a big metal spoon, whisk the yogurt mixture into the flour mixture until just mixed.
- Do not overmix the Ingredients. Stir in the cooked rhubarb gently (take care because you want the pieces to remain intact).
- Fill the muffin cups two-thirds of the way with batter. Bake until golden brown and a toothpick inserted in the middle of a muffin comes out clean, 12 to 15 minutes. Cool for 5 minutes in the pan before turning out onto a wire rack to cool fully.

12. Ginger and Pecan Muffins

Prep time: 40 min | Serves: 12 | Difficulty: Moderate
Nutrition: Calories: 277kcal | Fat 8.7g | Protein 11g | Carbohydrate 29g

Ingredients
- 1 cup superfine white rice flour
- 1/2 cup tapioca flour
- 1/2 cup cornstarch
- 2 teaspoons gluten-free baking powder
- 1 teaspoon baking soda
- 1 teaspoon xanthan gum or guar gum
- 3 tablespoons unsalted butter, melted
- 3/4 cup gluten-free, low-fat vanilla yogurt
- 2 large eggs
- 1 1/4 cups superfine sugar
- 1/2 cup roughly chopped pecans
- 1/2 cup chopped crystallized ginger, plus 12 small pieces for garnish

Instructions
- Preheat oven to 325 degrees Fahrenheit (170 degrees Celsius) and line a 12-cup muffin tin with paper liners.
- In a large mixing bowl, sift together the rice flour, tapioca flour, cornstarch, baking powder, baking soda, and xanthan gum three times (or whisk in the bowl until well combined).
- In a medium mixing bowl, combine the melted butter, yogurt, eggs, sugar, pecans, and ginger. Add to the flour mixture and whisk until just mixed with a heavy metal spoon (do not overmix).
- Fill the muffin cups two-thirds full with batter, then top with a piece of crystallized ginger. Bake for 15–20 minutes, or until golden brown and a toothpick inserted in the center comes out clean.
- Cool for 5 minutes in the pan before turning out onto a wire rack to cool fully.

13. Cheesy Corn Muffins

Prep time: 40 min | Serves: 12 | Difficulty: Moderate
Nutrition: Calories: 218kcal | Fat 9g | Protein 11g | Carbohydrate 31g

Ingredients
- 1 cup superfine white rice flour
- 1/2 cup cornstarch
- 1/2 cup tapioca flour
- 2 teaspoons gluten-free baking powder
- 1 teaspoon baking soda
- 1 teaspoon xanthan gum or guar gum
- 3 tablespoons salted butter, melted
- 3/4 cup gluten-free, low-fat plain yogurt
- 3 large eggs
- 1/2 cup grated cheddar, plus twelve 1/3-inch cubes
- 1/2 cup finely grated Parmesan
- 4 to 6 lean bacon slices, cooked until crispy and crumbled (optional)
- 1 cup drained canned or thawed frozen corn kernels
- Pinch of salt and freshly ground black pepper

Instructions
- Preheat oven to 325 degrees Fahrenheit (170 degrees Celsius) and line a 12-cup muffin tin with paper liners.
- In a large mixing bowl, sift together the rice flour, cornstarch, tapioca flour, baking powder,

baking soda, and xanthan gum three times (or whisk in the bowl until well combined).

- In a medium mixing dish, combine the melted butter, yogurt, eggs, cheddar, Parmesan, bacon (if using), and corn. Stir the yogurt mixture into the flour mixture with a big metal spoon until everything is well blended (do not overmix).
- Salt & pepper to taste. Fill the muffin cups halfway with batter, then top with a cube of cheddar cheese.
- Fill the cups two-thirds full with the remaining batter. Bake for 15 to 20 minutes, or until a toothpick inserted into the middle of a muffin (avoiding the cheese filling) comes out clean. Cool for 5 minutes in the pan before turning out onto a wire rack to cool fully.

14. Spinach and Tomato Muffins

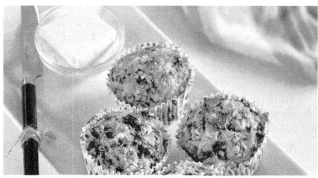

Prep time: 40 min | Serves:12 | Difficulty: Moderate
Nutrition: Calories: 200kcal | Fat 7g | Protein 9g | Carbohydrate 19g
Ingredients
- 1 cup superfine white rice flour
- 1/2 cup cornstarch
- 1/2 cup soy flour
- 2 teaspoons gluten-free baking powder
- 1 teaspoon baking soda
- 1 teaspoon xanthan gum or guar gum
- 5 tablespoons salted butter, melted
- 3/4 cup gluten-free, low-fat plain yogurt
- 3 large eggs
- 1 cup low-fat milk, lactose-free milk, or suitable plant-based milk
- 1 cup finely grated Parmesan
- 2 medium tomatoes, diced
- 2 ounces baby spinach leaves, rinsed, dried, and roughly chopped
- Pinch of salt and freshly ground black pepper
Instructions
- Preheat the oven to 325°F (170°C) and line a 12-cup muffin pan with paper liners.
- Sift the rice flour, cornstarch, soy flour, baking powder, baking soda, and xanthan gum three times into a large bowl (or whisk in the bowl until well combined).

- Combine the melted butter, yogurt, eggs, milk, Parmesan, tomatoes, spinach, and salt and pepper in a medium bowl. Add to the flour mixture and mix with a wooden spoon until just combined.
- Pour the batter evenly into the muffin cups until they are two-thirds full. Bake for 15 to 20 minutes, until firm to the touch and a toothpick inserted into the center of a muffin comes out clean.
- Cool in the pan for 5 minutes, then turn out onto a wire rack to cool completely.

15. High-Fiber Muffins with Zucchini and Sunflower Seeds

Prep time: 40 min | Serves: 12 | Difficulty: Moderate
Nutrition: Calories: 243kcal | Fat 8.8g | Protein 8.6g | Carbohydrate 29g
Ingredients
- 1 cup brown rice flour
- 1/2 cup cornstarch
- 1/2 cup soy flour
- 2 teaspoons gluten-free baking powder
- 1 teaspoon baking soda
- 1 teaspoon xanthan gum or guar gum
- 5 tablespoons salted butter, melted
- 1/2 cup low-fat milk, lactose-free milk, or suitable plant-based milk
- 3/4 cup gluten-free, low-fat plain yogurt
- 3 large eggs
- 3/4 cup (60 g) finely grated Parmesan
- 1/2 medium zucchini, grated
- 1/2 cup (75 g) roasted unsalted sunflower seeds
- 1/2 cup (60 g) rice bran
- 1/4 cup (25 g) walnuts, crushed
- 1/4 teaspoon freshly grated nutmeg
- Pinch of salt and freshly ground black pepper
Instructions
- Preheat the oven to 325°F (170°C) and line a 12-cup muffin pan with paper liners.
- Sift the rice flour, cornstarch, soy flour, baking powder, baking soda, and xanthan gum three times into a large bowl (or whisk in the bowl until well combined).
- Combine the melted butter, milk, yogurt, eggs, Parmesan, zucchini, sunflower seeds, rice bran, walnuts, nutmeg, and salt and pepper in a medium bowl and mix well.
- Add the flour mixture and mix with a wooden spoon for 2 to 3 minutes (be careful not to overmix). Pour the batter evenly into the muffin cups until they are two-thirds full.
- Bake for 15 to 20 minutes, until firm to the touch and a toothpick inserted into the center of a muffin comes out clean.
- Cool in the pan for 5 minutes, then turn out onto a wire rack to cool completely.

16. Chili-Cheese Muffins

Prep time: 40 min | Serves:12 | Difficulty: Moderate
Nutrition: Calories: 184kcal | Fat 7g | Protein 8g | Carbohydrate 14g

Ingredients
- 1 cup superfine white rice flour
- ½ cup cornstarch
- ½ cup soy flour
- 2 teaspoons gluten-free baking powder
- 1 teaspoon baking soda
- 1 teaspoon xanthan gum or guar gum
- 1 teaspoon chili powder
- 5 tablespoons salted butter, melted
- ¾ cup gluten-free, low-fat plain yogurt
- 3 large eggs
- ¾ cup low-fat milk, lactose-free milk, or suitable plant-based milk
- ¾ cup finely grated Parmesan
- 1 cup grated cheddar
- 2 heaping tablespoons finely chopped flat-leaf parsley
- Pinch of salt and freshly ground black pepper

Instructions
- Preheat oven to 325 degrees Fahrenheit (170 degrees Celsius) and line a 12-cup muffin tin with paper liners.
- In a large mixing bowl, sift together the rice flour, cornstarch, soy flour, baking powder, baking soda, xanthan gum, and chili powder three times (or whisk in the bowl until well combined).
- In a medium mixing bowl, combine the melted butter, yogurt, eggs, milk, Parmesan, cheddar, parsley, salt & pepper.
- Add to the flour mixture and whisk until just mixed with a heavy metal spoon. Fill the muffin cups two-thirds full with the batter. Bake for 15 to 20 minutes, or until the muffins are firm to the touch and a toothpick inserted in the center comes out clean.
- Cool for 5 minutes in the pan before turning out onto a wire rack to cool fully.

17. Smoothie Magic

Prep time: 10 min | Serves: 1 | Difficulty: Moderate
Nutrition: Calories: 176kcal | Fat 5.2g | Protein 4g | Carbohydrate 16g

Ingredients
- Half cup Strawberries
- 1 cup milk(Lactogen free)
- Frozen cubes

Instructions
- Blend all Ingredients together until smooth.

18. Golden French Toast

Prep time: 20 min | Serves: 5 | Difficulty: Moderate
Nutrition: Calories: 142kcal | Fat 8.6g | Protein 11g | Carbohydrate 17g

Ingredients
- 4 large eggs
- ½ cup lactose-free milk
- 1 teaspoon vanilla extract
- 8 ounces sourdough bread or low-FODMAP gluten-free bread
- 1 teaspoon ground cinnamon
- 1 tablespoon butter, or more if needed

Instructions
- In a 9 x 13-inch baking dish, whisk together the eggs, milk, and vanilla extract. Using the egg and milk combination, soak the bread pieces. Cinnamon should be liberally sprinkled.
- Melt a teaspoon of butter in a large, well-seasoned cast-iron frying pan or nonstick skillet over medium heat. Place a single layer of bread slices in the pan after the butter is boiling. Cook for 2 to 3 minutes, or until the bottoms of the bread pieces are golden brown. Flip and heat until golden brown on the other side.
- When done, the middle of each toast should puff out slightly. Repeat with the remaining bread slices and 2 teaspoons butter.
- Serve the French toast immediately, or keep it warm on an ovenproof tray in a 200°F oven until ready to eat.

19. Hummingbird Muffins

Prep time: 40 min | Serves: 5 | Difficulty: Moderate
Nutrition: Calories: 218kcal | Fat 9g | Protein 11g | Carbohydrate 31g

Ingredients
- 1 large egg
- ¼ cup packed light brown sugar
- ¼ cup neutral-flavored oil
- ¼ cup crushed pineapple, drained
- ¾ cup mashed ripe banana
- ¾ cup mashed ripe banana
- 1 tablespoon chia seeds
- ¼ cup/25g sorghum flour
- ½ cup/55g Authentic Foods Superfine Brown Rice Flour
- 2 tablespoons tapioca starch
- 1 tablespoon cornstarch
- 1 tablespoon arrowroot powder
- 2 teaspoons baking powder
- ¼ teaspoon salt
- 1 teaspoon ground cinnamon
- ¼ cup chopped walnuts
- Cooking spray
- 1 tablespoon coarse sugar crystals

Instructions
- Combine the egg, brown sugar, oil, pineapple, and banana in a large mixing dish.

- Stir the chia seeds into the egg mixture to incorporate them. Stir in the sorghum flour, rice flour, tapioca starch, cornstarch, arrowroot powder, baking powder, salt, and cinnamon until the dough is thick and spoon able.
- Add the walnuts and mix well. Allow 15 minutes for the batter to rest.
- Preheat the oven to 350 degrees Fahrenheit. Using cooking spray, coat a 6-cup muffin pan.
- Give the batter one more swirl before dividing it among the muffin cups. Sprinkle the sugar on top of each muffin. Preheat oven to 350°F and bake for 25–30 minutes, or until firm to the touch. Cool for a few minutes in the pan before removing it to cool entirely on a rack. Serve immediately, or keep refrigerated for up to 1 day or frozen for up to 6 months in an airtight container.

20. Sweet Potato Hash

Prep time: 30 min | Serves: 2 | Difficulty: Moderate
Nutrition: Calories: 178kcal | Fat 8g | Protein 7.4g | Carbohydrate 19g

Ingredients
- 1 medium sweet potato (¾ pound)
- 2 tablespoons garlic-infused olive oil
- 1 small onion, sliced
- 1 small summer squash (about ¾ pound), diced
- 10 medium radishes (about ½ pound), chopped
- ½ cup chopped scallion greens

Instructions
- Penetrate the sweet potato several times and microwave for 4 to 6 minutes on high, or until cooked enough to pierce with a fork. When the unpeeled sweet potato is cool enough to handle, slice it into bite-size pieces and set it aside.
- Warm the oil in a large skillet over medium heat. Remove and discard the onion after adding it and sautéing it until it is translucent.
- Sauté the squash and radishes for 3 minutes in the skillet. Allow 8 to 10 minutes for the sweet potato to brown on the bottom, stirring occasionally. Scrape the vegetable mixture from the bottom of the pan with a spatula, flip gently, and cook for another 5 minutes. Serve immediately with scallion greens as a garnish.

21. Breakfast Scones

Prep time: 45 min | Serves: 14 | Difficulty: Moderate
Nutrition: Calories: 297kcal | Fat 6.2g | Protein 9.8g | Carbohydrate 31g

Ingredients:
- 2 cups (300 g) cornstarch
- 2 cups (250 g) tapioca flour
- 1 cup (90 g) soy flour
- 2 teaspoons xanthan gum
- 1 tablespoon baking powder (gluten-free if following a gluten-free diet)
- ½ cup superfine sugar
- 10 tablespoons unsalted butter, at room temperature, cut into cubes
- 1 ¼ cups low-fat milk, plus 2 tablespoons (preferably cow's milk)
- 2 eggs
- Jam, optional
- Whipped cream, optional

Instructions:
- Preheat the oven to 400 degrees Fahrenheit (200 degrees Celsius). Dust a baking sheet with cornstarch and grease it.
- In a large mixing bowl, sift the cornstarch, tapioca flour, soy flour, xanthan gum, baking powder, and sugar three times (or mix with a whisk to ensure they are well combined). Add the butter and continue to cut until the mixture resembles fine bread crumbs.
- In a mixing dish, whisk together 1 cup of milk and the eggs. Stir into the flour mixture until the dough starts to come together. With your hands, gently pull the dough together and turn it out onto a lightly floured surface. Knead the dough four or five times until it is smooth.
- Roll out the dough to a thickness of 1 inch (3 cm). Use a 2-inch (5-cm) biscuit or cookie cutter to cut out the scones. Use a straight downward stroke with the cutter; if you twist it, the scones will rise unevenly. Using cornstarch to coat the cutter before each cut also helps.
- Place the scones approximately 12 inches (1 cm) apart on the baking sheet. Brush the remaining milk over the tops. Bake for 15 to 18 minutes, flipping the sheet halfway through until golden and cooked through.
- Remove the scones from the oven and wrap them in a clean kitchen towel right away (this gives them a soft crust). Serve the scones with jam and whipped cream, if preferred, after 5 minutes.

22. Hand-Milled Gluten-Free Breakfast Cereal

Prep time: 25 min | Serves: 4 | Difficulty: Moderate
Nutrition: Calories: 211kcal | Fat 5g | Protein 8g | Carbohydrate 22g

Ingredients:
- ¼ cup long-grain brown rice
- ¼ cup millet
- ¼ cup quinoa (red or white)
- ¼ cup walnut or other nut pieces, ground if nut pieces are irritating
- ¼ cup dried blueberries
- ½ teaspoon cinnamon
- Pinch of salt
- 1 ½ cups water

- 1 /4 cup organic whole milk or non-dairy milk (such as unsweetened Rice Dream)
- Grade B maple syrup (optional)
- Butter or coconut oil (optional)

Instructions:
- In a coffee/spice grinder or a robust blender, grind the rice, millet, and quinoa.
- Combine the ground grains, nuts, dried blueberries, cinnamon, salt, and water in a mixing bowl.
- Bring to a boil, then lower to low heat. Cover and cook for 10 to 15 minutes, stirring regularly and adding more water as needed to achieve the desired consistency.
- As desired, add the milk, syrup, and butter.

23. Caramelized Banana and Date "Porridge" (SCD)

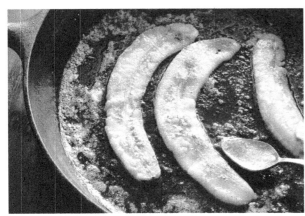

Prep time: 15 min | Serves: 2 | Difficulty: Moderate
Nutrition: Calories: 197kcal | Fat 4g | Protein 9.4g | Carbohydrate 19g
Ingredients:
- 1 banana
- 2 dates
- 1 teaspoon butter
- 1 /2 a head of cauliflower, pureed Dash of cinnamon
- 1 /2 to 1 tablespoon honey (optional)

Instructions:
- Cut the banana into slices. Dates should be pitted and sliced into small pieces.
- In a small frying pan, melt the butter over a medium-high flame.
- When the butter begins to melt, add the banana and dates and cook for 2 to 3 minutes, rotating frequently.
- Reduce the heat to medium and add the pureed cauliflower when the banana begins to turn golden. Heat to a high temperature.
- Sprinkle cinnamon on top and drizzle with honey if desired.

24. Soaked Oats Porridge

Prep time: 10 min | Serves: 1 | Difficulty: Moderate
Nutrition: Calories: 159kcal | Fat 2g | Protein 7.2g | Carbohydrate 17g
Ingredients:
- 2 cups organic oat groats
- 1 /4 cup dried figs
- 1 tablespoon walnuts
- 1 tablespoon shredded coconut
- 1 cup coconut juice or water to mix ingredients
- 4 ounces of coconut milk Pinch of cinnamon or nutmeg (optional)

Instructions:
- Place the oats, figs, almonds, and shredded coconut in a bowl the night before and cover with water to soak overnight.
- Rinse the ingredients thoroughly in fresh water in the morning to remove any residue.
- Blend the soaked mixture with the coconut juice or water in a blender or food processor until smooth.
- Pour the coconut milk over the mixed ingredients and season with a touch of cinnamon or nutmeg before serving (if desired).

25. Strawberries and Cream Oatmeal

Prep time: 5 min | Serves: 1 | Difficulty: Moderate
Nutrition: Calories: 195kcal | Fat 3.2g | Protein 6.2g | Carbohydrate 21g
Ingredients:
- 1 cup quick-cooking rolled oats
- 2 cups water
- 1 banana, cut up
- 5 strawberries, cut up
- 2 ounces coconut milk

Instructions:
- On a chilly stove, combine the rolled oats and water.
- Bring to a boil, then reduce to low heat and continue to cook for 5 minutes.
- In a mixing bowl, combine the banana and strawberries, then add the oats and coconut milk.

26. Cinnamon Pancakes with Ghee

Prep time: 20 min | Serves: 4 | Difficulty: Moderate
Nutrition: Calories: 292kcal | Fat 4.7g | Protein 8.5g | Carbohydrate 18g
Ingredients:
- 1 cup whole organic cashews
- 1 /2 teaspoon baking soda
- 3 eggs
- 1 tablespoon Kendall's SCD Dairy Yogurt
- Splash of vanilla
- Pinch of salt
- 2 tablespoons of honey
- 1 teaspoon cinnamon

- 1 tablespoon coconut oil

Instructions:
- Grind the cashews into a paste in a food processor.
- Blend together the baking soda, eggs, yogurt, vanilla, salt, honey, and cinnamon.
- Melt the coconut oil in a frying pan over medium-low heat in the oven.
- In 14-cup pools, pour the batter into the pan.
- When golden, flip.

27. Gratifying Ghee

Prep time: 10 min | Serves: 1 | Difficulty: Moderate
Nutrition: Calories: 188kcal | Fat 7g | Protein 4g | Carbohydrate 21g
Ingredients:
- 1 pound unsalted butter

Instructions:
- In a deep saucepan with a thick bottom, gradually melt the butter over low heat. Stirring is not allowed.
- Cook over low heat until the melted butter has turned into a clear golden liquid. If you have a deep enough pot, it will bubble and foam but not boil over. The milk solids will turn golden or light brown in color and may settle to the bottom of the pan. The heavy foam can be skimmed off and discarded.
- Remove the liquid from the heat when it has turned a clear gold color. Overdone ghee has a deeper hue.
- Place the 4 sheets of cheesecloth in a sieve and set it over a clean pot. Using the strainer, strain the still-hot ghee.
- Place the strained ghee in a clean jar with a tight-fitting cover.

28. Gluten-Free Pumpkin Spice Bread

Prep time: 43 min | Serves: 1 | Difficulty: Moderate
Nutrition: Calories: 142kcal | Fat 8.6g | Protein 11g | Carbohydrate 17g
Ingredients:
- 3 large eggs
- 2 cups sugar
- 1/2 cup grapeseed oil
- One 15-ounce can of organic pumpkin
- 2 teaspoons vanilla
- 2 cups gluten-free flour
- 1 1/2 teaspoons xanthan gum
- 1 teaspoon baking powder
- 1 teaspoon baking soda
- 2 teaspoons cinnamon
- 1/2 teaspoon ground cloves
- 3/4 teaspoon nutmeg
- 3/4 teaspoon ground ginger
- 1 teaspoon sea salt

Instructions:
- Preheat the oven to 350 degrees Fahrenheit.
- Set aside two loaf pans that have been sprayed with olive oil and lined with parchment paper.
- In a medium mixing basin, whisk the eggs with a hand mixer until foamy. Continue to beat in the sugar until it is completely smooth.
- Stir in the oil, pumpkin, and vanilla extract with a spatula.
- Combine the remaining ingredients in a separate bowl.
- Combine the dry and wet ingredients in a mixing bowl and stir to combine.
- Bake for 35 minutes, flipping the pans halfway through, after pouring the batter into the prepared pans. When a toothpick or wooden skewer pushed into the center of the loaf comes out clean, the bread is done. Allow cooling on a wire rack.

29. Banana Bread

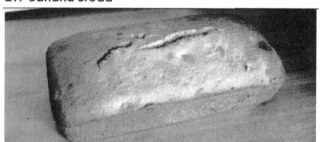

Prep time: 50 min | Serves: 1 | Difficulty: Moderate
Nutrition: Calories: 228kcal | Fat 8.5g | Protein 9g | Carbohydrate 26g
Ingredients:
- 2 cups finely ground almond flour
- 1/2 teaspoon baking soda
- 1/2 teaspoon salt
- 1/4 cup honey
- 1 large ripe banana, mashed
- 3 large eggs

Instructions:
- Preheat the oven to 300 degrees and grease and parchment paper a greased 9-x-5-inch loaf pan.
- In a mixing basin, combine the almond flour, baking soda, and salt.
- Mix the honey, mashed banana, and eggs together thoroughly.
- Pour the wet ingredients into the dry ingredients and whisk until everything is completely blended.
- Pour the batter into the prepared loaf pan and bake for 40 minutes, or until a knife inserted in the center comes out clean. Allow cooling.

30. Shannon's Non-Dairy "Yogurt."

Prep time: 1hr 5 min | Serves: 4 | Difficulty: Moderate

Nutrition: Calories: 211kcal | Fat 5g | Protein 11g | Carbohydrate 30g

Ingredients:
- 2 cups raw cashews
- Juice of 2 lemons (about 1/2 cup)
- 3 tablespoons agave or raw honey
- 1/2 teaspoon vanilla
- Pinch of sea salt

Instructions:
- Rinse the cashews after soaking them in water for 1 hour.
- In a blender or food processor, combine all of the ingredients and blend until smooth.

31. Kendall's SCD Dairy Yogurt

Prep time: 45 min | Serves: 1 | Difficulty: Moderate
Nutrition: Calories: 179kcal | Fat 3.5g | Protein 7.2g | Carbohydrate 30g

Ingredients:
- 1-quart organic whole milk
- 1 quart organic half and half (no carrageenan)
- One 10-gram package of Yogourmet starter

Instructions:
- Simmer the milk and half-and-half together. Remove the pot from the heat and cover it. Refrigerate for 25 to 30 minutes or until lukewarm. Pour a cup of the liquid through a strainer into the yogurt maker's inner bucket when it's lukewarm.
- Whisk 20 times in each direction with the contents of the starter packets. Into the bucket, strain the remaining milk mixture and whisk 10 times each way. Place the bucket's lid on top and 112 cups of water in the yogurt maker's outer container.
- Connect the machine and set the timer for 24 hours. After the 24-hour period has elapsed, remove the lid from the inner container and store it in the refrigerator for another 24 hours.

32. Herb Scramble

Prep time: 15 min | Serves: 4 | Difficulty: Moderate
Nutrition: Calories: 186kcal | Fat 9g | Protein 7.2g | Carbohydrate 18.7g

Ingredients:
- 1 bunch parsley, finely chopped 8 eggs
- 1/4 teaspoon salt
- 1/4 teaspoon freshly ground black pepper
- 1 tablespoon extra virgin olive oil

Instructions:
- Over high heat, bring a medium saucepan of water to a boil. Cook for 1 minute after adding the parsley (and any other herbs). Drain and rinse well with cold water.
- In a medium mixing basin, whisk together the eggs. Whisk together the parsley, salt, and several pinches of pepper.

- In a large nonstick or cast-iron skillet, heat the oil over medium heat. Pour in the eggs and whisk gently and consistently for 2 to 3 minutes, or until large curds form and the eggs are cooked to your liking. Serve right away.

33. Huevos Rancheros (Eggs Country-Style)

Prep time: 30 min | Serves: 3 | Difficulty: Moderate
Nutrition: Calories: 188kcal | Fat 3.1g | Protein 8.2g | Carbohydrate 31g

Ingredients:
- 6 eggs
- 1 teaspoon olive oil
- 1 small onion, finely chopped
- 1 Anaheim chili, deseeded and finely chopped
- 9 chives, finely chopped
- 10 snow peas, finely chopped
- 1 medium tomato, finely chopped
- 1/4 teaspoon oregano
- 1/4 cup fresh cilantro leaves, finely chopped
- 1/8 teaspoon each salt and pepper, or to taste
- 1/4 to 1/2 ounce grated Gruyère cheese

Instructions:
- Break the eggs into a bowl, whisk them together, and set them aside.
- In a nonstick pan, heat the olive oil over medium heat. Combine the onion and Anaheim chili in a mixing bowl. Allow 3 to 4 minutes for the onion and chiles to color. Cook for 1 minute together with the chives and snow peas in the pan.
- Cook for 2 to 4 minutes, or until the tomato is tender. Combine the oregano and the eggs in a mixing bowl. Toss in the cilantro right away. Season to taste with salt and pepper.
- Allow 3 to 5 minutes for the eggs to cook until they achieve the appropriate consistency, often stirring to avoid sticking to the pan. Add the grated cheese on top.

34. Cheese Omelet

Prep time: 10 min | Serves: 1 | Difficulty: Moderate
Nutrition: Calories: 200kcal | Fat 7.6g | Protein 11g | Carbohydrate 25g

Ingredients:
- 2 Eggs
- Salt and pepper to taste
- Low-fat cheese
- Butter

Instructions
- Butter the pan on medium heat.
- Meanwhile, beat the two eggs well with salt and pepper.
- Now pour the mix on the pan and place the cheese slices.
- Let it cook, then turn sides. Serve hot!

Chapter 5: Appetizers, Sides, and Snacks

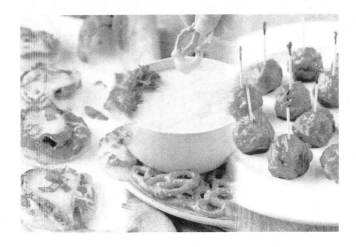

1. Cheese and Olive Polenta Fingers

Prep time: 40 min | Serves: 30 | Difficulty: Moderate
Nutrition: Calories: 122kcal | Fat 2.3g | Protein 2.5g | Carbohydrate 14g

Ingredients

- 3 cups gluten-free, onion-free chicken or vegetable stock*
- 1 cup coarse cornmeal (instant polenta)
- 1/3 cup pitted black olives, finely chopped
- 2 tablespoons salted butter
- 1/4 cup chopped flat-leaf parsley
- 1/2 cup grated Parmesan
- Freshly ground black pepper

Instructions

- Use parchment paper to line an 8-inch (20-cm) square baking dish.
- Fill a medium saucepan halfway with water and bring to a boil. Cook, stirring regularly, for 3 to 5 minutes over medium heat with the cornmeal.
- The polenta should be fairly thick at this point. Stir in the olives, butter, parsley, and half of the Parmesan until the butter and cheese are completely melted. With the black pepper, season to taste. Fill the baking dish halfway with polenta and smooth the top.
- Allow it to cool slightly before refrigerating for one hour. Preheat oven to 350 degrees Fahrenheit (180 degrees Celsius) and line a baking sheet with parchment paper. Cut the polenta into long, thin rectangles by turning it out onto a cutting board.
- Sprinkle the remaining Parmesan over the top and place it on the baking sheet. Bake for 10 to 15 minutes, or until the cheese has melted and the fingers have turned golden brown. Warm the dish before serving.

1. Crispy Noodle Cakes with Chili Sauce

Prep time: 30 min | Serves: 16 | Difficulty: Moderate
Nutrition: Calories: 179kcal | Fat 1.8g | Protein 6.5g | Carbohydrate 21g

Ingredients

- 1 pound dried flat rice noodles, broken into 2-to 4-inch
- lengths
- 3 to 4 heaping tablespoons chopped cilantro
- 2 teaspoons grated ginger
- 1/2 teaspoon Chinese five-spice powder
- 3 large eggs, lightly beaten
- 2 tablespoons sesame oil
- 2 teaspoons garlic-infused olive oil
- 1/3 cup (80 ml) gluten-free sweet red chili sauce*
- 2 heaping tablespoons cornstarch
- Salt
- Nonstick cooking spray

For Chili Sauce

- 1/2 cup gluten-free sweet red chili sauce
- 1 heaping tablespoon tomato puree
- 1/2 teaspoon gluten-free soy sauce

Instructions

- Fill a large mixing basin halfway with boiling water. Soak the noodles for 4 to 5 minutes or until they are softened. Drain, then rinse with cold water before returning to the dish.
- Combine the cilantro, ginger, five-spice powder, eggs, sesame oil, garlic-infused oil, chili sauce, cornstarch, and salt in a large mixing bowl. Over medium heat, heat a big heavy-bottomed frying pan.
- Cooking sprays the pan and the insides of the egg rings (use as many rings as will fit comfortably in the pan). Fill each ring with just enough noodle mixture to keep it from overflowing. Cook for 2 to 3 minutes on each side, or until golden brown on both sides.
- Remove the noodle cakes from the pan by running a knife along the inside of each ring. Place on a platter and loosely cover with foil to keep warm while you finish the rest of the cakes.
- In a mixing bowl, combine all of the Ingredients for the chili sauce. Serve the chili sauce beside the steaming noodle cakes.

2. Crispy Rice Balls with Parmesan and Corn

Prep time: 1h-15 min| Serves: 30| Difficulty: Moderate

Nutrition: Calories: 188kcal |Fat 1.7g| Protein 8.5g|Carbohydrate 23g

Ingredients

- 3 cups gluten-free, onion-free chicken or vegetable stock*
- 3⁄4 cup long-grain white or brown rice
- 3⁄4 cup grated Parmesan
- 3⁄4 cup canned corn kernels, drained
- 1 large egg, beaten
- 11⁄3 cups dried gluten-free, soy-free bread crumbs*
- Canola oil for pan-frying

Instructions

- Fill a big saucepan halfway with water and bring to a boil. Cook until the rice is soft, about 10 to 12 minutes for white rice and 45 to 50 minutes for brown rice.
- Return to the pan after draining. Stir in the Parmesan and corn while the rice is still heated. Set aside to chill to room temperature in a mixing bowl.
- Preheat the oven to 300 degrees Fahrenheit (150 degrees Celsius). Make 30 golf ball-sized balls out of the cooled rice mixture. Roll the balls in the bread crumbs after dipping them in the beaten egg.
- In a medium frying pan, heat a little canola oil over medium-high heat. Working in batches of ten, add the rice balls to the pan and cook until beautifully browned all over, flipping often.
- Place on a baking sheet and keep warm in the oven while you finish the rest of the recipe, adding extra oil if necessary. Warm the dish before serving.

3. Mediterranean Crustless Quiche

Prep time: 30 min| Serves: 6| Difficulty: Moderate

Nutrition: Calories: 215kcal | Fat 3.8g| Protein 8.5g|Carbohydrate 28g

Ingredients

- 2 teaspoons olive oil
- 2 tomatoes, chopped
- 1 tablespoon balsamic vinegar
- 1 large zucchini, thinly sliced into ribbons
- 1 cup grated cheddar
- 1/2 cup grated Parmesan
- 6 large eggs, lightly beaten
- 3 tablespoons basil leaves
- Salt and freshly ground black pepper

Instructions

- Preheat the oven to 350 degrees Fahrenheit (170 degrees Celsius). Line a 9-inch quiche dish or pie pan with parchment paper and grease it.
- In a nonstick frying pan, heat the olive oil over medium heat. Cook until the tomatoes and vinegar have softened.
- Place the tomatoes in a large mixing basin. Mix together the zucchini, cheddar, Parmesan, eggs, basil, salt & pepper. Fill the baking dish halfway with the quiche.
- Cook for 20 to 25 minutes, or until firm and golden brown.
- Allow for a 5-minute rest before slicing.

4. Roasted Vegetable Stacks

Prep time: 40 min| Serves: 4| Difficulty: Moderate

Nutrition: Calories: 302kcal|Fat 6.8g| Protein 11.5g|Carbohydrate 23g

Ingredients

- 1 large eggplant, cut lengthwise into 1/4-inch slices
- 1 red bell pepper, seeded and cut into 2-inch strips
- 2 large zucchinis, cut into 1/4-inch (5 mm) slices
- 1 small sweet potato, peeled (if desired) and cut into 1/4-inch (5 mm) slices
- Olive oil
- 3⁄4 cup grated Parmesan
- 4 ounces mozzarella, thinly sliced
- Salt and freshly ground black pepper
- 4 teaspoons Basil Pesto

Instructions

- Preheat oven to 350 degrees Fahrenheit (170 degrees Celsius) and line two baking sheets with parchment paper.
- On one sheet, arrange the eggplant and bell pepper in a single layer, and on the other, arrange the zucchini and sweet potato in a single layer. Bake for 15 to 20 minutes, until soft, after brushing with olive oil.
- To construct stacks, layer the eggplant slices with bell pepper, zucchini, and sweet potato on one of the baking pans. The majority of the Parmesan should be sprinkled over the stacks.
- Place the mozzarella on top of the stacks.
- Bake for 10 to 15 minutes, or until the cheeses have melted and the stacks are cooked through.
- Season with salt and pepper and top with the remaining Parmesan and a dollop of pesto.

5. Stuffed Roasted Bell Peppers

Prep time: 50 min| Serves: 4| Difficulty: Moderate

Nutrition: Calories: 169kcal |Fat 7.8g| Protein 12g|Carbohydrate 21g

Ingredients

- 4 red bell peppers
- 11⁄2 cups white rice
- 1 tablespoon garlic-infused olive oil
- 11⁄2 pounds lean ground beef

- 1 teaspoon smoked paprika
- Leaves from 8 thyme sprigs
- 3 large ripe tomatoes, peeled, seeded, and roughly chopped
- 1 teaspoon olive oil
- Splash of balsamic vinegar
- 1 heaping tablespoon pine nuts
- 1/2 cup grated Parmesan, plus more for sprinkling
- Salt and freshly ground black pepper

Instructions
- Over high heat, bring a large saucepan of water to a boil.
- Meanwhile, remove the stems and seeds from the bell peppers and chop off the tops. Hold a bell pepper over the heat of a gas burner with metal tongs to sear the exterior evenly all over.
- The skin will become black and start to bubble. (Alternatively, place all of the peppers on a foil-lined baking sheet and broil for 5 minutes, regularly rotating with tongs.) Place in a plastic bag and place somewhere warm to sweat.
- Rep with the rest of the bell peppers. At the same time, you're making the filling, set aside in the bag. Cook for 10 minutes or until the rice is soft in the boiling water, then reduce the heat to medium-high.
- Drain the water and set it aside. Preheat the oven to 350 degrees Fahrenheit (170 degrees Celsius). In a large frying pan, heat the garlic-infused oil over medium heat. Cook, constantly stirring, until the beef, paprika, and thyme are beautifully browned, breaking up any lumps as you go.
- Push the meat to the side of the pan and add the tomatoes and olive oil, cooking until the tomatoes are softened. Incorporate the sauce into the meat.
- Combine the rice, vinegar, pine nuts, and Parmesan cheese in a mixing bowl. Stir in the salt and pepper until everything is thoroughly combined.
- Peel the charred skin off the peppers after removing them from the plastic bag. It's acceptable if little shards of charred skin remain; they'll lend a delicious smoky taste to the meal.
- Fill the bell pepper shells evenly with the meat filling, lay them on a baking pan, and top with a bit additional Parmesan. Bake for 20 to 25 minutes, or until well cooked.

6. Spring Rolls

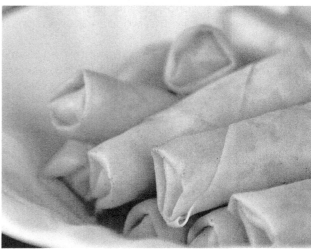

Prep time: 2h 15 min | Serves: 12 | Difficulty: Moderate
Nutrition: Calories: 241Kcal | Fats: 8g | Carbohydrates: 17g | Proteins: 8g

Ingredients
- 2 teaspoons garlic-infused olive oil
- 2 teaspoons rice bran oil, sunflower oil, or canola oil, plus enough for deep-frying
- 1 teaspoon finely grated ginger
- 2 teaspoons Chinese five-spice powder
- 2 tablespoons plus 2 teaspoons gluten-free soy sauce, plus more for serving (optional)
- 8 ounces ground pork
- 1/2 carrot, finely grated
- Half an 8-ounce can bamboo shoots, drained well and finely chopped
- 2 cups finely shredded cabbage
- Twelve 8-inch round spring roll wrappers

Instructions
- In a medium mixing bowl, mix together the garlic-infused oil, rice bran oil, ginger, five-spice powder, soy sauce, pork, carrot, bamboo shoots, and cabbage.
- To enable the flavors to mingle and the veggies to soften, cover and chill for at least 2 hours.
- Fill a big shallow dish halfway with hot water and set it aside. Soak a spring roll wrapper in water for about 1 minute or until it softens somewhat.
- Blot until completely dry with paper towels or a clean kitchen towel. Place 2 heaping teaspoons of the filling in a line approximately 112 inches (4 cm) long on the bottom third of the wrapper.
- Roll the wrapper once from the bottom over the filling and fold in the edges to cover the filling, then roll up firmly like a cigar.
- Place the rolls on a dish and cover with a damp towel while you finish the rest.
- Refrigerate for at least 2 hours before serving.
- Preheat the oven to 300 degrees Fahrenheit (150 degrees Celsius). Fill a deep-fryer or big heavy-bottomed saucepan halfway with rice bran oil

and heat to 350°F (180°C) over medium-high heat; a cube of bread placed in the oil will brown in 15 seconds, or little bubbles will form around the handle of a wooden spoon dipped in it.

- Add the spring rolls in small batches and deep-fry for 5 to 6 minutes, until crisp and golden. Drain on paper towels after removing with a slotted spoon.
- Warm in the oven while you finish the rest of the spring rolls. If preferred, serve with soy sauce.

7. Rice Paper Rolls with Dipping Sauce

Prep time: 15 min | Serves: 24 | Difficulty: Moderate
Nutrition: Calories: 200Kcal | Fats:8g | Carbohydrates:23g | Proteins:9g

Ingredients

- 2 cups gluten-free rice vermicelli, broken into 4-inch lengths
- 7 ounces boneless, skinless chicken thighs, thinly sliced
- 1/4 cup gluten-free sweet red chili sauce, plus more for serving
- Nonstick cooking spray
- Twenty-four 8-inch round rice paper wrappers
- 1 small head of butter lettuce (Boston or Bibb), leaves shredded
- 1 small carrot, thinly sliced into 1-inch-long strips
- A handful of cilantro leaves

Instructions

- Fill a large mixing basin halfway with boiling water. Soak the noodles for 4 to 5 minutes or until they are softened. Drain and rinse under cold water before draining one more.
- Toss the chicken strips in the sweet chili sauce in the meantime. Cook for 1 to 2 minutes over medium heat, until the chicken is cooked through, in a frying pan sprayed with cooking spray. Allow cooling before serving.
- Fill a big shallow dish halfway with hot water and set it aside. Soak a spring roll wrapper in water for about 1 minute or until it softens somewhat.
- Using paper towels or a clean kitchen towel, blot dry. On the bottom third of the wrapper, place a tiny handful of noodles, a little shredded lettuce, and two or three pieces of carrot and chicken in a line about 112 inches (4 cm) long.
- Garnish with a sprig of cilantro. Roll the wrapper once from the bottom over the filling and fold in the edges to cover the filling, then roll up firmly like a cigar.
- Place the rolls on a dish and cover with a damp towel while you finish the rest. If not serving right once, cover with plastic wrap and chill.
- Serve with a small cup of sweet chili sauce for dipping the rolls in.

8. Sushi

Prep time: 1h-25 min | Serves: 6-8 | Difficulty: Moderate
Nutrition: Calories: 202Kcal | Fat: 5g | Carbohydrates: 24g | Protein: 8g

Ingredients

- 2 1/2 cups short-grain (sushi) rice
- 1/3 cup seasoned rice vinegar
- 1 heaping tablespoon superfine sugar
- 1/2 teaspoon salt
- 6 nori sheets
- Gluten-free wasabi paste, toasted sesame seeds, and gluten-free soy sauce for serving

For Fillings Suggestions

Shrimp and avocado: Calories: 199kcal
- 12 peeled cooked shrimp (halved lengthwise), avocado slices, and toasted
- Sesame seeds

Vegetarian: Calories: 225kcal
- Avocado slices, baked or fried tofu strips, carrot matchsticks, shredded lettuce, cucumber strips, gluten-free mayonnaise, and toasted sesame seeds

Smoked salmon: Calories: 241kcal
- Smoked salmon strips or flaked canned tuna, avocado slices (optional), cucumber strips, and gluten-free mayonnaise

Instructions

- In a large saucepan, combine the rice and 4 cups (1 liter) of water.
- Bring to a boil, then lower to medium-low and simmer for 8 minutes, covered. Remove from the heat and let aside for 10 minutes, covered.
- In a small bowl, whisk together the vinegar, sugar, and salt until the sugar has dissolved. Transfer the rice to a large mixing basin, add the vinegar mixture, and gently whisk to combine the rice grains, keeping them separated but slightly sticky.
- Keep warm by covering with a moist kitchen towel. Do not store in the refrigerator. Place a sheet of nori, shiny-side down, on a sushi mat or piece of parchment paper with the long edge closest to you. Spread one-sixth of the cooked rice in an 18- to 14-inch-thick (3 to 5 mm) layer over the closest two-thirds of the nori sheet.
- Fill the middle of the rice layer with the filling of your choice. Using the sushi mat or parchment paper as a guide, roll the nori edge closer to you over the filling.
- Roll it tightly until the end of the sheet is reached. To seal the end, wet it with a little water and gently press it shut. Place the nori, rice, and fillings in a separate bowl, seam side down, and repeat with the remaining nori, rice, and contents.
- Cover with plastic wrap and refrigerate for 1 hour. Cut the rolls in half or into smaller pieces using a sharp knife. Wasabi paste, roasted

sesame seeds, and soy sauce are served on the side.

9. Dim Sims (Pork and Shrimp Dumplings)

Prep time: 15 min | Serves: 24 | Difficulty: Moderate
Nutrition: Calories: 211Kcal | Fats: 7.3g | Carbohydrates: 16g | Proteins: 29g

Ingredients
- 1-pound ground pork
- 5 ounces raw shrimp, peeled and deveined, finely chopped
- One 8-ounce can of bamboo shoots, drained and finely chopped (about 2/3 cup/160 ml)
- 1 cup finely chopped cabbage
- 1 large egg, lightly beaten
- 2 tablespoons plus 2 teaspoons gluten-free soy sauce, plus more for serving
- 2 teaspoons sesame oil
- 2 teaspoons garlic-infused olive oil
- 1 1/2 teaspoons finely grated ginger
- 1 heaping tablespoon cornstarch
- Twenty-four 6-inch round spring roll wrappers
- Canola, soybean, safflower, rice bran, or sunflower boil for deep-frying

Instructions
- Preheat the oven to 300 degrees Fahrenheit (150 degrees Celsius). In a medium mixing bowl, combine the pork, shrimp, bamboo shoots, and cabbage.
- In a small bowl, whisk together the egg, soy sauce, sesame oil, garlic-infused oil, ginger, and cornstarch until smooth. Mix the sauce into the pork mixture until everything is completely mixed. Fill a big shallow dish halfway with hot water and set it aside.
- Soak a spring roll wrapper in water for about 1 minute or until it softens somewhat. Using paper towels or a clean kitchen towel, blot dry.
- In the middle of the wrapper, place 2 teaspoons of the pork mixture. Using kitchen string, gather the wrapping in the center and tie it in a bow.
- Place on a serving tray and cover with a damp towel while you finish the rest of the dumplings.
- Fill a deep-fryer or big heavy-bottomed saucepan halfway with canola oil and heat to 350°F (180°C) over medium-high heat; a cube of bread placed in the oil will brown in 15 seconds, or little bubbles will emerge around the handle of a wooden spoon inserted in it.
- Deep-fry a small batch of dumplings for 5 minutes, or until golden and crisp. Drain on paper towels after removing with a slotted spoon.
- Untie the string and place the dumplings in the oven to keep warm while you finish the remainder. Serve with soy sauce on the side.

10. Salmon and Shrimp Skewers

Prep time: 3h | Serves: 4 | Difficulty: Moderate
Nutrition: Calories: 382kcal | Fats: 11g | Proteins:10g | Carbohydrates:19g

Ingredients
- 1 1/4 pound boneless, skinless Atlantic salmon steaks or fillet, cut into 3/4-inch cubes
- 24 large raw shrimp, peeled and deveined, tails intact
- 1/4 cup olive oil
- 2 tablespoons plus 2 teaspoons fresh lime juice
- 2 to 3 teaspoons finely grated lime zest
- 1/4 teaspoon cayenne pepper
- 1/2 teaspoon salt
- Freshly ground black pepper
- Green salad, for serving

Instructions
- In a glass or ceramic dish, combine the salmon and shrimp.
- In a small bowl, combine the olive oil, lime juice and zest, cayenne pepper, salt, and pepper.
- Toss the salmon and shrimp in the sauce to mingle.
- To marinate, cover, and chill for 2 to 3 hours. To avoid burning, soak wooden skewers in water for about 10 minutes before using them (you will need eight skewers for this recipe).
- On the skewers, alternate chunks of salmon and shrimp. Cook the skewers in a pan, on the broiler, or on the grill until the seafood is just done (no longer translucent). Serve alongside a crisp green salad.

11. Sesame Shrimp with Cilantro Salad

Prep time: 40 min | Serves: 4 | Difficulty: Moderate
Nutrition: Calories: 366kcal | Fats: 9.4g | Proteins:14g | Carbohydrates:21g

Ingredients
- 1 large egg
- 1/4 cup sesame seeds, toasted
- 1 1/4 cups cornstarch

For Cilantro Salad
- 3 cups roughly chopped lettuce leaves
- 1/2 English cucumber, diced
- 2 celery stalks, thinly sliced
- 1/2 green bell pepper, seeded and diced
- A handful of cilantro leaves
- A small handful of mint leaves
- 2 tablespoons plus 2 teaspoons fresh lemon juice
- 1 tablespoon plus 1 teaspoon seasoned rice vinegar
- 2 teaspoons sugar
- 1/2 small chile pepper, seeded and finely chopped (optional)
- Canola, soybean, safflower, rice bran, or sunflower oil for deep-frying
- 16 large raw shrimp, peeled and deveined, tails intact

Instructions

- In a medium bowl, whisk together the egg, sesame seeds, 1 cup (150 g) cornstarch, and 2/3 cup (170 ml) water. Make sure there are no lumps in the mixture.
- Refrigerate for 30 minutes before serving. In a large mixing bowl, add the lettuce, cucumber, celery, bell pepper, cilantro, and mint.
- In a small bowl, combine the lemon juice, vinegar, sugar, and chile (if using). Separately refrigerate the salad and dressing until shortly before serving. Heat oil to 350°F (180°C) in a deep-fryer or big heavy-bottomed saucepan over medium-high heat; a cube of bread put in the oil will brown in 15 seconds, or little bubbles will emerge around the handle of a wooden spoon inserted in it.
- Take the batter out of the fridge and give it a good stir. Shake off any leftover cornstarch before tossing the shrimp in the remaining cornstarch. In small batches, dip the shrimp in the batter and drop them into the hot oil.
- Cook for 3–4 minutes, or until the batter has become crispy. While you cook the remainder, remove the shrimp with a slotted spoon and drain on paper towels.
- Pour the dressing over the salad and gently toss to coat while the last set of shrimp cooks. Serve the prawns beside the salad right away.

12. Salt-nd-Pepper Calamari with Garden Salad

Prep time: 4h-15 min | Serves: 4 | Difficulty: Moderate
Nutrition: Calories: 475kcal | Fats:12g | Proteins:13g | Carbohydrates:29g
Ingredients
- 8 medium squid bodies, well cleaned and cut into quarters
- 1 tablespoon garlic-infused olive oil
- 2 tablespoons olive oil
- 1/2 teaspoon salt
- Freshly ground black pepper

For Garden Salad
- 3 cups roughly chopped lettuce leaves
- 1/2 English cucumber, thinly sliced
- 1 avocado, pitted, peeled, and sliced (optional)
- 2 celery stalks, thinly sliced
- 1/2 green bell pepper, seeded and sliced
- 1 cup snow pea shoots or bean sprouts

For Dressing
- 1/4 cup olive oil
- 2 tablespoons fresh lemon juice
- 1 tablespoon garlic-infused olive oil
- 1/2 teaspoon brown sugar
- Salt

Instructions
- Score the squid pieces in a 13-inch (1 cm) crisscross pattern with a sharp knife.

- Make sure you don't cut all the way through—about three-quarters of the way through. When the squid is cooked, it will curl as a result of this. In a large mixing bowl, combine the garlic-infused oil, olive oil, salt, and pepper. Toss in the squid pieces to coat.
- Refrigerate for 3 to 4 hours, covered. Prepare the salad just before you're ready to dine. In a large mixing bowl, combine the lettuce, cucumber, avocado (if using), celery, bell pepper, and snow pea shoots.
- To prepare the dressing, whisk together all of the Ingredients in a small screw-top jar until thoroughly combined. Preheat the grill to high temperature (or place a ridged grill pan or cast-iron skillet over high heat). Cook for 3 to 4 minutes, until the squid is curled and faintly brown.
- If the dressing has split, re-shake it and sprinkle it over the salad, tossing gently to coat.
- Arrange the squid on top of the mixture in separate dishes. Serve right away.

13. San Choy Bow (Asian Pork Lettuce Wraps)

Prep time: 15 min | Serves: 6 | Difficulty: Moderate
Nutrition: Calories: 301kcal | Fats: 9.5g | Proteins:17g | Carbohydrates: 26g
Ingredients
- 2 tablespoons sesame oil
- 1 tablespoon garlic-infused olive oil
- 2 teaspoons finely grated ginger
- 1-pound ground pork
- One 8-ounce can bamboo shoots, drained and finely chopped
- One 8-ounce can water chestnuts, drained and finely chopped
- 1 heaping tablespoon chopped cilantro
- 2 tablespoons plus 2 teaspoons fresh lemon juice
- 2 tablespoons gluten-free sweet red chili sauce*
- 1 teaspoon fish sauce, or 3/4 teaspoon soy sauce and a splash of lime juice
- 6 iceberg lettuce leaves, rinsed and dried

Instructions
- Preheat a wok over high heat. Heat the sesame oil and garlic-infused oil until they are nearly smoking.
- Stir in the ginger until it is barely caramelized. Stir-fry the pork for 3 to 4 minutes over high heat, until nicely browned, breaking up any lumps as you go.
- Stir-fry for another 2 minutes with the bamboo shoots, water chestnuts, cilantro, lemon juice, sweet chilli sauce, and fish sauce.
- Place the lettuce, convex side down, on a platter or individual plates (like cups). Spoon the pork filling into the lettuce cups with a slotted spoon and serve right away.

14. Oysters, Three Ways

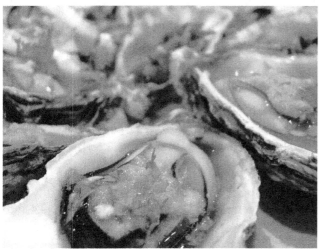

Prep time: 20 min| Serves: 12| Difficulty: Moderate
Nutrition: Calories: 291kcal |Fats: 9g| Proteins:15g | Carbohydrates: 21g

Ingredients
- 12 freshly shucked oysters, fully detached from and replaced on their shell

Cheese-Crusted   Calories: 38kcal
- 2 heaping tablespoons dried gluten-free, soy-free bread crumbs*
- 1 heaping tablespoon grated Parmesan
- 1 teaspoon finely chopped flat-leaf parsley
- 3 1/2 ounces Camembert, cut into 12 thin slices

Oysters Kilpatrick   Calories: 55kcal
- 3 to 5 lean bacon slices, finely chopped
- 1/4 cup gluten-free Worcestershire sauce
- Tomato and Chile
- 2 teaspoons garlic-infused olive oil
- 1/2 small red chile pepper, finely chopped
- 1/2 cup tomato puree

Tomato and Chile   Calories: 19kcal
- 2 teaspoons garlic-infused olive oil
- 1/2 small red chile pepper, finely chopped
- 1/2 cup tomato puree

Instructions
- Place the oysters in their shells on a baking sheet that has been lined with foil. Preheat the broiler to its highest setting. In a separate bowl, mix the bread crumbs, Parmesan, and parsley for the cheese-crusted oysters.
- On each oyster, place a piece of Camembert. Over the top, strew the bread crumb mixture. Cook the bacon till crisp for the oysters Kilpatrick.
- Using a paper towel, absorb any excess liquid. Heat the oil in a small frying pan over medium heat, add the chile pepper, and sauté until softened for tomato and chile oysters. Add the tomato puree and mix well.
- Pour the sauce over the oysters in an equal layer. Cook the oysters in the broiler for a few minutes until they are heated. Serve right away, but be careful since the shells are really hot.

15. Chicken Liver Pâté with Pepper and Sage

Prep time: 3h 15 min| Serves: 12| Difficulty: Moderate
Nutrition: Calories: 191kcal |Fats: 9.3g| Proteins:21g | Carbohydrates:17g

Ingredients
- 8 tablespoons salted butter, plus 3 tablespoons, melted butter
- 1 tablespoon garlic-infused olive oil
- 1 tablespoon olive oil
- 1 teaspoon finely chopped sage, plus more leaves for garnish
- 17 ounces chicken livers, rinsed and trimmed (about 10 livers)
- 1 heaping tablespoon freshly ground black pepper
- 1/2 cup light cream
- Gluten-free crackers, for serving

Instructions
- In a medium saucepan over medium heat, combine the 8 tablespoons butter, garlic-infused oil, and olive oil.
- Cook, stirring often, for 2 to 3 minutes after adding the sage. Cook until the chicken livers are lightly browned. Remove the pan from the heat and mix in the cream and pepper.
- Puree in a food processor or with an immersion blender until smooth. Blend in the melted butter until smooth. Serve in six 4-ounce (125-ml) ramekins or one 3-cup (700-ml) mould with sage leaves on top.
- Cover and chill for 3 hours, or until firm. With crackers on the side.

16. Crêpes with Cheese Sauce

Prep time: 35 min| Serves: 4| Difficulty: Moderate
Nutrition: Calories:317 kcal| Fat:8.6 g |Protein: 25 g| Carbohydrates:16 g

Ingredients
Crêpes
- 3/4 cup superfine white rice flour
- 1/2 cup cornstarch
- 1/3 cup soy flour
- 3/4 teaspoon baking soda
- 2 large eggs, lightly beaten
- 1 1/2 cups low-fat milk, lactose-free milk, or suitable plant-based milk
- 3 tablespoons salted butter, melted
- Nonstick cooking spray

Cheese Sauce
- 2 cups low-fat milk, lactose-free milk, or suitable plant-based milk
- 2 heaping tablespoons cornstarch
- 2 cups grated reduced-fat cheddar
- Salt and freshly ground black pepper

Ham and Spinach Filling   Calories: 670kcal
- Olive oil, for pan-frying
- 8 ounces baby spinach leaves, rinsed and dried

- 8 ounces thinly sliced gluten-free smoked ham

Tempeh and Rice Filling   Calories: 676kcal
- 1/2 tablespoon garlic-infused olive oil
- 12 ounces crumbled gluten-free tempeh
- 1/2 teaspoon smoked paprika
- Leaves from 4 thyme sprigs
- 3/4 cup cooked white rice
- 2 medium ripe tomatoes, peeled, seeded, and roughly chopped
- 1/2 teaspoon olive oil
- Splash of balsamic vinegar
- Salt and freshly ground black pepper to taste
- 1/4 cup pine nuts

Instructions
- Sift the rice flour, cornstarch, soy flour, and baking soda three times into a large mixing basin to make the crêpes (or whisk in the bowl until well combined).
- Make a well in the center, then add the eggs and milk and mix until smooth. Add the melted butter and mix well. Set aside for 20 minutes, covered in plastic wrap.
- Spray a heavy-bottomed frying pan or crêpe pan with cooking spray and heat over medium heat.
- Pour approximately 1/4 cup (60 ml) batter into the preheated pan and tilt to thinly coat the bottom. Cook until bubbles emerge, then carefully flip the crêpe and cook the other side for a few seconds.
- Transfer to a tray and cover loosely with foil to keep warm while you create the cheese sauce and continue with the remaining batter (for a total of 8 crêpes).
- To prepare the cheese sauce, mix a paste with 14 cup (60 ml) milk and the cornstarch. Whisk in the remaining milk, making sure there are no lumps. Pour the Ingredients into a small saucepan and cook, stirring constantly, until it thickens. (Do not allow it to boil.) Stir in the cheddar until it is completely melted.
- Season with salt and pepper to taste. While you prepare the filling of your choosing, keep warm. In a large frying pan, heat the olive oil over medium heat to prepare the ham and spinach filling. Stir in the spinach to coat it with the oil.
- Cover and simmer for 1 minute, then uncover, stir, cover, and cook for 1 minute longer, or until the spinach is barely wilted.
- Place the spinach in the middle of the crêpes and top with sliced ham. In a large frying pan, heat the garlic-infused oil over medium-high heat to prepare the tempeh and rice filling.
- Cook for 7 minutes, or until the crumbled tempeh, smoked paprika, and thyme are browned and crisp. Continue to sauté until the rice is completely warmed through.
- Remove the pan from the heat and add the tomatoes, olive oil, balsamic vinegar, and

seasonings. Distribute the contents evenly among the crêpes and finish with a sprinkling of pine nuts on top of each. Fold the crêpes in half and top with a sprinkle of cheese sauce and your filling of choice.
- Finish with a final grain of pepper and the leftover cheese sauce.

---

17. Spinach, Squash, and Sage Polenta Squares

Prep time: 3h-40min| Serves: 4| Difficulty: Moderate
Nutrition: Calories: 191kcal| Fats: 9.5g| Proteins:17g | Carbohydrates: 19g
Ingredients
- 14 ounces kabocha or other suitable winter squash, peeled, seeded, and cut into 3/4-inch cubes
- Garlic-infused olive oil
- 3 cups gluten-free, onion-free vegetable stock
- 1 cup coarse cornmeal (instant polenta)
- 2 tablespoons roughly chopped sage leaves
- 2 ounces baby spinach leaves, rinsed and dried
- Salt and freshly ground black pepper
- Green salad, for serving

Instructions
- Preheat the oven to 350 degrees Fahrenheit (180 degrees Celsius). Drizzle the oil over the squash pieces on a baking sheet.
- Bake for 30 to 40 minutes, or until brown and cooked through, flipping once. Set aside, covered with foil. In a medium saucepan over high heat, bring the stock to a boil.
- Reduce the heat to medium-low and cook the cornmeal for 2 to 3 minutes, stirring frequently. The polenta should be fairly thick at this point. Turn off the heat.
- Stir in 2 tablespoons oil, the sage, and the spinach until the spinach has wilted. Season with salt and pepper to taste.
- Arrange the squash pieces over the bottom of an 8-inch (20-cm) square baking dish lined with parchment paper. Pour the polenta on top and spread it out evenly.
- Allow it cool slightly before wrapping in plastic wrap and placing in the refrigerator for 2 to 3 hours, or until hard. Cut the polenta into pieces after turning it out onto a cutting board.
- Warm it in foil under the broiler for 3 to 5 minutes if you prefer it cold. It's also great warmed up in a ridged grill pan or cast-iron skillet on the stove. Serve with a fresh salad on the side.

18. Pesto Mini Pizzas

Prep time: 30 min | Serves: 6 | Difficulty: Moderate
Nutrition: Calories: 311kcal | Fats: 11.9g | Proteins:9.3g | Carbohydrates: 26g

Ingredients
- 2 cups gluten-free, soy-free bread mix
- 2 tablespoons Basil Pesto

For Chicken and Bacon   Calories: 514kcal
- 2 teaspoons garlic-infused olive oil
- 1 pound boneless, skinless chicken breasts, thinly sliced
- 8 ounces lean bacon slices, chopped
- 6 mozzarella bocconcini, sliced

For Tempeh And Red Pepper   Calories: 323kcal
- 2 teaspoons garlic-infused olive oil
- 1-pound gluten-free tempeh, crumbled and steamed
- 1/2 cup roasted red bell peppers, sliced

Instructions
- Preheat the oven to 250 degrees Fahrenheit (120 degrees Celsius). Use parchment paper to line one or two large baking sheets. Prepare the bread mix according to the package guidelines.
- Spread one-sixth of the bread mixture onto the parchment paper in a 6-inch (15-cm) circle with the back of a big metal spoon. If required, dip the spoon in water to aid in spreading.
- Rep with the rest of the mixture. Preheat oven to 350°F and bake for 15 minutes, or until gently browned. Remove the pan from the oven and raise the temperature to 350 degrees Fahrenheit (180 degrees Celsius). Meanwhile, heat the oil in a heavy-bottomed frying pan over medium heat for the chicken and bacon pizzas.
- Cook, tossing constantly, until the bacon is crispy and the chicken is golden brown. Drain on paper towels after removing with a slotted spoon.
- Heat the oil in a heavy-bottomed frying pan over medium heat for the tempeh and red pepper pizzas. Cook, stirring constantly, until the tempeh is crispy.
- Drain on paper towels after removing with a slotted spoon. Using 1 teaspoon of pesto, spread 1 teaspoon of pesto on each pizza dough.
- Alternatively, top with bacon and chicken, followed by mozzarella, or tempeh and roasted peppers. Bake for 15 minutes, or until the cheese is completely melted. Bake the pizzas directly on the oven rack for a crispier crust.

19. Vegetable-Tofu Skewers

Prep time: 3h-25 min | Serves: 4 | Difficulty: Moderate
Nutrition: Calories: 462kcal | Fats: 12g | Proteins:27g | Carbohydrates: 23g

Ingredients
- 1/2 cup gluten-free soy sauce
- 2 tablespoons sesame oil
- 1 teaspoon grated ginger
- 7 ounces firm tofu, pressed and cut into 1/2-inch cubes
- 18 ounces sweet potatoes, cut into 3/4-inch cubes
- 1 large eggplant, cut into 1/2-inch cubes
- 1 large zucchini, halved lengthwise and cut into 1/3-inch slices
- 2 green or red bell peppers, seeded and cut into 3/4-inch squares
- Olive oil (optional)
- 1/2 cup gluten-free sweet red chili sauce

Instructions
- In a small bowl, combine the soy sauce, sesame oil, and ginger. In a big container with a cover, place the tofu.
- Pour the marinade on top and gently toss to coat. Cover and chill for 2 to 3 hours, shaking regularly to ensure that the tofu is well coated in the marinade. A big pot of water should be brought to a boil.
- Cook for approximately 5 minutes, until the sweet potato is barely cooked, over medium-high heat. Drain the water and set it aside. To avoid burning, soak wooden skewers in water for about 10 minutes before using (you will need eight skewers).
- Prepare the broiler if broiling; if grilling, preheat the grill to medium. Alternate between threading the veggie and tofu pieces onto the skewers.
- Grill or pan-fry the skewers over medium heat, or broil them, flipping them frequently and spraying with olive oil if needed to keep them from sticking. Serve immediately with the sweet chilli sauce poured over top.

20. Chicken Drumsticks with Lemon and Cilantro

Prep time: 2h-30 min | Serves: 4 | Difficulty: Moderate
Nutrition: Calories: 235kcal | Fat 7.8g | Protein 11.5g | Carbohydrate 28g

Ingredients
- 1/4 cup gluten-free soy sauce
- 2 tablespoons plus 2 teaspoons light brown sugar
- 2 teaspoons garlic-infused olive oil
- 2 teaspoons olive oil
- 2 tablespoons plus 2 teaspoons fresh lemon juice
- 2 tablespoons plus 2 teaspoons sesame oil
- 8 chicken drumsticks
- 2 heaping tablespoons chopped cilantro

Instructions

- To create the marinade, in a large baking dish, whisk together the soy sauce, brown sugar, garlic-infused oil, olive oil, lemon juice, and sesame oil until the sugar has dissolved.
- Toss the chicken in the marinade and flip each drumstick to ensure that it is well covered. Refrigerate the dish for several hours or overnight.
- Preheat the oven to 350 degrees Fahrenheit (180 degrees Celsius) or the grill to medium-high. Bake or grill the drumsticks for 15 to 20 minutes, flipping regularly, until the juices flow clear when a toothpick is inserted into the thickest section of the drumsticks. Just before serving, garnish with cilantro.

21. Beef Kofta with Tahini Sauce

Prep time: 20 min| Serves: 4-6 | Difficulty: Moderate
Nutrition: Calories: 347kcal | Fat 8.9g| Protein 26g|Carbohydrate 19g
Ingredients
Tahini Sauce
- 1/2 cup gluten-free low-fat plain yogurt
- 2 teaspoons fresh lemon juice
- 2 tablespoons plus 2 teaspoons tahini
- 1 teaspoon garlic-infused olive oil
- 1 pound lean ground beef
- 2 large eggs, lightly beaten
- 1/3 cup dried gluten-free, soy-free bread crumbs*
- 1/4 cup finely chopped flat-leaf parsley
- 1 teaspoon ground cinnamon
- 2 tablespoons ground cumin
- 1/2 teaspoon cayenne pepper, or to taste
- 1 heaping tablespoon ground turmeric
- 1 1/2 teaspoons ground allspice
- Green salad or vegetables, for serving

Instructions

- To avoid burning, soak wooden skewers in water for 10 minutes before using (you will need 12 skewers). Preheat the grill if you're grilling. In the meantime, create the tahini sauce by mixing together all of the Ingredients in a small basin.
- Set aside for a few minutes to enable the flavours to mingle. In a large mixing basin, add the meat, eggs, bread crumbs, parsley, cinnamon, cumin, cayenne pepper, turmeric, and allspice, and mix thoroughly with your hands.
- Wrap each skewer in roughly a quarter cup (60 ml) of the meat mixture.
- Grill, broil, or pan-fry the kofta until it is evenly browned and cooked to your liking.
- Serve with tahini sauce and salad or veggies of your choice.

22. California Rice Pilaf

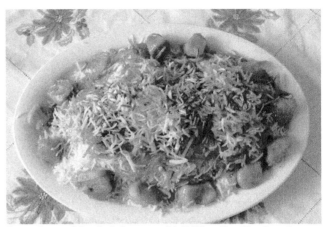

Prep time: 35 min| Serves: 8| Difficulty: Moderate
Nutrition: Calories: 212kcal| Fat 8g| Protein 7.5g|Carbohydrate 28g
Ingredients
- 2 cups uncooked jasmine rice
- 1 teaspoon salt
- 3 cups water
- 1 tablespoon grated lemon zest
- 1/4 cup fresh lemon juice (from 1 large lemon)
- 1/4 cup chopped walnuts
- 1 1/4 cups trimmed and chopped green beans, cut to the size of peas
- 1/4 cup extra-virgin olive oil
- 1/2 cup julienned sun-dried tomatoes
- 1/4 cup minced fresh parsley or basil
- 1/2 teaspoon freshly ground black pepper

Instructions

- Combine the rice, salt, and water in a medium saucepan. Bring to a boil over high heat, then lower to a low heat and cook for 20 minutes. Remove the pan from the heat, stir, cover, and let the rice to steam for another 10 minutes.
- Combine the lemon zest, lemon juice, walnuts, beans, oil, sundried tomatoes, parsley, and pepper in a large mixing bowl. Toss in the warmed rice.

23. Easy Caprese

Prep time: 10 min| Serves: 8| Difficulty: Moderate
Nutrition: Calories: 155kcal| Fat 3.8g| Protein 8.5g|Carbohydrate 17g
Ingredients
- 1/2 pound bite-size fresh mozzarella balls, drained
- 10 ounces grape or cherry tomatoes, cut in half
- 8 Kalamata olives, pits removed, cut in half
- 2 tablespoons extra-virgin olive oil
- 1 tablespoon balsamic vinegar
- 1/4 teaspoon salt
- 1/4 teaspoon freshly ground black pepper, plus more for serving
- 1/3 cup coarsely chopped fresh basil leaves

Instructions

- Combine the cheese, tomatoes, olives, oil, vinegar, salt, and pepper in a medium mixing bowl. Sprinkle the basil over top right before serving. If preferred, sprinkle with more freshly ground black pepper in serving dishes.

24. Quick and Easy Salsa

Prep time: 15 min | Serves: 10 | Difficulty: Moderate
Nutrition: Calories: 62kcal | Fat 3.8g | Protein 5.3g | Carbohydrate 25g

Ingredients

- 2 cups finely chopped ripe tomatoes
- 3 scallion greens, thinly sliced
- 2 tablespoons finely chopped fresh cilantro leaves
- 1 teaspoon garlic-infused olive oil
- ¼ teaspoon salt, or more if needed
- 2 tablespoons fresh lime juice (from 1 lime)

Instructions

- Combine the tomatoes, scallion greens, cilantro, oil, salt, and lime juice in a medium glass or ceramic bowl. To enable the flavors to mix, cover and chill for several hours.
- Warm or cold salsa can be offered. Refrigerate for up to 4 days, or until ready to use.

25. Rockin' Gravy

Prep time: 15min | Serves: 6 | Difficulty: Moderate
Nutrition: Calories: 343kcal | Fat 5.2g | Protein 9.5g | Carbohydrate 29g

Ingredients:

- 1/4 cup almond butter
- 1/2 cup filtered water
- 2 cups quartered portabella mushrooms
- 1 tablespoon minced onion
- 6 stalks celery, minced
- 1 teaspoon each garlic powder and onion powder
- 2 tablespoons Nama Shoyu
- 1/4 teaspoon fresh black pepper, or to taste
- 4 tablespoons finely chopped cremini mushrooms
- 1 tablespoon powdered flaxseed to thicken gravy

Instructions

- In a blender, puree the celery, garlic powder, onion powder, Nama Shoyu, and pepper until smooth. Place in a mixing basin.
- Cook until the mixture is thick and gravy-like, then add the chopped mushrooms and powdered flaxseed. Warm in a dehydrator on the warm setting or in an oven on the lowest heat with the door open (if desired)

26. Refrigerator Pickles

Prep time: 25 min | Serves: 8 | Difficulty: Moderate
Nutrition: Calories: 119kcal | Fat 3.2g | Protein 2.5g | Carbohydrate 23g

Ingredients

- 4 cups sliced or julienned vegetables, such as pickling cucumbers, carrots, radishes, green beans
- 8 sprigs of fresh dill
- 2 teaspoons mustard seeds
- 1 teaspoon salt
- 1 tablespoon sugar
- 1¼ cups apple cider vinegar
- ¾ cup water

Instructions

- Fill two 1-pint canning jars with the veggies. Continue filling until the jars are completely full, shaking them to settle the veggies. Place four dill sprigs in each jar. Distribute the mustard seeds evenly among the jars.
- Combine the salt, sugar, vinegar, and water in a small saucepan and stir until the salt and sugar are dissolved. Bring to a boil, then gently pour the vinegar mixture into the jars, dividing it equally. If required, add additional boiling water to fill the jars.
- Allow to cool. Cover the jars firmly after they've cooled enough to handle. Refrigerate the pickles for at least 3 hours, or up to 1 week, before serving.

27. Crispy-Tender Roasted Potato Wedges

Prep time: 25 min | Serves: 6 | Difficulty: Moderate
Nutrition: Calories: 207kcal | Fat 6.2g | Protein 6.5g | Carbohydrate 32g

Ingredients

- 2 pounds russet (baking) potatoes, unpeeled, cut into ¾-inch wedges
- 1 tablespoon garlic-infused olive oil
- ¼ teaspoon salt
- ¼ teaspoon freshly ground black pepper
- 1 teaspoon Italian seasoning
- 1¼ cups boiling water
- Fresh herbs such as dill or parsley, for garnish (optional)

Instructions

- Preheat the oven to 450 degrees Fahrenheit.
- Drizzle the oil over the potato wedges on a baking sheet with 1-inch sides. Stir to moisten the potatoes, then arrange them in a single layer and season with salt, pepper, and Italian seasoning. Cut sides down, arrange the potato wedges in a single layer. Avoid washing the spice off the potatoes by pouring 34 cup of hot water around them.
- 30 minutes of roasting Remove the baking tray from the oven, flip the potatoes, and fill the baking pan with the remaining 12 cup water.

Return the pan to the oven for another 45 to 60 minutes, or until the potato wedges are crisp on the edges and soft and fluffy on the inside. If desired, garnish with fresh herbs. Serve right away.

28. Spicy Hummus
Prep time: 45 min | Serves: 8 | Difficulty: Moderate
Nutrition: Calories: 189kcal | Fat 7.2g | Protein 5.2g | Carbohydrate 24.3g
Ingredients
- 1 15-ounce can chickpeas, drained and rinsed
- 3 tablespoons water
- 2 tablespoons fresh lemon juice (from 1 small lemon)
- 2 tablespoons peanut butter
- 3 tablespoons garlic-infused olive oil
- 1 teaspoon ground cumin
- ½ teaspoon salt
- 2 teaspoons sesame oil, plus more for serving if desired
- 1 small fresh chile, seeds removed, finely chopped (optional)
- 2 tablespoons finely chopped fresh cilantro, plus more for serving if desired
Instructions
- Combine the chickpeas, water, lemon juice, peanut butter, olive oil, cumin, salt, sesame oil, and chile in a blender or food processor. Grind at a low speed for a few seconds, then process on high until the necessary smoothness is achieved. Scrape down the sides as needed and add a teaspoon of water at a time to keep the hummus moving in the blender. Add the cilantro and mix well.
- Pour the hummus into a serving dish and top with more sesame oil and cilantro, if desired. Refrigerate until ready to serve.

29. Spinach Dip and Mini Sweet-Pepper Poppers
Prep time: 45 min | Serves: 14 | Difficulty: Moderate
Nutrition: Calories: 167kcal | Fat 4.2g | Protein 10g | Carbohydrate 26g
Ingredients
- 1 pound multicolored miniature sweet peppers
- 1 12-ounce package frozen chopped spinach
- ¼ cup mayonnaise
- ¼ cup grated Parmesan cheese (1 ounce)
- 4 ounces Neufchâtel cheese, softened
- ⅛ teaspoon salt
- ⅛ teaspoon salt
- ¼ teaspoon freshly ground black pepper
- ¼ cup shredded pepper jack cheese (1 ounce)
Instructions
- With a sharp knife, cut the peppers lengthwise, keeping in mind which side the peppers would naturally lay on, with the sliced side facing straight up. Using a sharp-edged spoon or melon baller, remove the seeds.
- Follow the package directions for cooking the spinach. Drain it in a strainer, carefully pushing out the excess water.
- Preheat the oven to 350 degrees Fahrenheit. Oil a baking sheet by brushing or spraying it.
- In a medium mixing bowl, combine the mayonnaise, Parmesan, Neufchâtel cheese, salt, and pepper. Stir in the spinach gently. Spoon the dip into the peppers and arrange them on the prepared baking sheet, dip side up. Top each one with a hefty amount of pepper jack cheese.
- Bake for 35 minutes, or until the cheese is melted and bubbling. Place the poppers on a dish and serve immediately.

30. Thai Summer Salad Rolls
Prep time: 45 min | Serves: 14 | Difficulty: Moderate
Nutrition: Calories: 201kcal | Fat 6g | Protein 12g | Carbohydrate 30g
Ingredients
- 4 ounces rice sticks or vermicelli
- 8 11-inch rice papers
- 2 cups shredded lettuce
- 1 cup fresh basil leaves
- ½ cup fresh cilantro leaves
- 2 medium carrots, shredded
- 1 medium cucumber, cut into matchsticks
- 16 medium shrimp (½ pound), peeled, deveined, and cooked
Instructions
- Rinse with cold water, and lay aside the rice sticks according to the package guidelines. (If the Instructions are unclear, boil the rice sticks for 2 minutes, then test for doneness, drain, and set away.) Place a moist towel on the counter and a big basin of extremely warm water next to it. Make sure you have all of the necessary components on hand.
- One rice paper at a time, dip it into the warm water and rotate it for approximately 5 seconds before spreading it out on the moist towel. The soaking duration will vary somewhat depending on the temperature of the water; after removed from the water, the rice paper will continue to soften.
- In the lowest third of the rice paper, make a 5- to 6-inch log-shaped mound with approximately one-eighth of the shredded lettuce, basil, cilantro, carrots, cucumbers, shrimp, and rice sticks. Fold the rice paper's bottom tightly over the contents. Overlap the 2-inch side flaps over the center. Finally, create a tight coil approximately 5 inches long by rolling the log toward the rear border of the rice paper. The sticky rice paper will attach to itself if it is moist. Set aside on a serving platter while you finish up

the rest of the Ingredients and rice sheets. Until ready to serve, keep the completed rolls covered with a clean, moist cloth.

- With a sharp knife, slice each summer roll once on the diagonal and serve immediately.

31. Bacon Deviled Eggs

Prep time: 45 min | Serves: 14 | Difficulty: Moderate
Nutrition: Calories: 198kcal | Fat 9g | Protein 13g | Carbohydrate 22g

Ingredients
- 2 thick slices of bacon
- 1 dozen large eggs
- 5 tablespoons mayonnaise
- ¼ teaspoon salt
- ¼ teaspoon freshly ground black pepper
- 2 teaspoons grainy mustard
- 2 tablespoons chopped fresh chives or scallion greens

Instructions
- Cook the bacon in a small pan over medium heat until crisp. Set aside after draining on a paper towel.
- Bring 2 quarts of water to a boil in a 3-quart saucepan. Using a spoon, carefully place the eggs into the boiling water one by one. Return the water to a boil, then reduce to a medium heat and cook for 12 minutes. Drain the eggs and place them in an ice bath to chill down. When the eggs are cold enough to handle, break them carefully and peel them. Using a sharp knife, cut each egg in half. Set the egg white halves cavity on a serving platter and collect the yolks in a medium bowl.
- Mash the yolks with a fork until smooth, then add the mayonnaise, salt, pepper, and mustard. The yolk mixture should be piped or spooned into the halved egg whites. Chop the bacon into small pieces to use as a garnish for the filled eggs; add the chives, cover, and refrigerate until ready to serve.

32. Hot Vegetable Pie

Prep time: 45 min | Serves: 4 | Difficulty: Moderate
Nutrition: Calories: 210kcal | Fat 3.2g | Protein 5.5g | Carbohydrate 37g

Ingredients
- 1 pie crust of your choice
- 1/2 cauliflower head
- 3 cups greens, stems removed (such as collards, spinach, or chard)
- 115 g fresh mushrooms
- 1 tablespoon canola oil or grapeseed oil, divided
- 1 sweet onion, diced
- 1 clove garlic, minced
- 2 cups oat milk

- 2/3 cup oats
- 3/4 cup crumbled goat cheese or sheep's milk cheese (strong flavor)
- 3 teaspoons caraway seeds

Instructions
- This is as comfortable as a blanket; a warm, chewy, wonderful blanket."
- Preheat the oven to 425°F (220°C, gas mark 7) and bake for 30 minutes.
- Prepare the pie dough by rolling it out and pressing it into the pie pan.
- Until the cauliflower and greens are tender, steam them. (If you're using a double pot steamer, bring the cauliflower closer to the boiling water; otherwise, steam the cauliflower for a few minutes before adding the greens.)
- Sauté the mushrooms in a frying pan. Set the cauliflower, greens, and mushrooms aside in the pie shell. Sauté the onions and garlic in the remaining oil in the frying pan until they begin to soften.
- Meanwhile, put the milk substitute and oats in a cup, then combine the mixture with the onions and garlic in the frying pan. To thicken, cook for 1 to 2 minutes, stirring regularly. Remove the pan from the heat and add the cheese. Over the veggies in the pie shell, pour the sauce. Bake for 25 to 30 minutes, uncovered. Serve with a sprinkling of caraway seeds on top.

33. Gnocchi Sweet Gnocchi

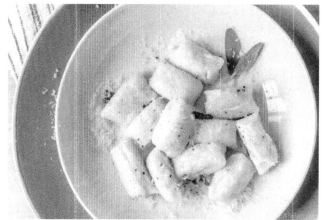

Prep time: 45 min | Serves: 4 | Difficulty: Moderate
Nutrition: Calories: 182kcal | Fat 5.2g | Protein 10g | Carbohydrate 29g

Ingredients
- 3 parsnips
- 13/4 cups buckwheat flour, divided
- 3/4 cup oat flour
- 1 teaspoon allspice
- 3 teaspoons cinnamon
- 1 can pumpkin puree
- 1/2 teaspoon salt

Instructions

- Preheat the oven to 400 degrees Fahrenheit (200 degrees Celsius, or gas mark 6)
- Each parsnip should have five to six sets of holes pierced with a fork. Bake the parsnips for approximately an hour, or until the flesh is extremely tender. To avoid scorching the skin, rotate the parsnips once or twice.
- Combine the 1 cup 010 g) buckwheat flour, oat flour, all spice, cinnamon, and pumpkin in a mixing bowl.
- Half-fill a saucepan with water, then add the salt and set it on top of the burner to use later.
- Remove the skin and scrape the meat away from the cores when the parsnips are done cooking; discard the cores and skins. Puree or crush the meat with your hands in a food processor. Combine the parsnips and pumpkin in a blender. To make the dough less sticky, add part of the saved buckwheat flour now.
- On a level surface, sprinkle some of the saved buckwheat flour. Bring the water to a boil in the saucepan. Roll out the dough into "logs" of about a half-inch (2 cm) thick. Pinch off little pieces and flatten with the back of a fork one side. Place 10 to 15 gnocchi in a pot of boiling water and cook for 2 minutes, or until they float to the top. Using a strainer spoon, remove the gnocchi from the water.

34. Mediterranean Tofu Scramble

Prep time: 45 min | Serves: 3 | Difficulty: Moderate
Nutrition: Calories: 210kcal | Fat 5.2g | Protein 9.5g | Carbohydrate 31g
Ingredients
- 1/2 cup low-sodium vegetable broth
- 1 12 ounces package soft tofu or 12-18 egg whites
- 1 bag (mixed red and green chard, stems removed (small leaves preferable)
- 1 teaspoon dark, unrefined sesame seed oil
- 2 tablespoons black sesame seeds, ground
- 3 ounces goat cheese or sheep's milk crumbles (optional)

Instructions
- Bring the vegetable broth to a boil in a saute pan over medium heat. Sauté the chard for 3 to 5 minutes, or until wilted.
- Continue to sauté, stirring often, as you add the tofu (crumbling with a fork) or egg whites. Reduce the heat to medium, then add the oil and the seeds, stirring constantly. Cover for about 3 minutes after adding the cheese, if using. Remove the pan from the heat and arrange the plates on top.

35. Saag-sationa

Prep time: 45 min | Serves: 4 | Difficulty: Moderate
Nutrition: Calories: 245kcal | Fat 4g | Protein 8.4g | Carbohydrate 27g
Ingredients
- 8 ounces frozen cauliflower, thawed
- 8 ounces frozen, chopped spinach, thawed
- 2 teaspoons ginger powder
- 1 teaspoon fennel seeds
- 1 teaspoon brown mustard seeds
- 1/2 teaspoon chili powder
- 3 teaspoons minced garlic
- 1 teaspoon salt
- 1 red onion, finely chopped
- 1/2 cup (120 ml) grapeseed oil
- 3 teaspoons cilantro
- 15-20 grape tomatoes, halved
- 2-3 tablespoons water

Instructions
- To eliminate extra water, pat the cauliflower dry. Place the spinach in a colander and squeeze out as much water as possible using the back of a mixing spoon.
- Grind the ginger, fennel seeds, mustard seeds, chili powder, garlic, and salt into a thick paste with a mortar and pestle (or the back of a spoon).
- Sauté the onion in the oil in a sauté pan until it softens greatly. Continue to sauté for a few minutes after adding the spice paste. Reduce the heat to low and mix in the spinach, cilantro, tomatoes, and cauliflower, as well as the water, until everything is well combined. (At this stage, the dish will need around 20 minutes to cook.) The cauliflower should crumble, and the completed dish should clump together with only a small amount of liquid.)

36. Crispy Rice Pizza

Prep time: 45 min | Serves: 4 | Difficulty: Moderate
Nutrition: Calories: 329kcal | Fat 7g | Protein 10g | Carbohydrate 33g
Ingredients
- 1/4 cup flaxseeds
- 1/3 cup water
- 3 cups cooked brown rice
- 1 red onion, diced
- 1 teaspoon oregano
- 1 teaspoon crushed garlic
- 2 cups crumbled goat's milk feta cheese or Parmesan cheese, divided
- 4 mild Italian chicken sausages, or zucchini
- 1 jar pizza sauce

Instructions
- Preheat the oven to 450 degrees Fahrenheit (230 degrees Celsius, gas mark 8) Spray a 13-by-9-inch (32.5-22.5-centimeter) baking pan with canola oil spray.

- Soak the flaxseeds in water for a few minutes in a large mixing basin. Then, to make a gel, stir them together.
- Combine the rice, onion, oregano, garlic, and 1 cup of the cheese in a large mixing bowl. Place the mixture in the baking pan that has been prepared. Form a crust by patting it down. Preheat oven to 350°F and bake for 20 minutes, or until gently browned.
- Meanwhile, sauté the sausages or zucchini in a pan over low heat, turning every few minutes. Remove the sausages or zucchinis from the pan when they are almost done and thinly slice them. Take the crust out of the oven. Make sure the oven is switched on. Spread the sauce up to 1/4 inch (6 mm) from the edge of the crust. On top of the sauce, equally distribute the remaining 1 cup of cheese. Over the sauce and cheese, arrange the sausage or zucchini. Cook for an additional 10 minutes. Allow it cool completely before cutting into 3-inch (7.5 cm) squares to serve.

37. Polenta -Broccoli -Pesto Pizza
Prep time: 45 min | Serves: 14 | Difficulty: Moderate
Nutrition: Calories: 289kcal | Fat 7.3g | Protein 11g | Carbohydrate 31g
Ingredients
- 2 cups uncooked polenta (do not use ready-made)
- 3 cups broccoli, steamed
- 1 cup pine nuts
- 3 tablespoons olive oil
- 2 cups sun-dried tomatoes in oil, diced

Instructions
- Preheat the oven to 3200 degrees Fahrenheit (Isoac, gas mark 4). Using cooking spray, lightly coat a baking sheet or a 13- by 9-inch pan. To make the polenta, follow the package guidelines. Using a narrow spatula, spread the polenta thinly over the preheated pan.
- Blend the broccoli, pine nuts, and oil in a food processor until finely ground.
- Distribute the mixture evenly over the polenta. Thinly put the tomatoes on top of the broccoli-pesto layer. Preheat oven to 200°F and bake for 15 to 20 minutes, or until gently browned. Allow to cool before cutting into squares.

38. Heart 'n Colon Porridge
Prep time: 35 min | Serves: 4 | Difficulty: Moderate
Nutrition: Calories: 199kcal | Fat 7.4g | Protein 9g | Carbohydrate 25g
Ingredients
- 2 cups water
- 1/2 teaspoon salt
- 1/2 cup whole barley (sprout able vs. pearl if available)
- 1/2 cup oat groats
- 1/4 cup maple syrup or agave nectar
- 3 cups blueberries
- 1 cup chopped almonds

Instructions
- Bring the water, salt, barley, and groats to a boil in a large sauce saucepan. Cover and cook for approximately 40 minutes, or until the grains are cooked and the liquid has been absorbed in part.
- (At this stage, the mixture should be slightly runny.) Cook for another 5 minutes after adding the syrup or nectar.
- Cook for another 3 minutes after adding the blueberries and almonds.

39. Barley Treat
Prep time: 45 min | Serves: 14 | Difficulty: Moderate
Nutrition: Calories: 189kcal | Fat 3.5g | Protein 13.7g | Carbohydrate 21g
Ingredients
- 1/2 cups barley grits
- 4 cups water
- 1 teaspoon salt
- 2 red onions, chopped
- 8 shallots, diced
- 1 cup canned fire-roasted tomatoes
- 1/2 cup cooked spinach
- 1 can chestnuts, drained
- 1 can water chestnuts, drained
- 1 can artichoke hearts, drained
- 1 teaspoon thyme
- 1 teaspoon ginger powder
- 2 tablespoons (28 ml) extra virgin olive oil

Instructions
- Place the barley in a dry saucepan over medium heat. Allow it to simmer for 3 minutes, stirring occasionally to prevent it from burning. Turn the heat off.
- Meanwhile, bring the water to a boil in a kettle.
- As you pour in the hot water, stir the barley until it froths. Toss in the salt. To bring the barley back to a boil, start cooking over high heat. Cover, decrease the heat to low, and cook for 10 minutes. Take the barley off the fire and set it aside for another 10 minutes. Meanwhile, sauté the onions and shallots in a sauté pan. Add the tomatoes and spinach once they've softened and continue to simmer, stirring often. The

chestnuts, water chestnuts, artichokes, thyme, and ginger are then added. Cook, stirring regularly to prevent sticking to the bottom of the pan, for approximately 15 minutes, or until well-combined and soft. Remove the vegetable combination from the heat and incorporate it into the barley along with the oil.

- Cooking spray the sauté pan in the meantime. Return the hash to the sauté pan, cover, and simmer for 8 to 10 minutes over medium-low heat. (Keep the temperature low to avoid burning the bottom of the hash.) Remove from the heat and set aside to cool for a minute. To loosen the hash, run a spatula over the edges and slightly below it. On top of the pot, place a baking sheet or another big, flat serving plate. Flip the pan over gently and place the flat surface on the counter top right away. To serve, cut the hash into wedges.

40. Rustic French toast

Prep time: 35 min | Serves: 4 | Difficulty: Moderate
Nutrition: Calories: 430kcal | Fat 9g | Protein 5.7g | Carbohydrate 34g
Ingredients
- 1 cup liquid egg whites
- 1 teaspoon cinnamon
- 3/4 cup light, unsweetened coconut milk
- 3/4 cup plain almond milk
- 1 loaf wheat-free bread, sliced thick
- Hemp-Berry Sauce
Instructions
- Whisk together the egg whites, cinnamon, coconut milk, and almond milk in a mixing basin. Place the bread in a shallow storage container with a lid and top with the egg white mixture.
- Allow the bread to soak for at least 4 hours (preferably overnight) in the refrigerator, rotating it once or twice. Preheat the oven to broil. Drain any excess moisture from the bread before placing it on a broiler pan. Broil for 5 minutes on each side, or until golden brown. Serve with a side of Hemp-Berry sauce or poured over each slice.

41. Fruit- Tata

Prep time: 35 min | Serves: 4 | Difficulty: Moderate
Nutrition: Calories: 397 kcal | Fat: 36 g | Protein: 10 g | Carbohydrates: 12 g
Ingredients
- 2 bags frozen berries, including cherries, thawed
- 1 package egg whites
- 2 tablespoons maple syrup
- 3 teaspoons cinnamon
- 2 cups oats
- 2 Fuji apples, peeled

- 2 cups raw almonds, finely chopped
- 2 teaspoons vanilla extract
Instructions
- Whisk together the egg whites, maple syrup, vanilla, and cinnamon in a mixing bowl until thoroughly blended. Refrigerate after folding in the oats. Meanwhile, cut the apples into 1/4 inch slices (6 mm). (A star form should appear in the centre of several slices.) Remove the seeds with care. Using cooking spray, coat a sauté pan. Over low heat, cook the apples until golden brown and tender, turning them a few times. Turn off the heat.
- Remove the egg mixture from the refrigerator and gently fold in the fruit; blend thoroughly. Coat a big saute pan with cooking spray and a lid. Arrange the apple slices in the pan to cover the bottom. Cover and simmer on low for 5 to 8 minutes after pouring the egg-fruit-oat mixture over the apples. Take off the lid. (At this time, the eggs should be solid, not runny.) Arrange the almonds on top in an equal layer.
- Cover and simmer for another 3 minutes, or until the egg mixture holds the almonds in place. Remove from the fire and let aside for a minute to cool. On top of the pot, place a flat serving dish or baking sheet. So that the fruit-tata settles apples up on the flat surface, flip the pot. Allow at least 10 minutes for cooling. Serve wedges cut into wedges.

42. Nixed -the-Noodles-far-Spaghetti Pad Thai

Prep time: 45 min | Serves: 4 | Difficulty: Moderate
Nutrition: Calories: 366 Kcal | Fat: 23 g | Protein: 20 g | Carbohydrates: 20 g
Ingredients
- 1 spaghetti squash
- 1/4 cup pad Thai sauce
- 3/4 cup almonds, chopped
- 1/4 cup mint leaves, julienned
- 1/2 cup liquid egg whites or 4 egg whites
- 2 teaspoons turmeric
Instructions
- Preheat the oven to 350 degrees Fahrenheit (180 degrees Celsius, gas mark 4) Using cooking spray, lightly coat a baking sheet. Squash should be cut in half. (If the squash is tough to chop raw, microwave it for a few minutes to soften it.) Remove the seeds using a spoon. Place the squash halves cut side down on the baking sheet that has been prepared. Bake for 45 to 60 minutes, covered. (The squash is done when it's soft enough to readily thread with a fork through the flesh.)
- These are going to be your "noodles." Allow the squash to cool before scraping the flesh into "noodles" using a fork. Toss the squash noodles with the sauce, almonds, and mint in a mixing

bowl. Cook over medium-low heat in a sauce pan coated with cooking spray.

- Combine the egg whites and turmeric in a mixing bowl. Scramble until the eggs are fully done. (The eggs should resemble orange-yellow crumbs.) Next, add the squash with a wooden spoon, being careful not to break the "noodles." Increase the heat to medium and stir-fry for 5 to 10 minutes, or until all of the ingredients are well mixed.

43. Lime Fish Kebabs

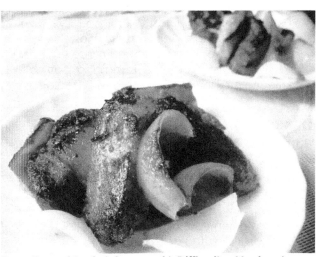

Prep time: 45 min | Serves: 4 | Difficulty: Moderate
Nutrition: Calories: 323 Kcal | Fat: 12 g | Protein: 11 g | Carbohydrates: 49 g
Ingredients
- Juice of three limes or 1/4 cup (60 ml) bottled lime juice
- 2 teaspoons black sesame seeds
- 2 clove garlic, minced
- 1 teaspoon coriander
- 1 teaspoon ground ginger
- 1 teaspoon soy sauce
- 4 wild cod, whitefish, or tilapia filets (about 5 ounces, or 140 g, each), cubed
- 2 zucchini, cut into '/4-inch (6 mm) slices
- 2 yellow squash, cut into '/4-inch (6 mm) slices

Instructions
- Combine lime juice, sesame seeds, garlic, coriander, ginger, and soy sauce in a mixing bowl. The fish, zucchini, and squash should all be rubbed with the mixture. Using skewers, skewer the fish and veggies. Place them in a baking dish with sides (to prevent dripping). Refrigerate the pan for at least an hour to enable the flavors to marinade. Preheat the grill or the oven to 350 degrees Fahrenheit (180 degrees Celsius, gas mark 4)
- Place the skewers on the grill and cook until the salmon becomes white, rotating the skewers every few minutes. If you're baking the fish in the oven and want it to look grilled, broil the skewers for about 3 minutes, flipping them every minute, after the fish is almost done (still transparent in the middle and mushy).

44. Feta, Pumpkin, and Chive Fritters

Prep time: 15 min | Serves: 4 | Difficulty: Moderate
Nutrition: Calories: 378 Kcal | Fat: 11 g | Protein: 17 g | Carbohydrates: 54 g
Ingredients:
- 10 ounces pumpkin or other winter squash, cut into 3⁄4-inch pieces (about 21⁄2 cups cubed)
- 1/3 cup (50 g) fine rice flour
- 2 tablespoons cornstarch
- 1/2 teaspoon xanthan gum
- 1/4 cup chopped chives
- 1/2 cup crumbled feta
- 2 eggs, lightly beaten
- 1/2 to 1 teaspoon ground cumin (to taste) Salt and freshly ground black pepper
- 2 tablespoons canola oil
- 3 tablespoons light sour cream.

Instructions:
- Cook the pumpkin for 8 to 10 minutes in a medium pot of boiling water, until tender. Drain and mash the potatoes. Allow to cool before serving.
- In a large mixing bowl, sift together the rice flour, cornstarch, and xanthan gum (or mix with a whisk to ensure they are well combined).
- Combine 2 tablespoons chives, feta, mashed pumpkin, eggs, and cumin in a large mixing bowl.
- Salt & pepper to taste. In a medium nonstick skillet, heat 1 tablespoon of the oil over medium heat.
- Cook for 2 to 3 minutes per fritter with 2 heaping teaspoons batter. Cook for a further 2 minutes, or until golden brown and cooked through, flipping and flattening slightly with the back of a spatula.
- If not eating right away, transfer the fritters to a platter and cover with foil to keep them warm (otherwise store them in the fridge for later).
- Repeat with the remaining batter and oil until all of the fritters have been fried.
- Combine the sour cream and the remaining 1 tablespoon of chives in a mixing bowl. Serve the fritters with salad and a dab of sour cream topping, if preferred.

45. Chicken Tikka Skewers

Prep time: 2hr-15min| Serves: 6| Difficulty: Moderate
Nutrition: Calories: 305 kcal| Fat: 27 g |Protein: 15 g | Carbohydrates: 2 g

Ingredients:
- 3⁄4 cup Greek yogurt (gluten-free if following a gluten-free diet)
- 1 tablespoon finely grated ginger
- 1 tablespoon garam masala
- 1⁄4 teaspoon ground cumin
- 1⁄4 teaspoon ground coriander
- 2 teaspoons turmeric
- 1⁄4 to 1⁄2 teaspoon chili powder (to taste) Salt and freshly ground black pepper
- 1.2 kg boneless skinless chicken breast, cut into 3⁄4-inch cubes
- Garden Salad.

Instructions:
- In a large mixing bowl, combine the yoghurt, ginger, garam masala, cumin, coriander, turmeric, and chile; season with salt and pepper.
- Stir in the chicken pieces until they are thoroughly coated. Refrigerate for 2 hours after wrapping in plastic wrap.
- Preheat the oven to broil. Using 18 skewers, thread the chicken.
- Place on a broiler pan or a baking sheet and broil for 6 to 8 minutes, rotating to cook on all sides, until golden brown and cooked through. Serve alongside a salad.

46. Tuna, Lemongrass, and Basil Risotto Patties

Prep time: 20min| Serves: 4| Difficulty: Moderate
Nutrition: Calories: 274 Kcal |Fat: 18 g| Protein: 23 g | Carbohydrates: 6 g

Ingredients:
- 3 cups onion-free chicken stock (gluten-free if following a gluten-free diet)
- 3⁄4 cup arborio rice
- One 5-ounce can oil-packed tuna, drained
- 2 tablespoons finely chopped lemongrass
- 2 tablespoons chopped basil
- 2 eggs, lightly beaten, divided
- 1 1⁄3 cups gluten-free bread crumbs Salt and freshly ground black pepper
- 1⁄2 cup cornstarch
- Canola oil
- Garden Salad

Instructions
- Fill a big saucepan halfway with water and bring to a boil. Cook for 10 to 12 minutes, or until the rice is soft.
- Any surplus liquid should be drained. Stir in the tuna, lemongrass, and basil while the sauce is still heated, until completely blended. Set aside to cool to room temperature in a medium mixing bowl.

- Preheat the oven to 300 degrees Fahrenheit (150 degrees Celsius). Season the chilled rice with salt and pepper and stir in 1 beaten egg and 1 3 cup (40 g) bread crumbs.
- Create 8 big balls out of the mixture, then flatten them to make patties. (Add extra bread crumbs if the mixture isn't stiff enough.)
- In three separate bowls, combine the cornstarch, remaining egg, and the remaining 1 cup (120 g) bread crumbs. Coat the patties with cornstarch, beaten egg, and then bread crumbs.
- Place on a platter and set away. In a medium skillet, heat a little oil over medium-high heat. Cook for 2 to 3 minutes, or until equally browned on both sides, in a pan with 4 patties.
- Transfer to a baking sheet and place in the oven to stay warm. Cook the remaining patties in a little more oil in the pan. Serve with a salad.

47. Cheese-and-Herb Polenta Wedges with Watercress Salad

Prep time: 30min| Serves: 4| Difficulty: Moderate
Nutrition: Calories: 241 Kcal |Fat: 18 g| Protein: 17 g| Carbohydrates: 4 g

Ingredients:
- 3 cups onion-free vegetable stock (gluten-free if following a gluten-free diet)
- 1 cup cornmeal
- 2 tablespoons butter
- 1⁄3 cup chopped flat-leaf parsley
- 1⁄3 cup chopped oregano
- Marjoram 1⁄2 cup grated

Parmesan Watercress Salad
- 4 cups watercress
- 1⁄2 small cucumber, halved lengthwise and thinly sliced
- 1⁄2 green bell pepper, cut into 3⁄4-inch strips
- 1⁄2 red bell pepper, cut into 3⁄4-inch strips
- 3 tablespoons alfalfa sprouts
- 3 tablespoons lemon-infused olive oil

Instructions:
- In a medium saucepan, bring the stock to a boil.
- Pour in the polenta and cook, stirring frequently, for 3 to 5 minutes over medium heat, until the mixture is quite thick. In a large mixing bowl, combine the butter, herbs, and 1 4 cup (20 g) Parmesan cheese.
- Use parchment paper to line an 8-inch (20-cm) square baking dish. Fill the dish halfway with polenta and smooth the top. Allow to cool slightly before refrigerating for 1 hour.
- Preheat oven to 350 degrees Fahrenheit (180 degrees Celsius) and line a baking sheet with parchment paper. Cut the polenta into 8 wedges or rectangles after turning it out onto a cutting board.

- Sprinkle the remaining Parmesan over the wedges on the baking sheet. Bake for 10 to 15 minutes, or until the cheese has melted and the wedges are golden brown.
- Broil for 5 to 7 minutes as an alternative. In a large mixing bowl, combine the watercress, cucumber, green and red bell peppers, and alfalfa sprouts to form the watercress salad.
- Toss in the lemon-infused oil until well combined.
- Warm polenta wedges are served alongside.

48. Caraway and Tofu

Prep time: 3hr | Serves: 4 | Difficulty: Moderate
Nutrition: Calories: 407 kcal | Fat: 35 g | Protein: 7 g | Carbohydrates: 6 g
Ingredients:
- 1 teaspoon ground caraway seeds
- 1/2 teaspoon freshly ground black pepper 1/2 teaspoon salt
- 1/4 teaspoon paprika
- 1/4 teaspoon ground allspice
- 1/3 cup vegetable oil
- 14 ounces puffed tofu pieces (about 2 x 2 inches/5 x 5 cm) Cooked rice
- Garden Salad

Instructions:
- In a small dish, combine the caraway seeds, pepper, salt, paprika, and allspice, then add 2 tablespoons of the oil.
- Transfer the tofu to a platter after brushing it with the spice mixtures. To enable the flavors to infuse, cover and chill for 2 to 3 hours.
- In a medium skillet, heat the remaining oil over medium-high heat.
- Cook for 1 to 2 minutes on each side, or until tofu is warmed through.
- Serve with salad and steaming rice.

49. Sweet Potato, Blue Cheese, and Spinach Frittata

Prep time: 45min | Serves: 4 | Difficulty: Moderate
Nutrition: Calories:317 kcal | Fat:8.6 g | Protein: 25 g | Carbohydrates:16 g
Ingredients:
- 1 1/2 tablespoons butter
- 2 small sweet potatoes, cut into 1/2-inch cubes
- 2 cups baby spinach leaves
- 1 cup crumbled strong blue cheese
- 8 eggs, lightly beaten
- Salt and freshly ground black pepper
- Garden Salad

Instructions:
- Preheat the oven to 350°F (180°C). Melt the butter in a 7-inch (18 cm) skillet, preferably one with an ovenproof handle, over medium heat.
- Add the sweet potato cubes and cook for 10 minutes, or until tender and golden brown. (If you don't have an ovenproof skillet, transfer the

sweet potatoes to a greased 9-inch springform pan.)
- Lightly whisk together the spinach, blue cheese, and eggs in a bowl. Pour over the sweet potatoes, then place the pan in the oven and bake for 20 to 25 minutes, until firm (test by gently shaking the pan).
- Remove from the oven, then let stand for 5 minutes before slicing. Serve with the salad.

50. Zucchini and Potato Torte

Prep time: 1hr-15min | Serves: 6-8 | Difficulty: Moderate
Nutrition: Calories:297 kcal | Fat:6.4 g | Protein:19 g | Carbohydrates:24 g
Ingredients:
- 3 russet potatoes, peeled
- 2 large zucchinis, grated
- 8 ounces bacon or prosciutto, diced, optional
- 1 1/2 cups grated low-fat Cheddar
- 1/2 cup cornstarch
- 2 tablespoons canola oil
- 6 eggs, lightly beaten
- Salt and freshly ground black pepper

Instructions:
- Preheat the oven to 350 degrees Fahrenheit (170 degrees Celsius). Grease an 8-inch square glass or ceramic baking dish lightly.
- In a saucepan, combine the potatoes and 8 cups mildly salted water. Bring to a boil, then reduce to a low heat and simmer for 10 to 15 minutes, or until the vegetables are soft. Drain.
- Cut into 18-inch (3 mm) slices once cold enough to handle. Arrange the potato slices in the baking dish's bottom layer.
- In a large mixing bowl, combine the zucchini, bacon, Cheddar, cornstarch, canola oil, eggs, and salt & pepper. Over the potato pieces, pour the mixture. Shake the dish to evenly spread the mixture over the potatoes.
- Bake for 45 to 50 minutes, or until golden brown and thoroughly done. Remove the cake from the oven and set aside to cool for 5 to 10 minutes before cutting and serving.

51. Shepherd's Pie

Prep time: 35min | Serves: 8 | Difficulty: Moderate
Nutrition: Calories:321 kcal | Fat:11 g | Protein: 25 g | Carbohydrates:17 g
Ingredients:
- 1 pound lean ground beef
- 1/3 cup frozen peas
- 1/3 cup frozen corn
- 1 medium carrot, grated
- 1/4 cup onion-free gravy powder (gluten-free if following a gluten-free diet)
- 1 cup water

- 4 large potatoes, peeled and quartered
- 2 tablespoons margarine
- 1/3 cup reduced-fat milk Salt and freshly ground black pepper

Instructions:
- Preheat the oven to 350 degrees Fahrenheit (180 degrees Celsius). Using nonstick cooking spray, coat an 8-inch (20-cm) square baking dish.
- Combine the ground beef, peas and corn, carrot, gravy powder, and water in a medium saucepan. Cook, stirring occasionally, until the ground beef is browned and the gravy has thickened, about 15 minutes. Meanwhile, cook the potatoes until soft in a saucepan of boiling water.
- Drain. Add the margarine and milk and mash well, making sure there are no lumps and that the consistency is smooth. Season to taste with salt and pepper. If necessary, add extra milk.
- Fill the baking dish halfway with the cooked beef mixture. Serve with mashed potatoes on top. Bake for 20 to 30 minutes, or until the tops of the mashed potatoes are golden brown.

52. Squash, Rice, and Ricotta Slice

Prep time: 1hr-20min | Serves: 4-6 | Difficulty: Moderate
Nutrition: Calories:219 kcal | Fat:6 g | Protein:15 g | Carbohydrates:36 g

Ingredients:
- 1/2 cup fresh gluten-free bread crumbs (made from day-old bread)
- 1/3 cup arborio rice
- 1 cup grated winter squash
- 1 large zucchini, grated
- 2 eggs, lightly beaten
- 1 1/4 cup firm fresh ricotta or feta
- 2/3 cup grated Parmesan
- Salt and freshly ground black pepper
- Garden Salad

Instructions:
- In a medium saucepan, bring 2 cups (500 ml) water to a boil. Cook for 12 to 15 minutes, until the rice is cooked, over medium-high heat. Drain.
- Return the rice to the pan and mix in the zucchini and squash grated. Set aside, covered.
- Season the eggs and cheeses with salt and pepper in a large mixing bowl. Stir in the rice mixture until everything is fully blended.
- Spoon the mixture into the prepared dish and top with the remaining bread crumbs. Bake for 45–55 minutes, or until firm when pushed on top.
- Remove from the oven and allow it cool for 5 to 10 minutes before slicing. If preferred, serve with a salad.

53. Goat's Cheese and Chive Soufflés

Prep time: 35min | Serves: 6 | Difficulty: Moderate
Nutrition: Calories:319 kcal | Fat:9 g | Protein:15 g | Carbohydrates:36 g

Ingredients:
- 3 tablespoons dried gluten-free bread crumbs
- 4 tablespoons dairy-free margarine
- 1/3 cup cornstarch
- 1 1/4 cups (300 ml) goat's milk, lactose-free milk, or suitable plant-based milk
- 3 large eggs, separated
- 1 cup (120 g) crumbled goat's cheese
- 2 teaspoons chopped chives
- 2 teaspoons finely chopped flat-leaf parsley
- Salt and freshly ground black pepper

Topping
- 2 tablespoons fresh gluten-free bread crumbs (made from day-old bread)
- 1 teaspoon chopped chives
- 3 tablespoons crumbled goat's cheese
- Salt
- 2 teaspoons dairy-free margarine, melted
- Garden Salad

Instructions:
- Preheat oven to 350 degrees Fahrenheit (180 degrees Celsius) and line a baking sheet with parchment paper. Lightly cover six 5-ounce (150 ml) soufflé pans or ramekins in gluten-free bread crumbs. Shake out any excess crumbs by inverting the bowls. Place the plates in a shallow baking dish of their own.
- In a medium saucepan over low heat, melt the margarine. Cook, stirring frequently, for 1 to 2 minutes after adding the cornstarch. Slowly drizzle in the goat's milk and stir until a smooth paste forms. Cook for another 2 to 3 minutes, stirring constantly, until the sauce has thickened.
- Place the ingredients in a medium mixing basin. Add the egg yolks one at a time, beating thoroughly between each addition with an electric mixer. Combine the goat's cheese, chives, and parsley in a mixing bowl. Salt & pepper to taste.
- Remove the beaters and clean them. In a large clean mixing basin, whisk the egg whites for 5 to 6 minutes, or until firm peaks form. Fold gently into the cheese mixture until everything is completely mixed. Fill the soufflé plates halfway with the mixture. Fill the baking dish with enough boiling water to come halfway up the edges of the dishes. Bake for 20 minutes, or until golden brown and thoroughly risen.
- In a separate bowl, mix the bread crumbs, chives, and goat's cheese to form the topping. Season with salt and continue to stir until the mixture is uniformly fine and crumbly.
- Remove the soufflés from the oven and lay them on the baking sheet that has been prepared. Using melted margarine, brush the top with the

topping. Bake for 7–8 minutes, or until puffed and a crisp crust has formed. If preferred, serve immediately with salad.

54. Feta, Spinach, and Pine Nut Crêpes

Prep time: 40 min | Serves: 6 | Difficulty: Moderate
Nutrition: Calories: 547 kcal | Fat: 38 g | Protein: 33.7 g | Carbohydrates: 19.8 g
Ingredients:
- 3⁄4 cup fine rice flour
- 1⁄2 cup cornstarch
- 1⁄3 cup soy flour
- 3⁄4 teaspoon baking soda
- 11⁄2 cups low-fat milk, lactose-free milk, or suitable plant-based milk
- 2 eggs, lightly beaten
- 3 tablespoons butter, melted

Feta, Spinach, And Pine Nut Filling
- 2 teaspoons canola oil
- 3 tablespoons pine nuts
- One 16-ounce package chopped frozen spinach, thawed squeezed and dry
- 4 cups crumbled reduced-fat feta
- 1 egg, lightly beaten
- Salt and freshly ground black pepper
- 1 cup tomato puree
- 1⁄2 cup grated low-fat Cheddar Garden Salad

Instructions:
- Make a well in the centre of a bowl by sifting the rice flour, cornstarch, soy flour, and baking soda three times (or mixing well with a whisk to ensure they are thoroughly incorporated). Blend in the milk and beaten eggs to make a smooth batter. Add the melted butter and mix well. Set aside for 20 minutes, covered in plastic wrap.
- Set a skillet over medium heat and coat it with cooking spray. Pour enough batter into the pan to cover the bottom when tilted, and cook until bubbles emerge. Cook the opposite side as well. Remove from the oven and keep warm. Continue with the remaining batter to create a total of 12 crêpes.
- Preheat the oven to 350 degrees Fahrenheit (180 degrees Celsius).
- In a large heavy-bottomed pan, heat the oil over medium-high heat to prepare the filling. Cook until the pine nuts are lightly toasted (watch carefully as they can burn easily). Stir in the spinach and feta cheese until everything is thoroughly mixed. Stir in the egg until it is just set. Season with salt and pepper to taste.
- Roll up each crêpe with a spoonful of the filling in the center. Place the rolled crêpes, seam-side down, in a single layer in one big or two small baking pans, and pour the tomato puree over the top evenly. Cheddar cheese should be sprinkled on top. Bake for 10 to 15 minutes, or

until the cheese is completely melted. If preferred, serve with a salad.

55. Beef and Bacon Casserole with Dumplings

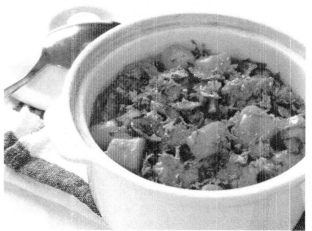

Prep time: 4hr-10min | Serves: 10 | Difficulty: Moderate
Nutrition: Calories: 281 kcal | Fat: 14 g | Protein: 26 g | Carbohydrates: 10 g
Ingredients:
- 2 tablespoons cornstarch
- Salt and freshly ground black pepper
- 21⁄2 pounds boneless beef blade steak, cut into 1-inch cubes
- 6 teaspoons garlic-infused canola oil
- 1⁄2-pound lean bacon slices, cut into thin strips
- 11⁄2 pounds new potatoes, Cut in half 1⁄2 cup brandy
- 2 tablespoons whole grain mustard
- 1⁄2 cup light cream
- 1 cup onion-free beef stock (gluten-free if following a gluten-free diet), or to taste
- 4 cups baby spinach leaves

Dumplings
- 2 large red-skin potatoes, peeled
- 3⁄4 cup low-fat milk, lactose-free milk, or suitable plant-based milk
- 3 tablespoons butter
- 3⁄4 cup fine rice flour
- 1⁄2 cup cornstarch
- 3 tablespoons tapioca flour
- 1⁄2 cup grated Parmesan
- 2 tablespoons chopped flat-leaf parsley, plus additional for garnish Salt and black pepper

Instructions:
- Preheat the oven to 280 degrees Fahrenheit (140 degrees Celsius).
- Season the cornstarch with salt and pepper in a large mixing basin. Toss in the steak and shake off any excess.
- In a Dutch oven, heat 2 tablespoons of the oil over medium heat. Cook, stirring occasionally,

for 6 to 8 minutes, or until the potatoes are golden and soft. Place in a mixing basin.

- In the Dutch oven, heat 2 tablespoons of oil. Cook, tossing periodically, for 2 minutes, or until the meat is browned all over. Place in a mixing basin. Continue with the remaining meat and oil. Return the steak to the saucepan, along with the potato mixture.
- Pour the brandy, mustard, cream, and stock into the saucepan together. Over medium heat, bring to a boil. Season with salt and pepper after removing from the fire. Bake for 2 hours with the lid on.
- Meanwhile, cover the potatoes with cold water in a big saucepan. Bring to a boil, then reduce to a low heat and simmer for 15 minutes, or until the potatoes are cooked. Set aside for 5 minutes after draining. Return the pan to the stove. Mash in the milk and butter until smooth. In a medium mixing bowl, sift the rice flour, cornstarch, and tapioca flour three times (or mix with a whisk so they are well combined). Toss the potatoes with the flour mixture, cheese, and parsley, and season with salt and pepper to taste. Make 12 dumplings out of the dough.
- Remove the dumplings from the Dutch oven, toss in the spinach, and return it to the oven. Bake for 20 minutes with the lid on. Remove the lid and bake for 15 to 20 minutes, or until the meat is cooked and the dumplings are golden. Serve garnished with parsley.

56. Pasta with Ricotta and Lemon

Prep time: 40 min| Serves: 6| Difficulty: Moderate
Nutrition: Calories: 217 kcal| Fat: 7.6 g |Protein: 25.7 g| Carbohydrates: 10.6 g
Ingredients:
- 1-pound gluten-free pasta
- 1 cup ricotta
- 3 cups baby spinach leaves
- 1/4 cup chopped flat-leaf parsley
- Grated zest of 1 lemon, plus additional thin strips of lemon zest for garnish, optional
- 3 tablespoons lemon juice
- Salt and freshly ground black pepper
Instructions:
- Cook the pasta according to package directions in a large saucepan of boiling water until just tender. Return to the pot after draining.
- In a mixing bowl, combine the ricotta, spinach, parsley, grated lemon zest, and lemon juice. Combine the heated pasta with the sauce. Season with salt and pepper to taste.
- Serve immediately, garnished with more lemon zest if preferred.

57. Parmesan Pasta

Prep time: 1hr-10 min| Serves: 6| Difficulty: Moderate
Nutrition: Calories: 410 kcal |Fat:30 g| Protein:14 g| Carbohydrates:35 g
Ingredients:
- 2 tablespoons garlic-infused olive oil
- 1 teaspoon crushed red pepper
- 1/3 cup sun-dried tomatoes packed in oil, drained and chopped
- 1 pound gluten-free pasta
- 7 ounces canned tuna in oil, drained and flaked
- 1/2 cup plus 2 tablespoons chopped kalamata olives
- 1/2 cup shredded basil
- 1/2 cup grated Parmesan
Instructions:
- Shake vigorously to incorporate the oil, crushed red pepper, and tomatoes in a jar.
- Allow 1 hour for preparation.
- Cook the pasta according to package directions in a large saucepan of boiling water until just tender.
- Return to the pot after draining. Combine the oil, tuna, olives, and half of the basil in a mixing bowl.
- Divide the spaghetti among six bowls and sprinkle with the remaining basil and Parmesan cheese.

58. Spinach and Pancetta Pasta

Prep time: 45 min| Serves: 6| Difficulty: Moderate
Nutrition: Calories:367 kcal |Fat: 29g| Protein:24 g| Carbohydrates:25 g
Ingredients:
- 1-pound gluten-free pasta
- 2 tablespoons garlic-infused olive oil, plus additional for serving, optional 8 ounces (225 g) thinly sliced lean pancetta
- 5 cups baby spinach leaves
- 1/4 cup pine nuts
- 1/2 cup grated Parmesan
- Salt and freshly ground black pepper
Instructions:
- Cook the pasta according to package directions in a large saucepan of boiling water until just tender. Return to the pot after draining. To remain warm, cover.
- In a large pan, heat the remaining 1 tablespoon of oil. Cook until the pine nuts are brown and the spinach has wilted, then add the pancetta, spinach, and pine nuts. Toss in the pasta and Parmesan until the cheese has melted over medium heat.
- Season with salt and pepper to taste, then drizzle with a little more oil if preferred.

59. Chicken and Pepper Pilaf

Prep time: 1hr 10 min | Serves: 6-8 | Difficulty: Moderate

Nutrition: Calories:367 kcal | Fat: 29g | Protein:24 g | Carbohydrates:25g

Ingredients:

- 2 cups basmati rice
- Small pinch of saffron threads
- 3 tablespoons garlic-infused canola oil
- 11⁄2 pounds boneless skinless chicken breasts, sliced 2 stalks celery, cut into thin slices.
- 1-inch piece cinnamon stick
- 2 green cardamom pods
- 2 cloves
- 1-star anise
- 20 fresh curry leaves
- 1 tablespoon chopped ginger
- 2 smalls red chile peppers, finely chopped
- 3 cups onion-free chicken stock (gluten-free if following a gluten-free diet) 1⁄2 red bell pepper, sliced
- 1⁄2 green bell pepper, sliced
- 1⁄2 yellow bell pepper, sliced

Instructions:

- Rinse the rice in cold water until it is completely clear. Fill a bowl halfway with cold water and soak the rice for 20 minutes.
- In a cup, combine the saffron with 1 tablespoon of boiling water and put aside to infuse.
- In a large skillet, heat 2 tablespoons of the oil over medium-high heat. Cook, tossing often, for 5 to 6 minutes, until the chicken is golden brown and the celery has softened, until the chicken is golden brown and the celery has softened. Place on a platter to cool.
- Reduce the heat to a low setting. Cook, stirring constantly, for 1 minute, or until aromatic, adding the remaining 1 tablespoon of oil, cinnamon, cardamom, cloves, star anise, curry leaves, ginger, and chile.
- Drain the rice and add it to the pan, swirling constantly to evenly coat it with the spice mixture.
- Raise the heat to high and add the saffron mixture, chicken, and stock. Bring to a boil, then lower to a low heat and simmer for 20 minutes, covered, or until the rice is cooked and the liquid has been absorbed.
- Stir in the bell peppers after removing the pan from the heat. Before serving, cover and leave aside for about 10 minutes. Remove the entire spices before serving if feasible; otherwise, tell people who will be eating the pilaf to avoid them.

60. Chinese Chicken on Fried Wild Rice

Prep time: 4hr-40 min | Serves: 6 | Difficulty: Moderate

Nutrition: Calories:467 kcal | Fat:30g | Protein:24g | Carbohydrates:33g

Ingredients:

- 3 tablespoons soy sauce (gluten-free if following a gluten-free diet)
- 2 teaspoons grated ginger
- 1 tablespoon garlic-infused canola oil
- 1 teaspoon Chinese five-spice powder
- Four 6-ounce boneless skinless chicken breasts

<u>Fried Wild Rice</u>

- 11⁄4 cups wild rice
- 2 teaspoons peanut oil
- 1⁄2 cup roasted peanuts, roughly chopped 2 eggs, lightly beaten
- 1 tablespoon soy sauce (gluten-free if following a gluten-free diet)
- 2 tablespoons coarsely chopped cilantro, plus additional for garnish Salt and freshly ground black pepper
- Steamed Asian greens

Instructions:

- In a small bowl, combine the soy sauce, ginger, garlic-infused oil, and five-spice powder. Pour the marinade over the chicken in a nonmetallic dish and toss to coat. Refrigerate for 2 to 3 hours after covering.
- Place the rice in a medium pot and cover with 334 cups (900 millilitre) cold water to begin making the fried rice. Bring to a boil, then reduce to a low heat and simmer, covered, for 45 minutes, or until the potatoes are soft and curling. Drain and allow aside to cool fully for 20 minutes.
- Preheat the oven to 350 degrees Fahrenheit (180 degrees Celsius).
- Spray a large nonstick pan with cooking spray, add the chicken, and cook for 2 minutes on each side over medium-high heat. Transfer to a roasting pan and bake for 20 to 25 minutes, rotating once, until cooked through. Remove the dish from the oven and set it aside to keep warm.
- In a wok or big pan, heat 1 teaspoon of the peanut oil. Cook, stirring regularly, until the peanuts are gently browned. Place on a platter to cool. In the same pan, heat the remaining oil. Cook, stirring constantly and breaking up the eggs into little pieces. Cook, stirring often, for 2 to 3 minutes, until the cooked wild rice, peanuts, and soy sauce are heated thoroughly. Turn off the heat. Season with salt and pepper to taste after adding the cilantro.
- Toss the chicken with the fried rice after cutting it into 12-inch (1-cm) pieces. Serve immediately with the steamed Asian greens, divided among six dishes and garnished with more cilantro.

61. Singapore Noodles

Prep time: 45 min | Serves: 4 | Difficulty: Moderate

Nutrition: Calories: 210 kcal | Fat: 27 g | Protein: 24 g | Carbohydrates:25 g

Ingredients:
- 1 cup rice vermicelli
- 2 tablespoons garlic-infused canola oil
- 2 tablespoons sesame oil
- 1 teaspoon grated ginger
- 1 small red chile, finely chopped
- 4 ounces peeled raw shrimp, deveined
- 5 small squid hoods, cleaned and thinly sliced
- 1 cup bean sprouts
- 8 ounces pork loin chops, thinly sliced
- 2 eggs, beaten
- 3 to 4 teaspoons curry powder (gluten-free if following a gluten-free diet)
- 1 tablespoon soy sauce (gluten-free if following a gluten-free diet)
- 2 teaspoons brown sugar
- 3 tablespoons onion-free chicken stock (gluten-free if following a gluten-free diet)
- Salt and freshly ground black pepper
- Chopped chives

Instructions:
- Allow the vermicelli noodles to soak in boiling water until soft. Drain and set aside after rinsing with cool water.
- In a wok or pan, heat both oils over high heat until extremely hot but not smoking. Stir in the ginger and chile for another 30 seconds.
- Reduce to medium-high heat. Stir-fry for 1 minute with the shrimp and squid. Stir in the bean sprouts and pork, and cook for another 2 minutes.
- In the center of the mixture, make a well. Pour in the beaten eggs and mix them softly with a fork.
- Stir in the curry powder, soy sauce, brown sugar, chicken stock, and cooked noodles until all of the liquid is gone. Season with salt and pepper to taste.
- Serve by dividing the mixture among four bowls and garnishing with chives.

62. Thai-Inspired Stir-Fry with Tofu and Vermicelli

Prep time: 45 min | Serves: 4 | Difficulty: Moderate

Nutrition: Calories:319 kcal | Fat:9 g | Protein:15 g | Carbohydrates:36 g

Ingredients:
- 8 ounces rice vermicelli
- 2/3 cup garlic-free sweet chili sauce
- 2 tablespoons fish sauce, or 1 teaspoon soy sauce (gluten-free if following a gluten-free diet)
- 2 teaspoons grated ginger
- 1 tablespoon cornstarch
- 1 cup warm water
- 1 teaspoon garlic-infused oil
- 1 teaspoon peanut oil

- One 14-ounce package firm tofu, pressed if desired, cut into thick slices
- 1/4 cup chopped cilantro, packed
- 1 cup chopped mint
- 2 tablespoons crushed peanuts

Instructions:
- Soak the vermicelli noodles in boiling water until they become soft. Drain after rinsing with cold water. Remove from the equation. In a small bowl, combine the sweet chilli sauce, fish sauce, and ginger.
- To prepare the sauce, make a paste with the cornstarch and roughly 2 tablespoons warm water in a cup. Mix with the remaining water thoroughly. Stir in the sweet chilli sauce until everything is fully blended.
- In a medium skillet, heat the oil over medium-high heat. Add the tofu and heat for 3 minutes, stirring once, or until golden brown. Stir in the sauce until it thickens, about 5 minutes.
- Combine the noodles, cilantro, and mint in a mixing bowl. Serve immediately with crushed peanuts as a garnish.

63. Pork with stir fried Veggies

Prep time: 40 min | Serves: 4 | Difficulty: Moderate

Nutrition: Calories:354 kcal | Fat:27g | Protein:32g | Carbohydrates:28g

Ingredients:
- 1 small red chile, thinly sliced
- 2 tablespoons dry sherry, or an additional 1 tablespoon brown sugar
- 2 teaspoons cornstarch
- 2 teaspoons brown sugar
- 2 teaspoons sesame oil
- 1 pound boneless pork chops, cut into thin strips
- 2 carrots, peeled and finely sliced on the diagonal
- 2 stalks celery, finely sliced on the diagonal
- 1/3 cup cilantro leaves
- Cooked white rice

Instructions:
- In a small jar, add the chile, sherry, cornstarch, and brown sugar and shake vigorously to incorporate.
- In a large wok or pan, heat 1 teaspoon of the oil over high heat. Toss in half of the pork strips until they are no longer pink. Place the pork on a platter and set aside. Rep with the rest of the pork strips.
- In the wok or pan, heat the remaining 1 teaspoon of oil. Stir-fry for 3 minutes, or until the carrots and celery are soft but beginning to crisp around the edges.
- Stir in the chile mixture and the pork strips for another 2 minutes. Remove the pan from the heat, mix in the cilantro, and serve over the rice right away.

64. Veggies, Rice and Parmesan

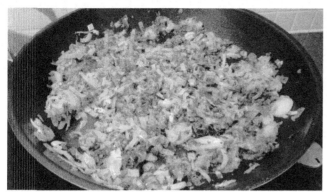

Prep time: 30 min | Serves: 6 | Difficulty: Moderate
Nutrition: Calories:310 kcal | Fat:27 g | Protein:18 g | Carbohydrates:35 g

Ingredients:
- 1 tablespoon garlic-infused olive oil
- 1 teaspoon saffron threads
- 2½ cups arborio rice
- 8 cups onion-free vegetable stock (gluten-free if following a gluten-free diet)
- ½ cup dry white wine, or additional vegetable stock
- ½ cup grated Parmesan
- ¼ cup chopped flat-leaf parsley Salt and freshly ground black pepper

Instructions:
- Heat the oil in a large saucepan. Add the saffron and stir over medium heat for 2 minutes. Add the rice and stir for 1 to 2 minutes, until the rice is well coated in the saffron mixture.
- Pour the stock into a medium saucepan over low heat and keep at a low simmer. Add the wine to the rice and cook until absorbed. Pour in 1 cup (250 ml) of the heated stock and cook, stirring, until absorbed.
- Add the remaining stock ½ cup (125 ml) at a time, reserving the last ½ cup (125 ml) of stock for later. Stir in the Parmesan and parsley.
- Pour in the reserved stock, stirring until completely absorbed. Taste, season with salt and pepper, and serve.

65. Tomato Chicken Risotto

Prep time: 35 min | Serves: 6 | Difficulty: Moderate
Nutrition: Calories:454 kcal | Fat:28g | Protein:29g | Carbohydrates:27g

Ingredients:
- 2 tablespoons garlic-infused olive oil
- Two 6-ounce boneless skinless chicken breasts, sliced
- 8 cups onion-free chicken stock (gluten-free if following a gluten-free diet)
- 2½ cups arborio rice
- ½ cup dry white wine, optional
- 2 cups (40 g) baby spinach leaves
- 1 cup canned chopped tomatoes
- ½ cup (40 g) grated Parmesan
- ¼ cup (15 g) chopped flat-leaf parsley, plus additional leaves for garnish Salt and freshly ground black pepper

Instructions:
- Heat 1 tablespoon of the oil in a small skillet over medium-high heat. Add the chicken and cook, tossing regularly, until lightly golden. Remove from the heat and set aside.
- Pour the stock into a saucepan over low heat and keep at a low simmer.
- Heat the remaining 1 tablespoon of oil in a large heavy-bottomed saucepan. Add the rice and stir for 1 to 2 minutes until the rice is well coated with oil. Pour in the wine and cook until absorbed. Add 1 cup (250 ml) of the heated stock and cook, stirring, until absorbed. Add all but ½ cup (125 ml) of the remaining stock, ½ cup (125 ml) at a time, cooking and stirring between each addition until the stock is absorbed.
- Add the chicken, spinach, tomatoes, Parmesan, and parsley, and stir until well combined. Pour in the reserved stock, stirring until completely absorbed. Season with salt and pepper, and serve garnished with extra parsley.

66. Poppy Seed, Pepper, and Cheese Sticks

Prep time: 1hr | Serves: 15-30 | Difficulty: Moderate
Nutrition: Calories:185 kcal | Fat:21g | Protein:12g | Carbohydrates:22g

Ingredients:
- One 8-ounce package cream cheese
- 5 tablespoons butter, softened
- ¾ cup grated Parmesan
- ½ cup fine rice flour
- 3 tablespoons cornstarch
- 3 tablespoons soy flour
- 1 teaspoon xanthan gum
- 2 tablespoons poppy seeds
- 1 teaspoon coarsely ground black pepper
- Extra virgin olive oil

Instructions:
- In a food processor, combine the cream cheese, butter, and ½ cup (40 g) Parmesan until smooth.
- In a large mixing bowl, sift the rice flour, cornstarch, soy flour, and xanthan gum three times (or mix with a whisk to ensure they are well combined). Add the poppy seeds and pepper to taste. Mix in the cream cheese mixture until it is completely blended. Make eight parts out of the dough. Roll each part into a 14-inch (35-cm) rope on a level surface, then cut in half or quarters to produce sticks.

- Using parchment paper, line a large baking sheet. Freeze the sticks for 20 minutes, or until solid, on a baking sheet.
- Preheat the oven to 350 degrees Fahrenheit (180 degrees Celsius). Divide the frozen sticks between the two baking sheets, allowing space between them, on a second baking sheet lined with parchment paper.
- Preheat the oven to 350°F and bake the sticks for 12 to 15 minutes, or until golden brown and cooked through. Remove from the oven and cool for 10 minutes on the baking sheets before transferring to another baking sheet.
- While still heated, spray or brush with olive oil and roll in the remaining Parmesan. Keep for up to 7 days in an airtight container.

67. Two-Pepper Cornbread

Prep time: 1hr-5 min| Serves: 10| Difficulty: Moderate
Nutrition: Calories: 178 Kcal |Fat: 13 g| Protein: 16 g| Carbohydrates:13 g
Ingredients:
- 1⁄2 cup fine rice flour
- 3 tablespoons cornstarch
- 3 tablespoons potato flour
- 2 teaspoons baking powder (gluten-free if following a gluten-free diet)
- 1 teaspoon baking soda
- 1 teaspoon xanthan gum
- 1 cup coarse cornmeal
- 1 teaspoon salt
- 2 eggs, lightly beaten
- 1 cup low-fat milk, lactose-free milk, or suitable plant-based milk
- 1 teaspoon olive oil
- 2 smalls red chile peppers, seeded and finely chopped 1⁄2 red bell pepper, seeded and finely diced 1 1⁄2 cups grated Parmesan

Instructions:
- Preheat the oven to 350 degrees Fahrenheit (180 degrees Celsius). Line an 8 x 4-inch (20 x 9 cm) loaf pan with parchment paper and lightly oil it.
- In a large mixing bowl, sift together the rice flour, cornstarch, potato flour, baking powder, baking soda, and xanthan gum three times (or mix with a whisk to ensure they are well combined). Combine the cornmeal and salt in a mixing bowl.
- Toss the flour mixture with the eggs, milk, oil, chile peppers, bell pepper, and three-quarters of the Parmesan cheese. To blend, whisk everything together thoroughly. Fill the loaf pan halfway with the mixture and top with the remaining cheese.
- Bake for 35–45 minutes, or until a toothpick inserted in the middle comes out clean. Remove from the oven and cool for 10 minutes in the pan

before transferring to a wire rack to finish cooling. Serve by cutting into slices.

68. Zucchini and Pumpkin Seed Cornmeal Bread

Prep time: 45 min| Serves: 12| Difficulty: Moderate
Nutrition: Calories:354 kcal |Fat:12g| Protein:23g|Carbohydrates:34g
Ingredients:
- 1 cup fine rice flour
- 3⁄4 cup potato flour
- 1⁄2 cup soy flour
- 2 teaspoons baking powder (gluten-free if following a gluten-free diet)
- 1 teaspoon baking soda
- 1 teaspoon xanthan gum
- 1 cup cornmeal
- 1 large zucchini, grated and drained on paper towel
- 1/3 cup raw or roasted pumpkin seeds
- 3⁄4 cup plus 2 tablespoons warmed low-fat milk, lactose-free milk, or suitable plant-based milk 3 tablespoons butter, melted
- 1 teaspoon salt
- 1⁄2 teaspoon freshly ground black pepper Olive oil
- Sea salt

Parsley Butter
- 4 tablespoons butter
- 1⁄4 cup chopped flat-leaf parsley

Instructions:
- Preheat oven to 400 degrees Fahrenheit (200 degrees Celsius) and line a baking sheet with parchment paper.
- In a mixing bowl, sift the flours, baking powder, baking soda, and xanthan gum three times (or mix with a whisk to ensure they are well combined). Combine the cornmeal, zucchini, and pumpkin seeds in a mixing bowl. In the middle, make a well and pour in the hot milk and melted butter. With a wooden spoon, combine the salt and pepper.
- To make a soft ball, gently bring the dough together with your hands. Turn out onto a clean, corn-starched surface and knead until smooth.
- Divide the dough in half and roll each half into two balls before placing them on the baking pan. Sprinkle with sea salt after brushing with a little oil. Cook for 20–25 minutes, or until golden brown and a toothpick inserted in the center comes out clean.
- In a bowl, combine the butter and parsley to produce the parsley butter. With the heated bread, serve.

69. Olive and Eggplant Focaccia

Prep time: 45 min | Serves: 6-8 | Difficulty: Moderate
Nutrition: Calories:204 kcal | Fat:7g | Protein:22g | Carbohydrates:31g

Ingredients:

- 3 tablespoons garlic-infused olive oil
- 2 teaspoons balsamic vinegar
- 1/4 teaspoon dried parsley
- 1/4 teaspoon dried oregano
- 1/4 teaspoon dried basil
- 1/2 small eggplant, cut into 1/2-inch slices
- 1 cup gluten-free bread mix
- 3 tablespoons garlic-free basil pesto (gluten-free if following a gluten-free diet)
- 1/2 cup sliced kalamata olives
- 1/2 cup grated Parmesan Salt and freshly ground black pepper
- Small basil leaves

Instructions:

- Combine the oil, vinegar, parsley, oregano, and basil in a large shallow dish. Turn the eggplant to evenly coat it, then set it aside to marinate while you make the bread.
- Preheat oven to 350 degrees Fahrenheit (180 degrees Celsius) and line a rimmed baking sheet with parchment paper. Follow the package directions to make the gluten-free bread mix and spread it onto the baking sheet. Spread the mixture out to cover the sheet with a spatula or the back of a spoon (it should be about 34 inch/2 cm thick).
- In a ridged grill pan or cast-iron skillet, heat a tiny quantity of the eggplant marinade over medium-high heat. Cook, rotating once, until the eggplant slices are faintly browned, 3 to 4 minutes.
- Using a spatula or the back of a metal spoon, spread the pesto evenly over the bread dough, dipping the spoon in water if necessary to avoid it from adhering to the dough. Season with salt and pepper before adding the olives, eggplant, and Parmesan. Preheat oven to 350°F and bake for 25–35 minutes, or until gently browned.
- Remove from the oven and cool on the baking sheet to room temperature. Serve heated, cut into pieces, and sprinkled with basil leaves.

70. Chia Seed and Spice Muffins

Prep time: 45 min | Serves: 12 | Difficulty: Moderate
Nutrition: Calories:289 kcal | Fat:12g | Protein:19g | Carbohydrates:27g

Ingredients:

- 1 cup brown rice flour
- 1/2 cup cornstarch
- 1/2 cup soy flour
- 2 teaspoons baking powder (gluten-free if following a gluten-free diet)
- 1 teaspoon baking soda
- 2 tablespoons pumpkin pie spice
- 1 tablespoon ground cinnamon
- 1 teaspoon xanthan gum
- 3 eggs
- 1/2 cup vegetable oil
- 1/2 cup low-fat milk, lactose-free milk, or suitable plant- based milk 1/3 cup chia seeds
- 1/2 cup hulled roasted sunflower seeds
- 2 tablespoons roasted pumpkin seeds
- 1/2 cup brown sugar

Instructions:

- Preheat the oven to 350 degrees Fahrenheit (170 degrees Celsius). Grease a 12-cup standard muffin tray with cooking spray.
- In a large mixing bowl, sift together the brown rice flour, cornstarch, soy flour, baking powder, baking soda, pumpkin pie spice, cinnamon, and xanthan gum three times (or mix with a whisk to ensure they are well combined).
- In a medium mixing bowl, whisk together the eggs, oil, milk, chia seeds, sunflower seeds, 12 cup (100 g) pumpkin seeds, and brown sugar until thoroughly blended. Pour into the sifted flours and stir thoroughly for 2 to 3 minutes with a wooden spoon.
- Fill the muffin cups two-thirds full with the batter, then sprinkle the 2 teaspoons of pumpkin seeds equally over the tops. Cook for 20–25 minutes, or until firm to the touch (a toothpick inserted into the center of the muffins should come out clean).
- Remove from the oven and cool for 5 minutes in the pan before transferring to a wire rack to finish cooling.

71. Pineapple Muffins

Prep time: 35 min | Serves: 12 | Difficulty: Moderate
Nutrition: Calories: 367 kcal | Fat: 19.7 g | Protein:25.5 g | Carbohydrates:16 g

Ingredients:

- 1 cup fine rice flour
- 1/2 cup cornstarch
- 1/2 cup potato flour
- 1 teaspoon baking soda
- 2 teaspoons baking powder (gluten-free if following a gluten-free diet)
- 1 teaspoon xanthan gum
- 1/2 cup superfine sugar
- 2 eggs
- 6 tablespoons unsalted butter, melted
- One 15.5-ounce can crushed pineapple, drained (liquid reserved)
- 3/4 cup suitable low-fat vanilla yogurt (gluten-free if following a gluten-free diet)
- 1 cup confectioners' sugar, sifted

Instructions:

- Preheat the oven to 350 degrees Fahrenheit (180 degrees Celsius). Using paper baking liners, line a

12-cup muffin tin. In a medium mixing bowl, sift the rice flour, cornstarch, potato flour, baking soda, baking powder, and xanthan gum three times (or mix with a whisk to ensure they are well combined). Mix in the sugar until everything is completely blended.

- Break the eggs into a mixing basin and whisk them together. Stir in the melted butter, pineapple, and yoghurt using a big spoon. Combine the flour, baking powder, and salt in a mixing bowl.
- Fill the muffin tins halfway with batter. Bake the muffins for 15 to 20 minutes, or until a toothpick inserted in the center comes out clean. Remove from the oven and cool for 5 minutes in the pan before transferring to a wire rack to finish cooling.
- To make a smooth, spreadable frosting, combine the confectioners' sugar with just enough of the saved pineapple juice. Serve with a drizzle over the cooled muffins.

72. Chocolate Chip Cookies

Prep time: 45 min | Serves: 18 | Difficulty: Moderate
Nutrition: Calories:367 kcal | Fat: 29g | Protein:24 g | Carbohydrates:25 g
Ingredients:
- 14 tablespoons unsalted butter, softened
- 3⁄4 cup brown sugar
- 2 eggs
- 1 1⁄4 cups fine rice flour 1⁄3 cup cornstarch
- 1⁄2 cup soy flour
- 1 teaspoon xanthan gum
- 1 cup chocolate chips (gluten-free if following a gluten-diet—white, milk, or dark, or use a mixture)

Instructions:
- Preheat oven to 350 degrees Fahrenheit (180 degrees Celsius) and line two cookie sheets with parchment paper.
- Using an electric mixer, beat together the butter and brown sugar until smooth. One at a time, add the eggs, beating thoroughly after each addition.
- In a mixing bowl, sift the rice flour, cornstarch, soy flour, and xanthan gum three times (or mix with a whisk to ensure they are well combined). Stir into the butter mixture until everything is fully mixed. Mix in the chocolate chips, then use your hands to gently pull the mixture together. Roll the dough into golf-ball-sized balls and space them 2 inches (5 cm) apart on the pans (to allow room for spreading). With the back of a spoon, flatten gently.
- Preheat oven to 350°F and bake for 12 to 15 minutes, or until golden brown. Allow to cool for 10 minutes on the cookie sheets before transferring to a wire rack to cool fully.

73. Almond Cookies

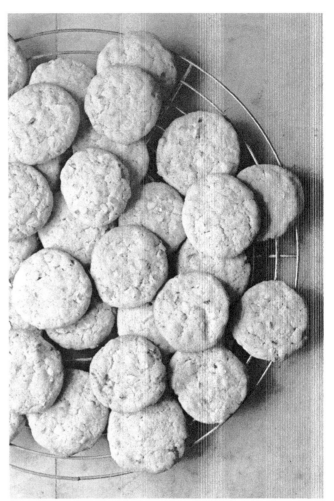

Prep time: 45 min | Serves: 40 | Difficulty: Moderate
Nutrition: Calories:284 kcal | Fat:9.7 g | Protein:18.5 g | Carbohydrates:18 g
Ingredients:
- 3⁄4 cup ground almonds, or natural almond flour
- 1⁄2 teaspoon baking powder (gluten-free if following a gluten-free diet)
- 1 egg white
- 1⁄2 cup superfine sugar
- 3 drops of almond extract
- 1 1⁄2 tablespoons unsalted butter, melted

Instructions:
- Preheat oven to 280 degrees Fahrenheit (140 degrees Celsius) and line two cookie sheets with parchment paper. In a small mixing bowl, combine the ground almonds and baking powder.
- With an electric mixer, beat the egg white in a separate bowl until soft peaks form when the beaters are raised. Gradually add the sugar and beat for another 5 minutes, or until firm peaks form. Stir together the ground almond mixture, almond extract, and melted butter.
- Make 2-teaspoon-sized balls out of the dough. Place about 2 inches (5 cm) apart on baking

sheets (to allow for spreading) and flatten slightly.
- Preheat oven to 350°F and bake for 25 minutes, or until golden brown. Allow to cool for 5 minutes on the baking sheets before transferring to a wire rack to cool fully.

74. Rice Cookies

Prep time: 30 min | Serves: 20 | Difficulty: Moderate
Nutrition: Calories: 281 kcal | Fat: 14 g | Protein: 26 g | Carbohydrates: 10 g
Ingredients:
- 9 tablespoons unsalted butter
- 3 tablespoons brown sugar
- 3 tablespoons superfine sugar
- 1 egg
- 1 teaspoon vanilla extract
- 2/3 cup (85 g) fine rice flour
- 1/2 cup cornstarch
- 3 tablespoons soy flour
- 1/2 teaspoon baking soda

Instructions:
- Preheat the oven to 350 degrees Fahrenheit (170 degrees Celsius) and oil two cookie sheets.
- In a mixing dish, cream together the butter and sugars using an electric mixer. In a separate bowl, whisk together the egg and vanilla extract.
- In a mixing bowl, sift the rice flour, cornstarch, soy flour, and baking soda three times (or mix with a whisk to ensure they are well combined). Add to the butter mixture and well combine.
- Place tablespoonfuls of dough on cookie sheets, spacing them about 2 inches (5 cm) apart (to allow for spreading), and bake for 8 to 10 minutes, or until golden brown.
- Remove from the oven and cool for 5 minutes on the baking sheets before transferring to a wire rack to finish cooling.

75. Lemon-Lime Bars

Prep time: 50 min | Serves: 20 | Difficulty: Moderate
Nutrition: Calories:187 kcal | Fat:7.7 g | Protein:19.5 g | Carbohydrates:9.8 g
Ingredients:
- 3/4 cup fine rice flour
- 1/2 cup soy flour
- 1/2 cup superfine sugar
- 2 teaspoons grated lemon zest
- 9 tablespoons cold unsalted butter, roughly chopped Confectioners' sugar

Topping
- 3 eggs
- 3/4 cup superfine sugar
- 3 tablespoons lemon juice
- 3 tablespoons lime juice
- 1 teaspoon grated lemon zest

- 3 tablespoons fine rice flour

Instructions:
- Preheat the oven to 320 degrees Fahrenheit (160 degrees Celsius). Using parchment paper, grease and line an 8-inch (18-cm) square cake pan.
- In a food processor, pulse the flours, sugar, and lemon zest until barely mixed. Pulse in the butter, one piece at a time, until the mixture forms into a ball. Remove from the pan and push into it. 10 minutes in the oven, or until gently browned. Reduce the oven temperature to 300 degrees Fahrenheit (150 degrees Celsius).
- To prepare the topping, whisk together the eggs and sugar until completely blended but not thickened. Stir in the lemon and lime juices, as well as the lemon zest and flours.
- Bake for 25 to 30 minutes, until the topping is brown. Allow it cool completely in the pan before slicing. Just before serving, dust with confectioners' sugar.

76. Strawberry Bars

Prep time: 5hr-20 min | Serves: 20 | Difficulty: Moderate
Nutrition: Calories:187 kcal | Fat:9.7 g | Protein:19.5 g | Carbohydrates:20 g
Ingredients:
- 7 ounces Simple Sweet Cookies, or other gluten-free vanilla cookies
- 6 tablespoons unsalted butter
- 1/2 cup brown sugar
- 1 egg, beaten

Filling
- 1/2 cup (75 g) cornstarch
- 2 cups (500 ml) low-fat milk
- 3/4 cup (185 ml) light whipping cream 1/3 cup (80 g) superfine sugar
- 2 teaspoons vanilla extract
- 2 egg yolks
- 2/3 cup strawberries, hulled and chopped

Topping
- 11/3 cups strawberries, hulled
- 2 teaspoons unflavored gelatin

Instructions:
- Use parchment paper to line a 9-inch (22-cm) square baking dish. In a food processor, crush the cookies.
- In a medium saucepan, combine the butter and brown sugar and whisk over low heat until the butter has melted and the sugar has dissolved. Stir in the egg until it has thickened. Mix in the cookie crumbs well. Set aside after pressing into the bottom of the baking dish.
- Mix the cornstarch with a little milk to produce a smooth paste for the filling. To mix, gradually whisk in the cream and remaining milk. Cook, stirring constantly with a wooden spoon, until the

mixture is smooth and thick, about 10 minutes over medium heat. Remove the pan from the heat and whisk in the egg yolks until well combined. Allow for cooling for 5 to 10 minutes. Add the diced strawberries and mix well. Fill the prepared crust with the custard filling. Refrigerate for 3 to 4 hours, or until the mixture is stiff.

- To prepare the topping, purée the strawberries until smooth in a food processor. In a small heatproof basin, add 3 tablespoons cold water and the gelatin, stirring constantly with a fork. Allow it to sit for 5 minutes, or until it starts to gel. Place the bowl in a bigger pot of boiling water and whisk regularly until the gelatin is completely dissolved. In a mixing bowl, combine the pureed strawberries and the remaining ingredients.
- Remove the dish from the refrigerator and top with the strawberry topping. Return the topping to the fridge for 2 to 3 hours, or until firm. Cut into bars using a heated knife.

77. Dark Chocolate Brownie Cake

Prep time: 4hr| Serves: 18-20| Difficulty: Moderate
Nutrition: Calories: 407 kcal |Fat: 35 g |Protein: 7 g | Carbohydrates: 6 g
Ingredients:
- 10 tablespoons unsalted butter
- 8 ounces dark chocolate chunks
- 1 1/2 cups firmly packed brown sugar
- 2/3 cup (130 g) fine rice flour
- 1/4 cup cornstarch
- 1 teaspoon xanthan gum
- 3 eggs, lightly beaten
- 1/2 cup dark chocolate chips (gluten-free if following a gluten-free diet)
- 1/2 cup light whipping cream
- 1 cup chopped pecans

Instructions:
- Preheat the oven to 320 degrees Fahrenheit (160 degrees Celsius). Grease and line a 7 x 11-inch (29 x 19-cm) baking pan with parchment paper.
- Melt the butter and dark chocolate pieces in a medium saucepan over low heat. Stir the ingredients until it is completely smooth. Stir in the brown sugar until it is completely dissolved. Allow the mixture to cool to room temperature in a large mixing basin.
- In a mixing bowl, whisk together the fine rice flour, cornstarch, and xanthan gum until thoroughly incorporated.
- One by one, whisk the eggs into the chocolate mixture. Combine the flours, chocolate chips, cream, and pecans in a mixing bowl. In the prepared baking pan, spread the mixture evenly.
- Preheat oven to 350°F and bake for 20 minutes. Bake for another 20 to 25 minutes, or until a

toothpick inserted in the middle comes out clean. Remove from the oven and set aside for 30 to 40 minutes to cool to room temperature in the pan.

- Refrigerate the pan for 2 to 3 hours, or overnight, until the brownies have firmed up. Remove the meat from the fridge and place it on a chopping board.
- Before serving, remove the squares from the parchment and cut them into squares.

78. Basic Chocolate Cake

Prep time: 1hr-15 min| Serves: 10-12| Difficulty: Moderate
Nutrition: Calories:319 kcal| Fat:9 g |Protein:15 g| Carbohydrates:36 g
Ingredients:
- 1 cup plus 2 tablespoons fine rice flour
- 1/2 cup cornstarch
- 1/2 cup potato flour
- 2/3 cup cocoa powder
- 2 teaspoons baking powder (gluten-free if following a gluten-free diet)
- 1 teaspoon baking soda
- 1 teaspoon xanthan gum
- 2 eggs
- 1 1/2 cups sugar
- 3 tablespoons unsalted butter, melted
- 3/4 cup vanilla yogurt (gluten-free if following a gluten-free diet)
- 2/3 cup low-fat milk, lactose-free milk, or suitable plant-based milk Confectioners' sugar
- Whipped cream

Instructions:
- Preheat the oven to 350 degrees Fahrenheit (170 degrees Celsius) and oil a 9-inch (23-cm) spring form pan.
- In a large mixing bowl, sift together the rice flour, cornstarch, potato flour, cocoa powder, baking powder, baking soda, and xanthan gum three times (or mix with a whisk so they are well combined).
- Whisk the eggs and sugar together until the mixture is thick and frothy. Stir in the melted butter, yoghurt, and milk until thoroughly mixed. Pour the mixture into the sifted flours and beat for 2 to 3 minutes with an electric mixer.
- Fill the pan halfway with batter and bake for 45 to 55 minutes, or until firm to the touch (a toothpick inserted into the center should come out clean). Halfway through baking, cover with foil to prevent overbrowning. Remove the cake from the oven and cool for 5 minutes in the pan before transferring to a wire rack to cool fully.
- Serve with a dollop of whipped cream and a dusting of confectioners' sugar.

79. Mocha Mud Cake

Prep time: 1hr-10 min | Serves: 12-14 | Difficulty: Moderate

Nutrition: Calories:298 kcal | Fat:15.7 g | Protein:11.5 g | Carbohydrates:32 g

Ingredients:
- 3 tablespoons strong coffee
- 7 ounces dark chocolate chips (gluten-free if following a gluten-free diet)
- 12 tablespoons butter, chopped
- 1 teaspoon vanilla extract
- 1/3 cup cocoa powder, plus additional for dusting, optional
- 1 cup superfine sugar
- 3 eggs
- 1/2 cup (65 g) fine rice flour 1/4 cup (45 g) potato flour
- 1/4 cup (40 g) cornstarch
- 1 teaspoon xanthan gum

Instructions:
- Preheat the oven to 320 degrees Fahrenheit (160 degrees Celsius). An 8-inch (20-cm) circular cake pan should be greased and lined.
- In a medium glass dish, combine the coffee, chocolate chips, butter, vanilla, and cocoa powder. Set over a pot of boiling water and whisk until the chocolate has melted and is thoroughly incorporated (make sure the bottom of the bowl does not touch the water).
- In a large mixing bowl, combine the sugar and eggs and beat on high for 3 to 5 minutes, or until light, fluffy, and doubled in volume. Gradually fold in the chocolate mixture with a spoon, stirring gently to incorporate.
- In a large mixing bowl, sift the rice flour, potato flour, cornstarch, and xanthan gum three times (or mix with a whisk to ensure they are well combined). Fold in the chocolate mixture gradually.
- Fill the pan halfway with batter and bake for 50–60 minutes, or until a toothpick inserted in the middle comes out clean. Remove from the oven and cool for 15 minutes in the pan before transferring to a wire rack to finish cooling. Serve with a dusting of cocoa powder, if preferred.

80. Vanilla Cake

Prep time: 50 min | Serves: 10-12 | Difficulty: Moderate

Nutrition: Calories: 281 kcal | Fat: 14 g | Protein: 26 g | Carbohydrates: 10 g

Ingredients:
- 1 cup fine rice flour
- 1/2 cup cornstarch
- 1/2 cup potato flour
- 2 teaspoons baking powder (gluten-free if following a gluten-free diet)
- 1 teaspoon baking soda
- 1 teaspoon xanthan gum
- 2 eggs
- 1 cup sugar
- 3 1/2 teaspoons vanilla extract 3 tablespoons butter, melted
- 3/4 cup vanilla yogurt (gluten-free if following a gluten-free diet)
- 2/3 cup low-fat milk, lactose-free milk, or suitable plant-based milk Confectioners' sugar

Instructions:
- Preheat the oven to 350 degrees Fahrenheit (170 degrees Celsius) and oil a 9-inch (23-cm) spring form pan.
- In a large mixing bowl, sift together the rice flour, cornstarch, potato flour, baking powder, baking soda, and xanthan gum three times (or mix with a whisk to ensure they are well combined).
- Whisk the eggs, sugar, and vanilla extract together until thick and frothy. Stir in the melted butter, yoghurt, and milk until thoroughly mixed. Pour into the sifted flours and beat for 2 to 3 minutes with an electric mixer.
- Fill the pan halfway with batter and bake for 30 to 35 minutes, or until firm to the touch (a toothpick inserted into the center should come out clean).
- Remove the cake from the oven and cool for 5 minutes in the pan before transferring to a wire rack to cool fully. Serve with a dusting of confectioners' sugar.

81. Carrot and Pecan Cake

Prep time: 1hr-15 min | Serves: 4 | Difficulty: Moderate

Nutrition: Calories: 310 kcal | Fat:11.7 g | Protein:17.5 g | Carbohydrates:22 g

Ingredients:
- 1 cup fine rice flour
- 1/2 cup cornstarch
- 1/2 cup tapioca flour
- 2 teaspoons ground cinnamon
- 1 teaspoon baking soda
- 2 teaspoons baking powder (gluten-free if following a gluten-free diet)
- 1 teaspoon xanthan gum
- 1 cup brown sugar
- 3/4 cup chopped pecans
- 2 small carrots, peeled and grated
- 1/2 cup vegetable oil 3 eggs, lightly beaten
- 1/2 cup low-fat milk, lactose-free milk, or suitable plant-based milk

Instructions:
- Preheat the oven to 350°F (170°C). Grease an 8 x 4-inch (20 x 9 cm) loaf pan and line with parchment paper.
- Sift the rice flour, cornstarch, tapioca flour, cinnamon, baking soda, baking powder, and xanthan gum three times into a medium bowl

(or mix with a whisk to ensure they are well combined). Stir in the brown sugar and chopped pecans. Add the grated carrots, oil, eggs, and milk, and mix well with a wooden spoon.

- Spoon the batter into the pan and smooth the surface. Bake for about 1 hour, or until golden brown (a toothpick inserted into the center should come out clean).
- Cover with foil halfway through baking to prevent overbrowning. Remove from the oven and allow to cool in the pan for 10 minutes before transferring to a wire rack to cool completely.

82. Asian Tempeh Kabobs

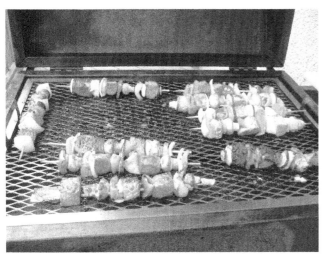

Prep time: 25min | Serves: 3 | Difficulty: Moderate
Nutrition: Calories:317 kcal | Fat:8.6 g | Protein: 25 g | Carbohydrates:16 g
Ingredients:
- One 83 /4-ounce package tempeh, cut into 1-inch cubes
- 3 tablespoons olive oil or high heat safflower oil
- Simmering Sauce
- Six 6-inch skewers
Simmering Sauce
- 1/4 cup tamari or soy sauce
- 2 tablespoons balsamic vinegar
- 2 tablespoons rice syrup, honey, or agave syrup
- 1 teaspoon ginger juice, or small piece of ginger, peeled and grated
- 1 tablespoon minced garlic, or 2 to 3 garlic cloves run through a garlic press
Instructions:
- In a frying pan, heat the oil over medium heat. Cook, flipping with tongs, until the tempeh is browned on both sides (approximately 2 minutes per side).
- Pour the simmering sauce into the frying pan and cook for 8 minutes, tossing the tempeh

regularly to ensure even absorption of the sauce.
- Remove the pan from the heat. Place 4 to 5 tempeh cubes on each skewer and serve on a platter.
- Serve with the remaining liquid from the pan drizzled over the skewers.
- Mix the tamari, vinegar, rice syrup, ginger juice, and garlic in a small bowl until the rice syrup has dissolved.

83. Oven-Baked Yam (or Potato) UnFries

Prep time: 1hr20min | Serves: 1 | Difficulty: Moderate
Nutrition: Calories: 139 kcal | Fat:21 g | Protein:24 g | Carbohydrates:35 g
Ingredients:
- 1 medium yam or potato, or 1 large handful new baby potatoes
- 1 /4 teaspoon sea salt
- 1 /2 teaspoon dried herbs of choice
Instructions:
- Preheat oven to 350 degrees Fahrenheit. Preheat oven to 350°F. Line two cookie sheets with parchment paper.
- Chop the yam/potatoes coarsely into pieces that are nearly the same size (so they cook evenly). Soak the yam/potato pieces for 30 minutes in cold water to remove excess starch and make them crispier.
- Remove the yams/potatoes from the water but do not allow them to dry. Instead, mix them with the sea salt and herbs right away.
- Spray the parchment paper lightly with cooking spray, then spread out the yams/ potatoes in a single layer. Don't pack them in because they won't cook as crisply and will take longer to cook.
- Bake for 15 minutes, then flip them over with a spatula and continue to bake for another 15 minutes.

84. Green Chicken Egg Bake

Prep time: 50min | Serves: 1 | Difficulty: Moderate
Nutrition: Calories: 547 kcal | Fat: 38 g | Protein: 33.7 g | Carbohydrates: 19.8 g
Ingredients:
- 4 ounces of chicken breast meat, diced
- 1 stalk of celery, diced
- 1 teaspoon olive or peanut oil
- 2 eggs
- 3 /8 cup water
- 1 cup spinach
- 1 /8 teaspoon each
- salt and pepper
- 1 /4 cup cheese, onions, peppers, bacon, or other leftovers (optional)

Instructions:

- Preheat oven to 400 degrees Fahrenheit. Set aside a loaf pan that has been greased.
- Heat the olive or peanut oil in a pan over medium heat. Cook for 1 to 2 minutes after adding the celery.
- Season the chicken with salt and pepper before putting it in the skillet with approximately a quarter cup of water. Remove the pan from the heat and continue stirring until the chicken is done.
- Whisk or beat the eggs and 1/8 cup of water with a fork in a separate bowl. Toss in the spinach, as well as any other optional additions (if desired).
- Cover the chicken/celery mixture with the egg/spinach mixture in the bottom of the loaf pan. Bake for 20 minutes, or until a knife inserted in the centre comes out clean.

85. Quick 'n' Easy Quiche

Prep time: 50min | Serves: 6 | Difficulty: Moderate
Nutrition: Calories: 210 kcal | Fat: 27 g | Protein: 24 g | Carbohydrates: 15 g
Ingredients:

- 3 egg whites, beaten with a fork
- 2/3 cup chicken broth, preferably organic
- 1/4 cup soy creamer
- 2 teaspoons fresh parsley, finely chopped
- 1/2 teaspoon salt
- 1/4 cup Parmesan cheese
- 1 cup mushrooms, cleaned and sliced
- 1/3 of a 10-ounce package frozen chopped spinach, thawed and drained
- 1/4 cup green onions (tops only), sliced thinly
- 9-inch frozen pie crust, unbaked

Instructions:

- Preheat oven to 450 degrees Fahrenheit.
- In a mixing bowl, whisk together the egg whites, broth, soy creamer, parsley, and salt. Remove from the equation.
- Poke holes in the bottom of the frozen pie crust with a fork. Remove the crust from the oven after 5 minutes of baking.
- Spread the spinach evenly across the bottom of the crust, then top with the green onions and mushrooms. Over the spinach, onions, and mushrooms, pour the egg mixture and top with the Parmesan.
- Bake for 10 minutes at 350°F, then reduce to 325°F and bake for another 25 minutes. When you can stick a knife in the middle of it and it doesn't come out with raw egg on it, you know it's done.

86. Nori Rolls

Prep time: 45min | Serves: 8 | Difficulty: Moderate
Nutrition: Calories:202 kcal | Fat:11 g | Protein:12 g | Carbohydrates:23 g
Ingredients:

- 4 sheets nori
- 1 cup Basic Nut or Seed Pâté or 1 cup Shannon's Quick Rice
- 1 carrot, julienned or grated
- 1 zucchini or cucumber, julienned
- 1 green onion, chopped
- 1/2 a green apple or pineapple, sliced thinly and julienned

Instructions:

- On a cutting board, lay out one sheet of nori at a time. Place the nut pâté on the nori sheet, then layer the veggies and fruit lengthwise on top.
- Form a cylinder out of the sheet and seal it with a damp finger. Allow it to rest for 30 minutes before slicing it into 6 pieces. Steps 1 and 2 should be repeated for the remaining nori sheets.

87. Tuna Cakes

Prep time: 6min | Serves: 1 | Difficulty: Moderate
Nutrition: Calories:317 kcal | Fat:8.6 g | Protein: 25 g | Carbohydrates:16 g
Ingredients:

- One 5-ounce can of tuna, drained
- 2 to 3 tablespoons almond meal
- 1 egg
- 1/8 teaspoon each salt and pepper, or to taste
- 1 to 2 teaspoons of olive oil, sunflower oil, or safflower oil, or ghee

Instructions:

- Combine the tuna, almond meal, egg, salt, and pepper in a small mixing dish. Remove from the equation.
- In a frying pan, heat the oil or ghee over high heat.
- Make little cakes out of the tuna mixture and place them in the frying pan. Cook for 3 to 4 minutes on one side, then flip and cook for another 3 minutes, or until crispy golden.

88. Tuna Salad, Hold the Mayo

Prep time: 13min | Serves: 1 | Difficulty: Moderate
Nutrition: Calories: 274 Kcal | Fat: 18 g | Protein: 23 g | Carbohydrates: 6 g
Ingredients:

- 1 hardboiled egg, diced small
- 1/4 of an avocado
- 2 to 3 tablespoons of Kendall's SCD Dairy Yogurt or any plain yogurt
- 1 teaspoon curry powder
- One 5-ounce can of tuna in water, drained

- 1/8 teaspoon each salt and pepper, or to taste

Instructions:
- In a small bowl, combine the egg and avocado. Add the yoghurt; if your yoghurt isn't very thick, you may only need 2 tablespoons. Curry powder should be added now (if desired).
- Combine the tuna, salt, and pepper in a mixing bowl.

89. Sardine Spread

Prep time: 2min | Serves: 2 | Difficulty: Moderate
Nutrition: Calories: 202 Kcal | Fat: 13 g | Protein: 16 g | Carbohydrates:13 g

Ingredients:
- One 3.75-ounce tin sardines
- 1 teaspoon Dijon mustard
- 2 tablespoons finely chopped red onion
- 1/2 teaspoon fresh lemon juice
- 2 pieces bread of your choice

Instructions:
- The sardines should be drained. Mash the sardines and mustard together in a bowl with a fork. Stir in the onion and lemon juice until everything is well combined.
- To prepare two open-faced sandwiches, spread generously on the bread.

90. Quinoa Vegetable Pilaf

Prep time: 45min | Serves: 4 | Difficulty: Moderate
Nutrition: Calories: 305 kcal | Fat: 27 g | Protein: 15 g | Carbohydrates: 2 g

Ingredients:
- 1 cup uncooked quinoa
- 2 cups vegetable stock or water
- 2 tablespoons olive oil
- 1 medium onion, finely diced
- 2 medium carrots, finely diced
- 5 to 6 button or cremini mushrooms, sliced (optional)
- 1/4 teaspoon each salt and pepper
- 2 teaspoons toasted sesame oil (optional)
- 1 teaspoon toasted sesame seeds

Instructions
- Set aside quinoa cooked according to package directions, using stock or water.
- In a medium frying pan over medium-high heat, heat the olive oil and sauté the onion and carrots. Add the mushrooms (if preferred) once the carrots have softened and continue to sauté until the mushrooms are done.
- Toss the quinoa into the frying pan with the vegetables and toss to combine. Season with salt and pepper to taste, then transfer to a serving plate. If desired, drizzle a little toasted sesame oil over the quinoa. Serve with toasted sesame seeds as a garnish.

91. Rainbow Vegetarian Quinoa

Prep time: 20min | Serves: 4 | Difficulty: Moderate
Nutrition: Calories:321 kcal | Fat:11 g | Protein: 25 g | Carbohydrates:17 g

Ingredients:
- 2 cups uncooked quinoa, rinsed
- 4 cups water
- 2 cups mix of chopped carrots, peas, and corn
- Dash of olive oil Dash of Braggs
  - Liquid Aminos, or Nama Shoyu, or miso, or pinch of salt

Instructions
- Bring the quinoa to a boil in a pot with the water. Reduce to a low heat, cover, and cook for 15 minutes, or until the quinoa is frothy.
- Place the vegetables in the pot, turn off the heat, and let aside for 5 minutes, or until heated.
- Finish with a drizzle of olive oil and a sprinkle of Braggs Liquid Aminos, Nama Shoyu, miso, or salt.

92. Oven-Baked UnFried Rice

Prep time: 20min | Serves: 4 | Difficulty: Moderate
Nutrition: Calories:319 kcal | Fat:9 g | Protein:15 g | Carbohydrates:36 g

Ingredients:
- 2 cups long grain rice, uncooked
- 1 small onion, chopped into small pieces
- 1 cup chicken broth
- 1/4 cup olive oil 1/4 cup tamari, or low-sodium soy sauce
- 1/3 cup fresh parsley, chopped

Instructions
- Preheat oven to 350 degrees Fahrenheit.
- To obtain the look of true fried rice, spray a small frying pan with cooking spray and quickly cook the egg white, breaking it into bits as it cooks for 1 or 2 minutes (if desired).
- In a casserole dish, combine all of the ingredients (including the egg, if desired). Bake for one hour, covered in tinfoil.

93. Shannon's Quick "Rice"

Prep time: 20min | Serves: 4 | Difficulty: Moderate
Nutrition: Calories: 305 kcal | Fat: 27 g | Protein: 15 g | Carbohydrates: 2 g

Ingredients:
- 1 cup parsnips, scrubbed, peeled, and chopped
- 1 cup chopped cauliflower
- 1 cup pine nuts
- 1 clove of garlic
- 1 tablespoon lemon juice
- 1 tablespoon Nama Shoyu (organic soy sauce)
- 1 to 2 tablespoons olive oil
- 1 tablespoon agave, or 2 dates, pitted (optional)

Instructions

- In a food processor, combine all of the ingredients and process until the mixture resembles rice in texture.

94. Brown Rice Powder Stuffing

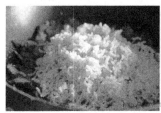 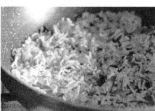

Prep time: 20min | Serves: 6 | Difficulty: Moderate
Nutrition: Calories: 311 kcal | Fat: 7.1 g | Protein: 14 g | Carbohydrates: 46 g
Ingredients:

- 1/2 cup ground flaxseeds
- 1 /2 cup brown rice protein powder
- 1 teaspoon sea salt
- 1 /2 cup flaxseed oil
- 5 tablespoons water
- 2 to 3 tablespoons olive or coconut oil
- 1 medium onion, chopped
- 2 to 3 cloves garlic
- 1 /2 cup pecans or walnuts, soaked 3 celery stalks, diced
- 3 apples, peeled, cored and diced
- 4 Swiss chard leaves, chopped
- 1 to 2 teaspoons nutmeg
- 3 to 4 teaspoons Italian herb mixture
- 2 to 3 teaspoons maple syrup
- 2 teaspoons freshly squeezed lemon juice, or to taste
- 1 /4 teaspoon each celery
- salt and pepper, or to taste
- Fresh oregano and mint to garnish (optional)

Instructions

- In a large mixing bowl, combine the ground flaxseeds, brown rice protein powder, and sea salt. Set aside the flaxseed oil and enough water to make a dry, doughy mixture.
- 2 to 3 tablespoons olive oil or coconut oil, heated in a large skillet, sauté the onion, garlic, nuts (if desired), celery, and apples over medium heat until almost soft. Continue to sauté the Swiss chard until all of the vegetables are soft.
- Combine the protein powder, nutmeg, Italian herbs, maple syrup, lemon juice, celery salt, and pepper in a mixing bowl with the produce mixture. Serve with fresh oregano and mint as a garnish (if desired).

95. Green Beans Almandine

Prep time: 15min | Serves: 4 | Difficulty: Moderate
Nutrition: Calories: 274 Kcal | Fat: 18 g | Protein: 23 g | Carbohydrates: 6 g
Ingredients:

- 1 pound fresh green beans, trimmed
- 2 to 4 tablespoons sliced or slivered almonds
- 1 teaspoon butter
- 1 1/4 teaspoon each salt and pepper, or to taste

Instructions

- Over high heat, bring a large saucepan of water to a boil. While you're waiting for it to boil, roast the almonds in a pan over medium heat, stirring regularly, for 5 to 7 minutes. When the almonds are toasted, remove them from the fire and set them aside.
- Cook the green beans for a few minutes in boiling water, until they're crisp.
- Drain the beans and combine them with the almonds, butter, and a pinch of salt and pepper in a mixing bowl.

96. Creamed Spinach

Prep time: 20min | Serves: 4 | Difficulty: Moderate
Nutrition: Calories:62 kcal | Fat:3 g | Protein: 5 g | Carbohydrates:12 g
Ingredients:

- 1 pound fresh spinach, or two 10-ounce boxes frozen spinach, drained and chopped
- 2 cloves of garlic, or 1 large clove of elephant garlic
- 1 teaspoon olive oil
- 1 /4 cup plain soy milk
- 1 /4 teaspoon each salt and pepper, or to taste
- 2 teaspoons grated Parmesan cheese to garnish

Instructions

- Over medium-low heat, sauté the garlic until it becomes translucent.
- Toss in the spinach. Mix the frozen spinach with the garlic until everything is well blended. With a large spoon, toss fresh spinach into the pan with the garlic until it wilts to a quarter of its original size.
- Stir in the soy milk to warm it up and cover the spinach. Season with salt and pepper to taste, then top with Parmesan and serve immediately.

97. Ginger Carrots

Prep time: 20min | Serves: 4 | Difficulty: Moderate
Nutrition: Calories:187 kcal | Fat:1.6 g | Protein:5 g | Carbohydrates:26 g
Ingredients:

- 4 tablespoons olive oil One 3-inch piece of ginger, peeled and diced
- 1 clove of garlic, peeled and chopped
- 2 pounds carrots, cut into matchsticks or 1 /4-inch rounds

- 1 cup Vegetable Stock (see the recipe in Chapter 9) or low-sodium canned vegetable broth
- 1 tablespoon butter
- 1/2 cup parsley, chopped

Instructions
- Heat the olive oil in a large sauté pan over high heat. To release the aroma, add the ginger and garlic and sauté for a few seconds. Stir in the carrots to evenly coat them.
- Bring the broth to a boil, then remove from the heat. Cover and reduce the heat to medium-low. Cook for about 20 minutes, or until the carrots are soft.
- Remove the cover, stir in the butter and parsley, and serve hot.

---

98. Marinated Kale

Prep time: 65min| Serves: 6| Difficulty: Moderate
Nutrition: Calories:98 kcal| Fat:1 g |Protein:3 g| Carbohydrates:7 g

Ingredients:
- 3 large leaves organic green leaf kale
- 1/4 of a sweet onion
- 3 tablespoons fresh tarragon
- 3 tablespoons fresh basil Juice of 1 lemon (about 1/4 cup)
- 3 tablespoons olive oil
- 1 1/2 teaspoons salt
- 1/4 teaspoon cayenne, or to taste
- 1 teaspoon raw agave
- 1 /4 teaspoon each garlic powder and chili powder, or to taste

Instructions
- Gently pulse or chop the kale in a food processor and then transfer it to a bowl.
- Add the rest of the ingredients to the kale. Toss, allow to marinate for 1 hour, and serve.

---

99. Savoring Sourdough Bread

Prep time: 2to8hrs| Serves: 13| Difficulty: Moderate
Nutrition: Calories: 281 kcal| Fat: 14 g |Protein: 26 g| Carbohydrates: 10 g

Ingredients:
- 4 teaspoons sugar
- 2 teaspoons salt
- 2 tablespoons olive oil, soft butter, or ghee (see the recipe in Chapter 6)
- 2 cups sponge (fermented starter; see the following recipes)
- 3 cups unbleached all-purpose flour, or more as necessary

Instructions
- Toss the sponge with the sugar, salt, and oil. Mix thoroughly, then mix in the flour 12 cup at a time, using as much flour as you need to form a good, elastic bread dough (using your hands, a bread machine, or a food processor).
- If the dough isn't already in a bowl, place it in one, cover it with a cloth, and keep it warm (70 to 80 degrees; 100 degrees is too warm). Allow the dough to double in size until you can poke a hole with your finger that doesn't spring back (this process may take 1 to 2 hours).
- Knead the bread once more, then shape it into a loaf in a 9-x-5-inch loaf pan lightly oiled with olive or coconut oil. Cover it with a moist towel or paper towel and set it aside to rise for another 40 minutes to an hour, or until it has doubled in size.
- Place the loaf pan in a cold oven and bake for 45 to 50 minutes, or until the crust is golden; if preferred, turn the loaf out on a cooling rack to check for doneness, poking the bottom with a toothpick to see if it comes out clean. Allow for 1 hour of cooling time before cutting.

---

100. Fresh Fries with Raw Jicama

Prep time: 5min| Serves: 2| Difficulty: Moderate
Nutrition: Calories: 274 Kcal |Fat: 18 g| Protein: 23 g |Carbohydrates: 6 g

Ingredients:
- 1 medium jicama
- 1 tablespoon olive oil
- 1 teaspoon sea salt
- 1 teaspoon onion and/or garlic powder
- 1/2 teaspoon chili powder

Instructions
- Peel the jicama and use a mandoline or a sharp knife to slice it into your favorite French fry shape.
- Toss the fries in the olive oil with the salt, onion/garlic powder, and chili powder.

---

101 Curried Spice-Baked Sweet Potatoes

Prep time: 80min| Serves: 4| Difficulty: Moderate
Nutrition: Calories:319 kcal| Fat:9 g |Protein:15 g| Carbohydrates:36 g

Ingredients:
- 2 medium sweet potatoes, washed and pierced in the center with a fork
- 1 teaspoon of fresh ginger, finely grated
- 1/2 to 1 teaspoon mild curry powder
- 1/2 teaspoon turmeric Pinch of cinnamon
- 1/8 teaspoon salt, or to taste
- 1 teaspoon coconut oil or extra virgin olive oil

Instructions
- Preheat oven to 400 degrees Fahrenheit. Remove the sweet potatoes from the oven and set aside to cool in a low-sided roasting pan for 30 to 45 minutes, or until tender.
- Cut the cooled potatoes in half lengthwise and scoop out the center flesh, leaving a 14-inch rim

of sweet potato connected to the skin to keep it together.

- In a mixing bowl, combine the meat and the remaining ingredients until smooth and creamy.

Fill the potato skins with the flesh mixture, lay them on a baking sheet, and return to the oven for another 25 minutes, or until heated through and slightly golden on top. Serve immediately.

Chapter 6: Mains

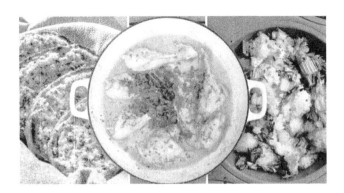

1. Baked Macaroni and Cheese
Prep time: 55 min| Serves: 12| Difficulty: Moderate
Nutrition: Calories: 323 Kcal |Fat: 12 g| Protein: 11 g | Carbohydrates: 49 g
Ingredients
- 1 pound uncooked corn/quinoa elbow macaroni
- ¼ cup cornstarch
- 1 teaspoon salt
- 1½ teaspoons dry mustard
- ½ teaspoon freshly ground black pepper
- 3½ cups lactose-free milk
- 4 cups grated extra-sharp white Cheddar cheese (1 pound)
- 1 teaspoon red pepper flakes (optional)
- ½ cup gluten-free or Toasted Bread Crumbs
- ½ teaspoon sweet paprika

Instructions
- Preheat the oven to 350 degrees Fahrenheit. Oil a 9 x 13-inch baking dish by brushing or spraying it.
- Cook the macaroni according to package directions in a 6- to 8-quart saucepan, 1 to 2 minutes undercooked (macaroni will cook some more in the oven).
- Drain the water and set it aside.
- In the same saucepan, combine the cornstarch, salt, mustard, and black pepper. Stir in the milk until it is completely smooth. Bring the mixture to a boil over medium heat, stirring frequently. Combine the cheese and red pepper flakes in a mixing bowl. Stir in the spaghetti until everything is nicely combined.
- Place the mixture in the baking dish and sprinkle the bread crumbs on top. Paprika should be lightly sprinkled on top. Bake for 25 minutes, or until the top is gently browned and bubbling. Allow 5 to 10 minutes to cool before serving.

2. Pesto -Baked Chicken
Prep time: 45 min| Serves: 6| Difficulty: Moderate
Nutrition: Calories: 378 Kcal |Fat: 11 g |Protein: 17 g |Carbohydrates: 54 g
Ingredients
- 1½ pounds boneless, skinless chicken breasts or cutlets
- ½ cup Basil Pesto
- ⅓ cup shredded mozzarella cheese

Instructions
- Preheat the oven to 450 degrees Fahrenheit. Set aside a 9 x 13-inch baking dish that has been oiled.
- Spread the pesto on top of the chicken pieces in the baking dish. Bake for 20 to 30 minutes, or until a quick-read thermometer inserted in the thickest part of the chicken registers 165 degrees Fahrenheit. Remove the pizza from the oven and top with mozzarella.
- Allow the cheese to melt for a few moments before serving.

3. Chana Masala
Prep time: 25 min| Serves: 4| Difficulty: Moderate
Nutrition: Calories: 305 kcal| Fat: 27 g |Protein: 15 g |Carbohydrates: 2 g
Ingredients
- 2 tablespoons garlic-infused olive oil
- 1 tablespoon minced fresh ginger
- 1 small red or green chile, minced
- Large pinch of garam masala
- 2 teaspoons curry powder
- ½ teaspoon salt
- ½ teaspoon salt
- 2 cups diced fennel bulb
- 1 ripe medium tomato, diced
- 1 tablespoon lemon juice
- 2 tablespoons water
- 1 14.5-ounce can chickpeas, drained and rinsed
- ¼ cup plain lactose-free yogurt or kefir

Instructions
- To make a smooth paste, add the oil, ginger, chile, garam masala, curry powder, and salt in a medium mixing bowl. In a large skillet, stir-fry the Ingredients for 3 minutes over low heat. Fennel, tomato, lemon juice, and water are added to the pan.
- Raise the heat to medium low and cook, covered, for approximately 10 minutes, or until the fennel is soft.

- Cook for another 5 minutes after adding the chickpeas. Add the yoghurt and mix well. Serve right away.

4. Chicken Korma

Prep time: 45 min | Serves: 6 | Difficulty: Moderate
Nutrition: Calories: 311 kcal | Fat: 7.1 g | Protein: 44 g | Carbohydrates: 16 g

Ingredients
- 3 tablespoons garlic-infused olive oil
- 5 cardamom pods, lightly crushed (optional)
- 2 tablespoons minced fresh ginger
- 1 tablespoon ground turmeric
- 1 red chile, fresh or dried, minced
- ½ teaspoon garam masala
- 4 teaspoons curry powder
- 1½ teaspoons salt
- 1½ teaspoons salt
- 1¾ pounds boneless, skinless chicken thighs, cubed
- 1 cup water or Low-FODMAP Chicken Stock
- 2 medium white turnips (about 1 pound), diced
- 1¾ cups diced tomatoes, fresh or canned
- 1 teaspoon light brown sugar
- 1 cup plain lactose-free yogurt
- 6 tablespoons almond flour
- ½ cup chopped fresh cilantro (optional)

Instructions
- Warm the oil in a big, heavy pan over medium-high heat until aromatic. Stir in the cardamom, ginger, turmeric, chile, garam masala, curry powder, and salt for 1 to 2 minutes, or until aromatic. Remove the cardamom from the skillet and set aside the rest of the spices.
- Add the chicken and cook, tossing periodically and flipping, over medium-high heat until browned on both sides, about 10 minutes. Combine the chicken stock, turnips, tomatoes, and brown sugar in a large mixing bowl. Reduce the heat to low and cook for 30 to 40 minutes, uncovered, or until the turnips are soft.
- While the stew cooks, pour 3 tablespoons of whey from the yoghurt onto a paper coffee filter (supported by a strainer) and let aside for 10 minutes, stirring several times. Whey should be discarded.
- Cook for a few minutes after adding the almond flour to the stew. Stir in the strained yoghurt and reheat slightly to integrate when ready to serve. If preferred, top the chicken with a dusting of cilantro.

5. Asian-Style Chicken Noodle Soup

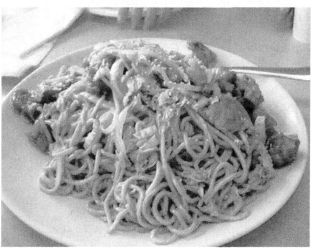

Prep time: 45 min | Serves: 3 | Difficulty: Moderate
Nutrition: Calories: 274 Kcal | Fat: 18 g | Protein: 23 g | Carbohydrates: 6 g

Ingredients
- 4 ounces uncooked rice noodles
- 1 tablespoon garlic-infused olive oil
- 2 teaspoons toasted or spicy sesame oil
- 1 tablespoon minced fresh ginger
- 2 large carrots, chopped
- 1 bunch scallion greens, thinly sliced
- 1 quart Low-FODMAP Chicken Stock
- 2 tablespoons fresh lemon juice (from 1 small lemon)
- 1 tablespoon reduced-sodium soy sauce
- ½ teaspoon salt, or more as needed
- 2 cups coarsely chopped fresh green beans
- 2 cups diced cooked chicken
- ½ cup chopped fresh cilantro, basil, or parsley

Instructions
- Place the noodles in a large mixing basin and cover with warm water to soak. To keep them from sticking together, stir them every now and again.
- Heat the oils in a 3- to 4-quart pot until aromatic. Combine the ginger, carrots, and scallion greens in a large mixing bowl. 7 to 8 minutes over medium heat, until the veggies begin to brown.
- Toss the veggies with the stock, lemon juice, soy sauce, and salt. Cover, bring to a boil, then lower to a low heat and continue to cook for about 10 minutes.
- Drain the noodles and add them to the boiling pan after the carrots are cooked.
- Continue to boil, stirring occasionally, until the green beans are gently cooked and the rice noodles are soft but still chewy, about 10 minutes. If desired, garnish the soup with cilantro.

6. Company Roast Chicken

Prep time: 45 min | Serves: 6 | Difficulty: Moderate
Nutrition: Calories: 241 Kcal | Fat: 18 g | Protein: 17 g | Carbohydrates: 4 g

Ingredients
- 1 tablespoon olive oil
- 1 roasting chicken, about 6 pounds
- ½ fresh lemon
- ½ teaspoon freshly ground black pepper
- ½ teaspoon crushed thyme leaves

Instructions
- Preheat the oven to 450 degrees Fahrenheit. Oil a roasting pan by brushing or spraying it.
- Remove any excess liquid from the chicken. Remove the giblets from the cavity and place them in the roasting pan after unwrapping them. Do not rinse or dry the chicken; lay it breast side up in the roasting pan, according to the current USDA food safety regulations.
- Squeeze half of the lemon over the chicken and tuck it into the cavity. Place the chicken on the center rack of the oven and season with pepper and thyme.
- Roast for 15 minutes, then reduce to 350°F and continue roasting for another 90 minutes, or until a thermometer inserted in the chicken registers 165°F (test many locations, avoiding bone). Immediately transfer the chicken to a serving platter and serve.

7. Easy Chicken Enchilada Casserole

Prep time: 45 min | Serves: 6 | Difficulty: Moderate
Nutrition: Calories: 293 Kcal | Fat: 18 g | Protein: 27 g | Carbohydrates: 14 g

Ingredients
- 1 tablespoon cornstarch
- 1 tablespoon ground ancho chile
- 1½ teaspoons ground cumin
- ¼ teaspoon sweet smoked paprika
- ½ teaspoon salt
- 3 tablespoons garlic-infused olive oil
- 1 28-ounce can finely chopped or crushed tomatoes
- 1 cup water
- 1¾ pounds chicken tenders or chicken breast, sliced ½ inch thick
- 8 6-inch fresh corn tortillas
- 1 large orange bell pepper, seeded and diced
- 2 cups shredded pepper jack cheese (½ pound)
- 1 bunch scallion greens, thinly sliced

Instructions
- Combine the cornstarch, ground chile, cumin, paprika, and salt in a medium saucepan. Add the oil, mix well, and cook until bubbling over medium heat.
- Toss in the tomatoes and some water. Bring to a boil, covered, stirring periodically.

- Reduce the heat to low and cook the chicken, stirring occasionally, for about 15 minutes, or until it is cooked through. Remove the chicken from the heat and set it aside to cool for a few minutes.
- Preheat the oven to 350 degrees Fahrenheit. Set aside a 9 x 13-inch baking dish that has been oiled.
- Using two forks, shred the chicken.
- 12 cup of the heated sauce should be spread on the bottom of the baking dish. Layer the tortillas, chicken, sauce, pepper, and cheese, starting with the cheese and finishing with the cheese.
- Bake for 35 minutes, or until the cheese on top has melted and the casserole has started to bubble. Allow it cool for 10 minutes before serving with the scallion greens.

8. Baked Eggplant Parmesan

Prep time: 45 min | Serves: 8 | Difficulty: Moderate
Nutrition: Calories: 181 Kcal | Fat: 5 g | Protein: 12 g | Carbohydrates: 24 g

Ingredients
- ⅓ cup garlic-infused olive oil
- 2 medium eggplants
- Marinara Sauce warmed
- 1 cup shredded mozzarella cheese
- ¾ cup grated Parmesan cheese
- ½ cup gluten-free or Toasted Bread Crumbs
- ½ cup chopped fresh basil or parsley

Instructions
- Preheat the oven to 450 degrees Fahrenheit. Brush a little oil on two baking sheets and a 9 x 13-inch baking dish.
- Unpeeled eggplant should be cut into 12-inch-thick strips or circles. Brush the eggplant slices with oil and arrange them in a single layer on the two baking sheets. Bake for 30 minutes, or until golden brown. Remove the pan from the oven and lower the temperature to 350°F.
- Half cup of the heated sauce should be spread in the bottom of the baking dish. Starting with the eggplant, layer the eggplant, sauce, and cheeses in that order, finishing with a layer of sauce. Bake for 30 minutes, then top with bread crumbs and finish in the oven for another 20 minutes. Allow it cool for 15 minutes before serving, then garnish with fresh basil.

9. Italian Wedding Soup

Prep time: 45 min | Serves: 5 | Difficulty: Moderate
Nutrition: Calories: 229 kcal | Fat: 7.7 g | Protein: 32.2 g | Carbohydrates: 8.3 g

Ingredients

- 12 ounces lean ground turkey or beef
- 1 large egg
- 2 tablespoons quick-cooking oats
- 1 tablespoon grated Parmesan cheese, plus additional for garnish if desired
- ½ teaspoon dried basil
- 2 teaspoons garlic-infused olive oil
- 1½ quarts Low-FODMAP Chicken or Beef Stock 2 medium carrots, diced
- ½ cup uncooked brown rice
- 4 cups tightly packed chopped kale
- ½ teaspoon salt, or more if needed
- ¼ teaspoon freshly ground black pepper

Instructions

- Combine the turkey, egg, oats, Parmesan, and basil in a medium mixing bowl. Using your hands or a tiny scoop, make 1-inch balls.
- Heat the oil in a large skillet over medium heat until fragrant. Brown the meatballs on both sides until no longer pink in the center, about 10 to 12 minutes; drain any extra fat if needed.
- Bring the stock to a boil in a 4-quart saucepan. Combine the carrots and rice in a mixing bowl. Cover the saucepan and cook for approximately 40 minutes, or until the carrots and rice are soft; check after 30 minutes. Cook for a few minutes, until the kale has wilted, then add the meatballs, salt, and pepper. Garnish with more Parmesan cheese if desired.

10. Polenta Pizza Squares

Prep time: 45 min | Serves: 6tfc | Difficulty: Moderate
Nutrition: Calories: 202 Kcal | Fat: 13 g | Protein: 16 g | Carbohydrates:13 g

Ingredients

- 1 tablespoon olive oil
- 3 cups water
- 1 cup coarsely ground cornmeal
- ⅛ teaspoon salt
- ¼ teaspoon crushed dried rosemary leaves
- 1 tablespoon garlic-infused olive oil
- ⅛ teaspoon red pepper flakes (optional)
- 1 cup grated Parmesan cheese (4 ounces)
- 1 cup Marinara Sauce, warmed
- 4 ounces fully cooked sweet Italian chicken sausage, sliced into ¼-inch rounds
- 1 cup grated mozzarella cheese (4 ounces)

Instructions

- Preheat the oven to 350°F. Liberally oil a 9-inch square baking dish.
- In a medium saucepan over medium-high heat, bring the water, cornmeal, and salt to a boil. Reduce the heat, cover, and simmer for 6 to 8

minutes, or until the grains are tender and the polenta has thickened. Polenta sputters as it cooks, so remove the pan from the heat for stirring and then re-cover promptly to continue cooking.

- Stir the oil, red pepper flakes, and Parmesan into the polenta, and spoon into the baking dish. Spread evenly in the bottom of the pan. Cover with the sauce, then distribute the sausage slices evenly across the sauce. Sprinkle the mozzarella on top and bake for 30 to 40 minutes, until the sauce is bubbly and the cheese is golden brown.

11. Portuguese Fisherman's Stew

Prep time: 45 min | Serves: 8 | Difficulty: Moderate
Nutrition: Calories: 185 kcal | Fat: 8 g | Protein: 3 g | Carbohydrates: 20 g

Ingredients

- 1 5-gram packet bonito flakes
- 3 cups boiling water
- ½ pound chard
- 2 tablespoons garlic-infused olive oil
- ½ pound lean ground pork
- 1 tablespoon Goya or Cholula Original hot sauce, or more to taste
- 1 fennel bulb, diced
- 1 yellow bell pepper, seeded and diced
- 1 pound small potatoes, unpeeled, cut into ½-inch slices
- 1 14.5-ounce can diced tomatoes
- 2 cups dry white wine, such as Sauvignon Blanc
- ½ teaspoon salt
- 2 teaspoons sweet smoked paprika
- 2 pounds white fish fillets, such as cod, haddock, or pollock
- ½ pound raw shrimp, peeled and deveined
- 1 bunch fresh cilantro, coarsely chopped
- Freshly ground black pepper

Instructions

- To make a fish stock, put the bonito flakes and boiling water in a medium basin.
- Remove the chard leaves from the stalks. Slice the leaves into 12-inch-thick strips and finely chop the stems.
- Warm the oil in a 6- to 8-quart saucepan over medium heat. Brown the pork for 7 to 8 minutes, breaking it up with a spatula as it cooks; drain extra fat if desired. Sauté for 10 minutes, stirring regularly, with the spicy sauce, chard stems, fennel, and bell pepper.
- Using a mesh strainer, filter the fish stock into the saucepan. Combine the potatoes, tomatoes, wine, salt, and paprika in a large mixing bowl. Bring to a boil, then lower to a low heat and cook for 10 minutes, uncovered.
- Arrange the fish fillets on top of the stew, cover, and poach for 5 to 15 minutes at a low heat.

After 5 minutes, check the fish with two forks to see whether it flakes. It will be opaque (solid white) rather than transparent when finished. Stir in the shrimp and chard leaves after breaking the fish into bite-size pieces. Cover and continue to cook for another 2 minutes; do not overcook.

- Before serving, ladle the stew into bowls and top with cilantro and a dusting of pepper.

12. Shrimp Fried Rice

Prep time: 45 min| Serves: 8| Difficulty: Moderate
Nutrition: Calories: 189 Kcal |Fat: 8 g| Protein: 7 g| Carbohydrates: 24 g

Ingredients

- 1 tablespoon brown sugar
- ¼ cup low-sodium soy sauce
- 2 tablespoons rice vinegar
- 2 tablespoons dark or spicy sesame oil
- ¼ teaspoon freshly ground black pepper
- ½ teaspoon hot sauce (optional)
- 2 large eggs
- 1 teaspoon water
- 2 tablespoons garlic-infused olive oil
- 1 cup chopped carrots
- 1 cup chopped carrots
- 1 tablespoon minced fresh ginger
- 4 cups chopped bok choy
- 3 cups cooked white or brown rice
- 2 cups cooked shrimp
- 1 cup pineapple chunks
- ½ cup unsalted peanuts
- 1 bunch scallion greens, thinly sliced

Instructions

- Combine the brown sugar, soy sauce, vinegar, sesame oil, pepper, and spicy sauce, if using, in a small bowl.
- Combine the eggs and water in a separate small bowl.
- 12 tbsp olive oil, heated over medium high heat in an extra-large skillet or wok Cook, stirring regularly, for approximately 2 minutes, or until the eggs are firm but not browned. Cut the eggs into strips after removing them from the skillet.
- In the same skillet, heat the remaining 112 tablespoons oil until it spatters when a drop of water is placed in. Over medium-high heat, sauté the carrots, ginger, and bok choy until soft. Transfer the rice to the skillet and cook for 5 to 10 minutes, turning periodically, until the rice is cooked through and gently crisped in spots. Stir in the shrimp, pineapple, egg strips, and soy sauce mixture until everything is cooked through, stirring periodically from the bottom.
- Serve immediately with the peanuts and scallion greens as a garnish.

13. Skillet Buffalo Chicken and Spinach Salad

Prep time: 25 min| Serves: 5| Difficulty: Moderate
Nutrition: Calories: 311 kcal |Fat: 7.1 g| Protein: 44 g| Carbohydrates: 16 g

Ingredients

- 3 tablespoons cornstarch
- 1 pound chicken tenders or boneless, skinless chicken breast, sliced into ¾- inch strips
- 1 tablespoon olive oil
- 1 tablespoon olive oil
- 2 tablespoons butter
- ¼ cup Cholula Original or Goya Hot Sauce
- 10 ounces baby spinach
- 1 cup carrot matchsticks
- Blue Cheese Dressing

Instructions

- Toss the chicken pieces in a medium basin with the cornstarch to coat them. Heat the oil in a large skillet over medium heat. Transfer the chicken pieces to the skillet when the oil is heated enough to make a drop of water sizzle. Cook the chicken over medium heat, rotating once, until an internal temperature of 165°F is reached, as measured by a quick-read thermometer. To avoid losing the crust, scrape the bottom of the frying pan with the spatula as you flip the chicken.
- In a microwave-safe bowl, melt the butter and whisk in the spicy sauce. Pour the mixture over the chicken while keeping your face away from the vapour created when the spicy sauce hits the skillet. Remove the chicken from the bottom of the pan, along with its crust, and mix to coat with sauce. Tear the chicken into bite-size pieces using two forks.
- Toss the spinach, carrots, and dressing together in a large salad bowl.
- Serve the salad immediately after dividing it into serving dishes and topping it with the chicken pieces.

14. Maple -Bourbon Baked Salmon

Prep time: 25 min| Serves: 6| Difficulty: Moderate
Nutrition: Calories: 407 kcal |Fat: 35 g |Protein: 7 g |Carbohydrates: 6 g

Ingredients

- 1½ pounds salmon fillet
- 2 tablespoons 100% pure maple syrup
- 1 tablespoon olive oil
- 1 tablespoon olive oil
- ¼ teaspoon sweet smoked paprika
- ½ teaspoon salt
- 2 tablespoons bourbon

Instructions

- Combine the maple syrup, oil, paprika, salt, and bourbon in a bowl the size of your salmon fillet. Place the salmon skin side up in the marinade, then turn it skin side down. Marinate for 8 to 10 hours, well covered.

- Preheat the oven to 400 degrees Fahrenheit. Foil the bottom and half of the sides of a baking dish large enough to contain the fish. Place the salmon skin side down in the pan. Brush the fish with the hot pan juices after approximately 10 minutes and bake for 15 minutes, until the salmon is opaque when flaked with a fork.

15. Spaghetti and Meatballs

Prep time: 35 min | Serves: 5 | Difficulty: Moderate
Nutrition: Calories: 202 Kcal | Fat: 13 g | Protein: 16 g | Carbohydrates: 13 g

Ingredients

- 1 pound lean ground pork
- 1 pound lean ground beef
- ¾ cup chopped fresh parsley
- ¼ cup grated Parmesan cheese (1 ounce), plus more for serving if desired
- 1 large egg
- 1½ teaspoons Italian seasoning
- 1 teaspoon salt
- ½ teaspoon red pepper flakes (optional)
- ¼ cup quick-cooking oats
- Marinara Sauce
- 1 pound low-FODMAP spaghetti

Instructions

- Preheat the oven to 400 degrees Fahrenheit.
- Gently combine the pork, beef, parsley, cheese, egg, seasoning, salt, red pepper flakes, if using, and oats in a large mixing basin. To contain the drippings, form the meatballs into sixteen 2-inch balls with your hands and lay on two large baking pans with at least 1-inch edges.
- Bake for 40 to 45 minutes, or until the meatballs are browned and a quick-read thermometer reads 165°F. The heated fat should be drained and discarded.
- Warm the sauce in a 3- to 4-quart saucepan over medium heat. Return the meatballs to the pan and keep them heated until ready to serve.
- Follow the manufacturer's Instructions for cooking and draining the spaghetti.
- Fill serving dishes halfway with pasta and top with heated meatballs and sauce. If desired, top with more Parmesan cheese.

16. Marinated Steak Kebabs

Prep time: 35 min | Serves: 8 | Difficulty: Moderate
Nutrition: Calories: 202 Kcal | Fat: 13 g | Protein: 16 g | Carbohydrates: 13 g

Ingredients

- 2 pounds boneless steak, cut into 2-inch cubes
- 3 tablespoons garlic-infused olive oil
- 1½ teaspoons sea salt
- 1 teaspoon ground ancho chile
- 1 teaspoon ground cumin
- ½ teaspoon sweet smoked paprika
- ½ teaspoon sweet smoked paprika
- 2 tablespoons fresh lime juice
- 2 small zucchini (about 1 pound), sliced into ¾-inch rounds
- 1 pint cherry tomatoes
- 1 medium red bell pepper, seeded and cut into 1-inch pieces
- 1 medium yellow bell pepper, seeded and cut into 1-inch pieces

Instructions

- Preheat the oven to 400 degrees Fahrenheit.
- Gently combine the pork, beef, parsley, cheese, egg, seasoning, salt, red pepper flakes, if using, and oats in a large mixing basin. To contain the drippings, form the meatballs into sixteen 2-inch balls with your hands and lay on two large baking pans with at least 1-inch edges.
- Bake for 40 to 45 minutes, or until the meatballs are browned and a quick-read thermometer reads 165°F. The heated fat should be drained and discarded.
- Warm the sauce in a 3- to 4-quart saucepan over medium heat. Return the meatballs to the pan and keep them heated until ready to serve.
- Follow the manufacturer's Instructions for cooking and draining the spaghetti.
- Fill serving dishes halfway with pasta and top with heated meatballs and sauce. If desired, top with more Parmesan cheese.

17. Taco Salad Deluxe

Prep time: 35 min | Serves: 4 | Difficulty: Moderate
Nutrition: Calories: 305 kcal | Fat: 27 g | Protein: 15 g | Carbohydrates: 2 g

Ingredients

- 5½ ounces mixed salad greens
- ¼ cup finely chopped fresh cilantro, plus more for garnish if desired
- 1 medium orange bell pepper, seeded and chopped
- ½ bunch scallion greens, thinly sliced
- 1 large ripe tomato, diced
- ½ pound lean ground beef or turkey
- 1 tablespoon Taco Seasoning Mix
- 2 tablespoons water
- ½ cup grated Cheddar cheese (2 ounces)
- 1 cup coarsely crushed tortilla chips
- 1 recipe Smoky Ranch Dressing

Instructions

- Combine the salad greens, cilantro, bell pepper, scallion greens, and tomato in an extra-large salad dish.
- Crumble and brown the ground beef in a large pan over medium-high heat until cooked thoroughly, about 10 minutes. If desired, remove any surplus fat. Cook and stir for another 2

minutes, until the meat is completely covered in sauce, then add the spice mix and water.
- Add the heated meat, cheese, tortilla chips, and dressing to the salad dish right before serving and mix everything together completely. If desired, top with more chopped cilantro.

18. Traffic Light Chili

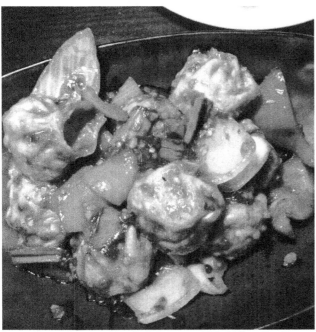

Prep time: 1 hour 10 min | Serves: 10 | Difficulty: Easy
Nutrition: Calories: 241 Kcal | Fat: 18 g | Protein: 17 g | Carbohydrates: 4 g
Ingredients
- 1 tablespoon garlic-infused olive oil
- 1¼ pounds extra-lean ground turkey or beef
- ½ pound carrots, chopped
- 3 cup chopped butternut squash (from 12 ounces squash)
- 1 large green bell pepper, seeded and chopped
- 1 large yellow bell pepper, seeded and chopped
- 1 large red bell pepper, seeded and chopped
- 1 tablespoon ground ancho chile
- 2 tablespoons ground cumin
- 1 teaspoon salt, or more as needed
- ½ teaspoon sweet smoked paprika
- ¼ teaspoon red pepper flakes (optional)
- 2 14.5-ounce cans lentils, drained and rinsed
- 1 28-ounce can diced tomatoes
- 1 cup water or Low-FODMAP Chicken Stock
- 1 avocado, chopped

Instructions
- Warm the oil in a big, heavy saucepan over medium heat. Add the turkey and cook, breaking it up into tiny pieces with a spatula, for 8 to 10 minutes, until browned. Carrots, squash,

bell peppers, ground chile, cumin, salt, paprika, and red pepper flakes, if used, should all be added at this point. Cook for about 10 minutes over medium heat, stirring periodically. Combine the lentils, tomatoes, and their juices, as well as the water. Reduce the heat to low and cook for 50 to 60 minutes, covered.
- To serve, ladle into bowls and top with diced avocado. Serve fresh.

19. Veggie Burger of Your Dreams
Prep time: 35 min | Serves: 8 | Difficulty: Easy
Nutrition: Calories: 256 kcal | Fat: 8 g | Protein:11 g | Carbohydrates:32 g
Ingredients
- 1 small eggplant (about ¾ pound), peeled and cubed
- ⅔ cup water
- 1 tablespoon chia seeds
- 1 cup cooked brown rice
- 1 cup drained canned lentils
- ½ cup finely chopped scallion greens
- ½ cup finely chopped scallion greens
- ½ cup red bell pepper, seeded and finely chopped
- ½ teaspoon sweet smoked paprika
- 1 teaspoon ground cumin
- ½ teaspoon salt
- 1 teaspoon crushed dried thyme leaves
- ¾ cup gluten-free or Toasted Bread Crumbs
- 2 tablespoons coconut oil

Instructions
- In a medium saucepan, bring the eggplant and water to a boil. Reduce the heat to low, cover, and cook for approximately 25 minutes, or until the eggplant is very soft.
- With a potato masher, mash the eggplant until it resembles chunky applesauce.
- Stir in the chia seeds until they are evenly distributed. In a large mixing bowl, add the rice, lentils, scallion greens, bell pepper, paprika, cumin, salt, and thyme. Stir in 12 cup of the bread crumbs. Add a spoonful of bread crumbs at a time until the mixture resembles mashed potatoes.
- 1 tablespoon coconut oil, heated over medium-high heat in a large cast-iron or heavy pan Spoon 4 big mounds of burger mixture (approximately half the quantity) onto the skillet when it is shimmering and aromatic, and flatten into patties with the back of a spoon. Cook, flipping halfway through, for approximately 10 minutes, or until the burgers are golden and crisp on the exterior and completely cooked on the inside. Keep heated while you finish the second half of the mixture with the remaining tablespoon of coconut oil. Serve atop a bed of

lettuce or lowFODMAP bread that has been toasted.

20. West African Sweet Potato Soup

Prep time: 35 min | Serves: 5 | Difficulty: Moderate
Nutrition: Calories: 192 kcal | Fat: 10 g | Protein: 13 g | Carbohydrates: 17 g

Ingredients
- 1 tablespoon garlic-infused olive oil
- 1¾ pounds boneless, skinless chicken thighs, cubed
- 3 tablespoons minced fresh ginger
- 1 small eggplant (½ pound), diced
- 2 small summer squash (1 pound total), diced
- 2 small sweet potatoes (1 pound total), unpeeled, diced
- 1 teaspoon ground coriander
- 2 tablespoons ground ancho chile
- 2 tablespoons ground cumin
- ½ teaspoon red pepper flakes (optional)
- 1 teaspoon salt
- 4 cups water
- 1 cup creamy-style natural peanut butter
- 1 cup chopped ripe tomatoes
- ½ cup thinly sliced scallion greens
- ½ cup roasted salted peanuts, chopped

Instructions
- Heat the oil in a 4- to 6-quart heavy pot or Dutch oven over medium-high heat. Brown the chicken for around 8 to 10 minutes after adding it to the pan. Sauté for 1 minute with the ginger before adding the eggplant, squash, and sweet potatoes.
- Combine the coriander, ground chile, cumin, red pepper flakes (if using), salt, and water in a large mixing bowl. Bring to a boil over high heat, then lower to a medium heat and let the stew simmer for 20 minutes.
- Cook for another 20 minutes, or until the eggplant is soft, after adding the peanut butter and tomatoes. As the stew cooks, it will thicken somewhat.
- Serve immediately by ladling the soup into dishes and garnishing with scallion leaves and chopped peanuts.

21. Pasta with Fresh Tomato, Olives, and Pecorino

Prep time: 20 min | Serves: 4-6 | Difficulty: Moderate
Nutrition: Calories: 277 kcal | Fat:11 g | Protein:16 g | Carbohydrates: 30.3 g

Ingredients
- 1-pound gluten-free pasta
- 2 tablespoons olive oil
- 1/4 cup pine nuts
- 4 ounces baby spinach leaves rinsed and dried
- 1 cup of kalamata olives, pitted
- 6 Roma tomatoes, chopped

- 1/4 cup basil leaves
- 1/4 cup flat-leaf parsley leaves
- 2½ ounces pecorino, shaved (about 2/3 cup), plus more for serving

Instructions
- A big pot of water should be brought to a boil. Cook the pasta according to the package directions until it is barely tender.
- Drain, then return to the saucepan to keep warm. In a large heavy-bottomed saucepan, heat the olive oil over medium heat, then add the pine nuts and stir until brown. Cook until the spinach has wilted, then add the olives, tomatoes, basil, and parsley.
- Heat the pecorino until it is slightly melted and warmed thoroughly. Season with salt and pepper to taste, then mix in the drained pasta.
- Serve with additional pecorino on top.

22. Creamy Blue Cheese and Spinach Pasta

Prep time: 20 min | Serves: 4-6 | Difficulty: Moderate
Nutrition: Calories: 367 kcal | Fat: 12 g | Protein:11 g | Carbohydrates:34 g

Ingredients
- 1-pound gluten-free pasta
- 1 tablespoon olive oil
- 2 teaspoons garlic-infused olive oil
- 1/3 cup light cream
- 1/3 cup white wine
- 1/4 cup of crumbled blue cheese
- 3½ ounces baby spinach leaves, rinsed and dried
- 1/4 cup roughly chopped flat-leaf parsley
- Salt and freshly ground black pepper

Instructions
- Bring a large pot of water to a boil. Add the pasta and cook according to package directions, until just tender.
- Drain, return to the pot, and cover to keep warm. Meanwhile, heat the olive oil and garlic-infused oil in a large heavy- bottomed frying pan over medium heat.
- Add the cream and wine and simmer, stirring occasionally, for 5 to 7 minutes, until the liquid has reduced and thickened. Add the blue cheese and stir until melted.
- Remove the pan from the heat. Add the drained pasta, spinach, and parsley and gently toss to coat. Allow the spinach leaves to wilt.
- Season to taste with salt and pepper and serve.

23. Speedy Spaghetti Bolognese

Prep time: 20 min | Serves: 6-8 | Difficulty: Moderate
Nitrition: Calories: 202 Kcal | Fat: 13 g | Protein: 16 g | Carbohydrates:13 g

Ingredients

- 2 12-ounce (or three 8-ounce packages gluten-free spaghetti
- 2 teaspoons olive oil
- 2 teaspoons garlic-infused olive oil
- 2 pounds (900 g) extra-lean ground beef
- 8 ounces (225 g) lean bacon slices, diced
- 2-2/3 cups (670 ml) tomato puree
- 2 teaspoons cayenne pepper
- 1/2 teaspoon chili powder (optional)
- Salt and freshly ground black pepper
- Grated Parmesan, for serving

Instructions

- A big pot of water should be brought to a boil. Cook the spaghetti according to the package directions until it is barely tender.
- Drain, then return to the saucepan to keep warm. Meanwhile, in a big heavy-bottomed frying pan, heat the olive oil and garlic-infused oil over medium heat.
- Cook until the steak is beautifully browned, breaking out any lumps as you go with the beef and bacon.
- Simmer for 10 minutes, stirring periodically, with the tomato puree, cayenne, and chilli powder (if using). Season with salt and pepper to taste.
- Spoon the Bolognese sauce over the pasta in four separate dishes.
- Serve immediately with a parmesan garnish.

24. Penne with Meatballs

Prep time: 45 min | Serves: 6 | Difficulty: Moderate
Nutrition: Calories:380 kcal | Fat:7 g | Protein:24 g | Carbohydrates:33 g

Ingredients

Meatballs
- 2 pounds extra-lean ground beef
- 1 cup cooked long-grain rice
- 3/4 cup grated Parmesan
- 1 large egg, beaten
- 2 teaspoons garlic-infused olive oil
- 2 teaspoons olive oil
- 3 to 4 heaping tablespoons finely chopped basil
- 1/4 cup finely chopped flat-leaf parsley
- 1/2 teaspoon cayenne pepper
- Salt and freshly ground black pepper
- Olive oil, for pan-frying
- One and a half 12-ounce (340 g) packages gluten-free penne (18 ounces/510 g total)
- 2 cups (500 ml) tomato puree
- 1/4 cup (5 g) roughly chopped basil
- Grated Parmesan, for serving
- Extra basil leaves, for serving (optional)

Instructions

- A big pot of water should be brought to a boil. To prepare the meatballs, in a large mixing bowl, add the beef, rice, Parmesan, egg, garlic-infused oil, olive oil, finely chopped basil and parsley, cayenne, salt, and pepper.
- Shape into golf ball–size balls using moist hands. In a large frying pan over medium heat, heat the olive oil, then add the meatballs and cook until beautifully browned on both sides and cooked through. Meanwhile, add the pasta to the boiling water and cook until barely tender, according to package recommendations.
- Drain, then return to the saucepan to keep warm. Pour the tomato puree over the meatballs and top with the basil, which has been finely chopped. Bring to a boil, then lower to a low heat and continue to cook for 2 to 3 minutes, or until well warmed.
- Distribute the penne into four bowls and top with the meatballs and sauce.
- Serve immediately with a dusting of Parmesan and additional basil leaves, if preferred.

25. Seafood Pasta with Salsa Verde

Prep time: 45 min | Serves: 4 | Difficulty: Moderate
Nutrition: Calories: 373 kcal | Fat: 12 g | Protein: 44 g | Carbohydrates: 24 g

Ingredients

- 1-pound (450 g) gluten-free pasta
- 1/2 cup (130 g) Salsa Verde
- 2 teaspoons olive oil
- 2 teaspoons garlic-infused olive oil
- 2 small squid bodies, cleaned and sliced into rings
- 8 ounces (225 g) boneless, skinless firm white fish fillets, cut into cubes
- 1 pound (450 g) raw large shrimp, peeled and deveined, tails intact
- 1 pound (450 g) fresh shelled mussel meats
- 1/2 cup (125 ml) light cream
- 2 tablespoons plus 2 teaspoons dry white wine
- Salt and freshly ground black pepper

Instructions

- A big pot of water should be brought to a boil. Cook until the pasta is barely soft, according to the package guidelines.
- Return to the pot after draining. Cover and keep heated by stirring in the majority of the Salsa Verde. Meanwhile, in a large nonstick frying pan, heat the olive oil and garlic-infused oil over medium-high heat.
- Cook for 2 minutes, tossing gently with the squid, fish, and shrimp. Reduce the heat to low and cook for 3 to 4 minutes, until the mussel flesh, cream, and wine are softly cooked through.
- Season with salt and pepper to taste.

- Distribute the spaghetti into four bowls and top with the seafood sauce.
- Serve immediately with tiny dollops of the leftover Salsa Verde.

26. Smoked Salmon Pasta in White Wine Sauce

Prep time: 30 min | Serves: 4 | Difficulty: Moderate
Nutrition: Calories: 712 kcal | Fat: 26.7 g | Protein: 45.1 g | Carbohydrates: 69.9 g

Ingredients
- 1-pound (450 g) gluten-free pasta
- 1/4 cup (60 ml) olive oil
- 1/2 cup (125 ml) dry white wine
- 1 garlic clove, peeled and halved
- 3/4 cup (60 g) grated Parmesan
- Heaping 1/4 cup (20 g) roughly chopped flat-leaf parsley
- 1 teaspoon freshly ground black pepper, plus more if needed
- 1 teaspoon finely grated lemon zest
- 4 ounces (113 g) smoked salmon, cut into thin strips
- Salt

Instructions
- Bring a large pot of water to a boil. Add the pasta and cook according to package directions, until just tender.
- Drain, return to the pot, and cover to keep warm. Meanwhile, combine the olive oil, wine, and garlic in a large frying pan and bring to a boil over high heat, stirring constantly.
- Reduce the heat to medium and simmer, stirring occasionally, for 5 to 6 minutes, until the sauce has thickened slightly.
- Remove from the heat and remove and discard the garlic. Add the Parmesan, parsley, pepper, and lemon zest and stir until the cheese has melted.
- Add the sauce and smoked salmon to the pasta and toss to combine.
- Season to taste with salt and pepper and serve.

27. Vegetable Pasta Bake

Prep time: 45 min | Serves: 6-8 | Difficulty: Moderate
Nutrition: Calories: 250 kcal | Fat: 8 g | Protein: 32 g | Carbohydrates: 11 g

Ingredients
- 8 ounces (225 g) gluten-free pasta spirals
- 14 ounces (400 g) peeled and seeded kabocha or other suitable winter squash, cut into 1/3-inch (1 cm) cubes
- 1/2 cup (60 g) dried gluten-free, soy-free bread crumbs*
- 1/2 cup (2 ounces/60 g) grated cheddar
- One 14.5-ounce (425 g) can crush tomatoes
- 2 medium zucchinis, grated

- 5 large eggs, lightly beaten
- 1/2 cup (11/2 ounces/40 g) grated Parmesan
- 1/4 cup (15 g) roughly chopped flat-leaf parsley
- 1 heaping tablespoon ground cumin
- 1 heaping teaspoon ground mustard
- Salt and freshly ground black pepper

Instructions
- Prepare two big pots of water by bringing them to a boil. Preheat the oven to 350 degrees Fahrenheit (180 degrees Celsius).
- Using cooking spray, grease an 8 × 8-inch (2-liter) baking dish. In a separate pot, boil the pasta according to the package directions until just tender.
- Drain and rinse well with cold water. Drain once again. Meanwhile, in the second pot, cook the squash until it is barely soft. Drain the water and set it aside.
- Set aside the bread crumbs and cheddar cheese. In a large mixing bowl, combine the pasta, squash, tomatoes, zucchini, eggs, Parmesan, parsley, cumin, and mustard.
- Season with salt and pepper to taste.
- Spread the mixture in the baking dish and top with the cheddar and bread crumbs. Preheat oven to 350°F and bake for 30 minutes, or until golden brown.

28. Tuna Macaroni and Cheese Bake

Prep time: 45 min | Serves: 6-8 | Difficulty: Moderate
Nutrition: Calories:461 kcal | Fat: 18 g | Protein: 44 g | Carbohydrates: 34 g

Ingredients
- 8 ounces (225 g) gluten-free macaroni
- 1/3 cup (40 g) dried gluten-free, soy-free bread crumbs*
- 1/3 cup (25 g) grated Parmesan
- 21/4 cups (560 ml) low-fat milk, lactose-free milk, or suitable plant-based milk
- 1/3 cup (50 g) cornstarch
- 2 cups (81/2 ounces/240 g) grated reduced-fat cheddar
- Salt and freshly ground black pepper
- One 12-ounce (340 g) can tuna packed in water, drained

Instructions
- Bring a large pot of water to a boil. Preheat the oven to 350°F (180°C).
- Using cooking spray, grease an 8 × 8-inch (2-liter) baking dish. Add the pasta to the boiling water and cook until just cooked, according to the package recommendations.
- Return the saucepan to the heat and cover to keep it heated. Set aside the bread crumbs and Parmesan cheese.
- In a medium mixing bowl, make a paste with 14 cup (60 ml) milk and cornstarch. Whisk in the

remaining 2 cups of milk, making sure there are no lumps.

- Pour into a saucepan and cook over medium heat, stirring constantly, until thickened but not boiling. Stir in the cheddar and season with salt & pepper to taste, then add the tuna.
- Mix the cheese sauce into the spaghetti until everything is well incorporated.
- Top with the Parmesan cheese and bread crumbs in the baking dish. Bake for 15 to 20 minutes, or until brown and bubbling.

29. Lasagna

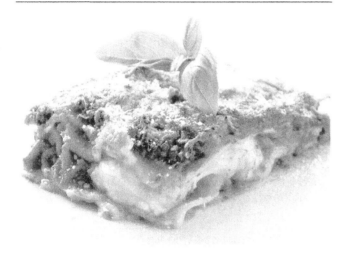

Prep time: 50 min| Serves: 8| Difficulty: Moderate
Nutrition: Calories: 371 kcal |Fat: 7.1 g| Protein: 14 g| Carbohydrates: 46 g
Ingredients
- 2 tablespoons olive oil
- 2 teaspoons garlic-infused olive oil
- 2 pounds (900 g) extra-lean ground beef
- 4 ounces (113 g) lean bacon slices, diced
- 2 teaspoons cayenne pepper
- 1/2 teaspoon chili powder (optional)
- One 28-ounce (794 g) can tomato puree
- 1 carrot, grated
- Salt and freshly ground black pepper
- 4 cups (1 liter) skim milk, lactose-free milk, or suitable plant-based milk
- 3 tablespoons cornstarch
- 3 cups (12 ounces/360 g) grated reduced-fat cheddar
- 1-pound (450 g) gluten-free lasagna sheets

Instructions
- Add the beef and bacon and cook until the beef is nicely browned, breaking up any lumps as you go. Spoon off any excess fat, then add the cayenne, chili powder (if using), tomato puree, and carrot.
- Season with salt and pepper. Simmer over medium heat for 10 minutes, stirring

occasionally, until the flavors meld. Blend 1/4 cup (60 ml) of the milk with the cornstarch in a medium bowl to form a paste.
- Add the remaining 33/4 cups of milk, whisking well to remove any lumps. Pour into a saucepan and stir over medium heat until thickened—don't let it boil.
- Add the cheddar and stir until melted. Season to taste with salt and pepper. Prepare the lasagna sheets according to the package directions. Place a layer of one third of the lasagna sheets over the bottom of an 11 x 7-inch (28 x 18 cm) baking pan, breaking them to fit if necessary.
- Spread half of the meat mixture evenly over the top. Spread one third of the cheese sauce over the meat.
- Repeat with another layer of lasagna sheets, the remaining meat mixture, and half the remaining cheese sauce.
- Finish with a final layer of lasagna sheets and the rest of the cheese sauce.
- Bake for 20 minutes or until bubbling and golden. Let sit for a few minutes before cutting.

30. Smoked Tuna Risotto

Prep time: 45 min| Serves: 6| Difficulty: Moderate
Nutrition: Calories: 354 kcal| Fat: 12 g| Protein: 24 g| Carbohydrates: 44 g
Ingredients
- 8 cups (2 liters) gluten-free, onion-free chicken or vegetable stock*
- 2 teaspoons olive oil
- 2 teaspoons garlic-infused olive oil
- 2 saffron threads
- 21/2 cups (500 g) Arborio rice
- 1/2 cup (125 ml) white wine
- 13.5 ounces (385 g) canned or packaged smoked tuna, drained and flaked
- 1 cup (120 g) frozen peas
- 2 medium zucchinis, halved lengthwise and sliced
- 1/2 cup (11/2 ounces/40 g) grated Parmesan
- 1/4 cup (15 g) roughly chopped flat-leaf parsley
- Salt and freshly ground black pepper

Instructions
- In a medium saucepan, pour the stock. Over low heat, cover and bring to a soft simmer.
- Meanwhile, in a large heavy-bottomed saucepan, heat the olive oil and garlic-infused oil over medium heat. Cook, stirring constantly, for 2 minutes after adding the saffron.
- Stir in the rice until it is thoroughly covered in the oil and saffron. Cook until the wine has been absorbed into the rice. Cook, stirring constantly, until 1 cup (250 ml) of the hot stock has been absorbed.
- Repeat the process, adding 1/2 cup (125 ml) of stock at a time, until there is only 1/2 cup (125

ml) of stock left. Stir in the tuna, peas, zucchini, Parmesan, and parsley until everything is thoroughly mixed.

- Pour in the remaining stock and stir until the liquid has almost completely evaporated and the rice is soft.
- Season with salt and pepper to taste and serve.

31. Beef Risotto with Whole Grain Mustard and Spinach

Prep time: 45 min | Serves: 8 | Difficulty: Moderate
Nutrition: Calories:612 kcal | Fat: 24.7 g | Protein: 41.1 g | Carbohydrates:59g

Ingredients

- 2 teaspoons garlic-infused olive oil
- 1 pound (450 g) lean beef, cut into strips
- 8 ounces (225 g) baby spinach leaves (8 cups), rinsed and dried
- 8 cups (2 liters) gluten-free, onion-free beef stock*
- 2 teaspoons olive oil
- 2 1/2 cups (500 g) Arborio rice
- 3/4 cup (2 ounces/60 g) grated Parmesan
- 1/3 cup (95 g) gluten-free whole grain mustard
- 2 heaping tablespoons roughly chopped flat-leaf parsley, plus sprigs for garnish

Instructions

- Preheat the oven to 350 degrees Fahrenheit (180 degrees Celsius).
- In a large heavy-bottomed frying pan, heat the olive oil and garlic-infused oil over medium heat. In a medium saucepan, pour the stock.
- Over low heat, cover and bring to a soft simmer. Meanwhile, in a large heavy-bottomed saucepan, heat the olive oil and garlic-infused oil over medium heat.
- Cook, stirring constantly, for 2 minutes after adding the saffron. Stir in the rice until it is thoroughly covered in the oil and saffron.
- Cook until the wine has been absorbed into the rice. Cook, stirring constantly, until 1 cup (250 ml) of the hot stock has been absorbed. Repeat the process, adding 1/2 cup (125 ml) of stock at a time, until there is only 1/2 cup (125 ml) of stock left. Stir in the tuna, peas, zucchini, Parmesan, and parsley until everything is thoroughly mixed.
- Pour in the remaining stock and stir until the liquid has almost completely evaporated and the rice is soft.
- Season with salt and pepper to taste and serve.

32. Asian Duck and Pea Risotto

Prep time: 4hr | Serves: 8 | Difficulty: Moderate
Nutrition: Calories: 547 kcal | Fat: 38 g | Protein: 33.7 g | Carbohydrates: 19.8 g

Ingredients

- Eight 6-ounce (170 g) duck leg quarters (leg and thigh)
- 1/2 cup (125 ml) gluten-free soy sauce
- 2 teaspoons garlic-infused olive oil
- 2 teaspoons grated ginger
- 2 tablespoons sesame oil
- Salt and freshly ground black pepper
- 8 cups (2 liters) gluten-free, onion-free chicken stock*
- 2 celery stalks, sliced
- 2 1/2 cups (500 g) Arborio rice
- 1 cup (120 g) frozen peas

Instructions

- Toss in the duck strips and remaining quarters to coat. Refrigerate for 3 to 4 hours or overnight, covered.
- Preheat the oven to 350 degrees Fahrenheit (180 degrees Celsius). In a medium saucepan, pour the stock. Over low heat, cover and bring to a soft simmer. Place the duck quarters in a baking dish, reserving the strips and marinade.
- Roast for 25 to 30 minutes, or until well done (liquid should run clear when a thigh is pierced with a toothpick in the thickest part).
- Keep warm by covering loosely with foil. While the duck quarters are roasting, in a large heavy-bottomed saucepan, heat the remaining 1 tablespoon sesame oil over medium heat, add the celery, and cook until soft and slightly caramelized.
- Stir in the rice until it is thoroughly covered in the oil and celery. Combine the duck strips and any remaining marinade in a mixing bowl. Cook, stirring constantly, until 1/2 cup (125 ml) of the hot stock has been absorbed.
- Repeat the process until the rice is soft, adding 1/2 cup (125 ml) of stock at a time.
- Cook until the liquid is nearly absorbed and the peas are thawed and warmed through, then add the peas with the remainder of the stock. To taste, season with salt and pepper.
- Distribute the risotto among six dishes, then top each with a roasted duck quarter and a pinch of black pepper.

33. Lamb and Eggplant Risotto with Middle Eastern Spices

Prep time: 45 min | Serves: 6 | Difficulty: Moderate
Nutrition: Calories: 673 kcal | Fat:32 g | Protein: 64 g | Carbohydrates: 54 g

Ingredients
- 11 ounces (300 g) peeled and seeded kabocha or other suitable winter squash,
- cut into 3⁄4-inch (2 cm) cubes
- 1 medium-small (100 g) eggplant
- Garlic-infused olive oil
- 11⁄2 teaspoons ground cumin
- 1 teaspoon ground coriander
- 1 teaspoon ground turmeric
- 1⁄4 teaspoon ground cardamom
- 1⁄4 teaspoon ground sumac, or 1⁄4 teaspoon paprika plus 1⁄2 teaspoon grated lemon zest
- 1 pound (450 g) lean lamb, cut into strips
- 101⁄2 cups (2.5 liters) gluten-free, onion-free beef stock*
- 21⁄2 cups (500 g) Arborio rice
- 1⁄3 cup (50 g) pine nuts, toasted
- 1⁄2 cup (11⁄2 ounces/40 g) grated Parmesan, plus more for serving (optional)
- 2 handfuls of baby spinach leaves, rinsed and dried

Instructions
- Preheat the oven to 350 degrees Fahrenheit (180 degrees Celsius). Place the eggplant on one baking sheet and the squash on the other.
- Brush them each with garlic-infused oil and bake for 20 to 30 minutes, or until soft and browning.
- Allow the squash to cool before wrapping the eggplant in foil and sweating it for 10 minutes. Take the eggplant out of the foil and cut it coarsely. Remove from the equation.
- In a large heavy-bottomed saucepan, heat 1 tablespoon garlic-infused oil over medium heat. Cook until aromatic, then add the cumin, coriander, turmeric, cardamom, and sumac.
- Toss in the lamb strips to coat them with the spices. Cook the lamb until it is just cooked through, stirring occasionally.
- Place the lamb in a mixing basin and set aside. The saucepan should not be washed. In a medium saucepan, pour the stock.
- Over low heat, cover and bring to a soft simmer. Cook the rice in the same pan as the meat for 2 to 3 minutes over medium heat, stirring occasionally.
- Cook, stirring constantly, until nearly all of the stock has been absorbed, about 1 cup (250 ml).
- Repeat the process, adding ½ cup(125 ml) of stock at a time, until there is only 1/2 cup(125 ml) left. Combine the lamb, squash, eggplant, pine nuts, Parmesan, and spinach in a large mixing bowl.
- Cook, stirring constantly, until the remaining liquid is practically absorbed and the rice is soft.
- Serve in 6 servings with an additional dusting of Parmesan cheese on top, if preferred.

34. Grilled Snapper on Lemon and Spinach Risotto

Prep time: 45 min | Serves: 4 | Difficulty: Moderate
Nutrition: Calories: 328 kcal | Fat:15 g | Protein: 43 g | Carbohydrates:34 g

Ingredients
Lemon and Spinach Risotto
- 4 cups (1 liter) gluten-free, onion-free chicken or vegetable stock*
- 2 tablespoons olive oil
- 2 teaspoons garlic-infused olive oil
- 1⁄3 cup (80 ml) fresh lemon juice
- 1 heaping tablespoon finely grated lemon zest
- 2⁄3 cup (130 g) Arborio rice
- Handful of baby spinach leaves, rinsed and dried
- 1⁄3 cup (1 ounce/25 g) grated Parmesan
- 2 heaping tablespoons finely chopped flat-leaf parsley
- Salt and freshly ground black pepper
- Four 7-ounce (200 g) snapper or barramundi fillets
- 1⁄4 cup (35 g) cornstarch
- Green salad, for serving

Instructions
- Pour the stock into a medium pot to cook the risotto.
- Over low heat, cover and bring to a soft simmer. In a large heavy-bottomed saucepan, boil the olive oil, garlic-infused oil, lemon juice, and zest over medium heat. Stir in the rice until it is evenly covered.
- Cook, stirring constantly, until 1 cup (250 ml) of the hot stock has been absorbed. Repeat the process, adding 1/2 cup (125 ml) of stock at a time, until there is only 1/2 cup (125 ml) of stock left.
- Combine the spinach, Parmesan, and parsley in a mixing bowl.
- Cook, stirring constantly, until the remaining liquid is practically absorbed and the rice is soft. Season with salt and pepper to taste.
- Keep warm by covering. Preheat the broiler to high while adding the spinach to the risotto.
- Cornstarch should be used to coat the snapper fillets.
- Broil for 4 to 6 minutes, or until golden brown.
- Broil the other side until it is barely cooked through.
- Serve the snapper with a fresh green salad and risotto.

35. Chicken Risotto with Roasted Squash and Sage

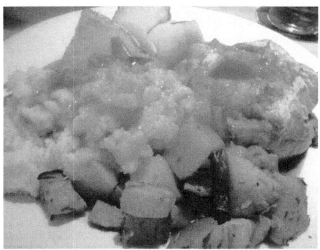

Prep time: 45 min | Serves: 6 | Difficulty: Moderate
Nutrition: Calories: 411 kcal | Fat: 12.1 g | Protein: 44 g | Carbohydrates: 16 g

Ingredients

- One 2-pound (1 kg) kabocha or other suitable winter squash, peeled, seeded, and
- cut into 3⁄4-inch (2 cm) cubes
- 2 tablespoons olive oil
- 61⁄2 cups (1.5 liters) gluten-free, onion-free chicken or vegetable stock*
- 2 teaspoons garlic-infused olive oil
- 12 ounces (340 g) boneless, skinless chicken breasts, diced
- 12 sage leaves, roughly chopped
- 2 cups (400 g) Arborio rice
- 1⁄2 cup (11⁄2 ounces/40 g) grated Parmesan
- 2 heaping tablespoons roughly chopped flat-leaf parsley
- Salt and freshly ground black pepper

Instructions

- Preheat the oven to 400 degrees Fahrenheit (200 degrees Celsius). Brush the squash with a little olive oil and spread it out on a baking sheet.
- Preheat oven to 350°F and bake for 30 minutes, or until soft and golden. Remove the pieces from the oven and choose four beautiful ones for the garnish.
- In a medium saucepan, pour the stock. Over low heat, cover and bring to a soft simmer.
- In a large heavy-bottomed saucepan, boil the remaining olive oil and the garlic-infused oil over medium heat.
- Cook, stirring occasionally, for 2 minutes after adding the chicken and sage. Stir in the rice until it is well covered in the oil and sage. Add 1 cup (250 mL) boiling stock and the squash (excluding the garnish bits) and simmer, stirring constantly, until the liquid is totally absorbed.
- Repeat this procedure until the rice is soft, adding half cup (125 ml) of liquid at a time.

- Stir in the Parmesan and parsley until well blended and the cheese begins to melt.
- Season with salt and pepper to taste, and serve with the squash pieces that were set aside.

36. Chicken Fried Rice

Prep time: 45 min | Serves: 4 | Difficulty: Moderate
Nutrition: Calories:612 kcal | Fat: 24.7 g | Protein: 41.1 g | Carbohydrates:59g

Ingredients

- 2 cups (400 g) white or brown long-grain rice
- 2 teaspoons garlic-infused olive oil
- 2 teaspoons olive oil
- 11⁄2 teaspoons Chinese five-spice powder
- 1⁄2 teaspoon ground cumin
- 1 heaping tablespoon grated ginger
- 1 pound (450 g) boneless, skinless chicken breasts, thinly sliced
- 1 large carrot, cut into matchsticks
- 1⁄2 cup (60 g) fresh or frozen peas
- 1⁄2 red bell pepper, seeded and cut into matchsticks
- One 8-ounce (225 g) can bamboo shoots, drained
- 1 cup (80 g) bean sprouts
- 2 large eggs, lightly beaten
- 1⁄4 cup (60 ml) gluten-free soy sauce
- 1 tablespoon toasted sesame oil
- Cilantro leaves, to garnish

Instructions

- Cook the rice according to the package directions until it is barely tender.
- Drain carefully and refrigerate for many hours or overnight, if possible.
- In a large frying pan or wok, heat the garlic-infused oil and olive oil over medium heat. Cook until aromatic, then add the five-spice powder, cumin, and ginger.
- Stir in the chicken and simmer for 4 to 5 minutes, or until it is just cooked through.
- Toss together the carrots, peas, bell pepper, bamboo shoots, and bean sprouts.
- Make a well in the center, crack the eggs into it, and stir until just done, breaking them up as you go.
- Cook until the carrots and bell peppers are soft, then add the rice and stir to blend.
- Stir in the soy sauce and sesame oil just before serving. Serve immediately with a garnish of cilantro leaves.

37. Pizza Crust

Prep time: 30 min | Serves: 4 | Difficulty: Moderate
Nutrition: Calories: 185 kcal | Fat: 8 g | Protein: 3 g | Carbohydrates: 20 g

Ingredients
- 1 cup (280 g) gluten-free, soy-free bread or pizza mix
- 2 teaspoons olive oil

Instructions
- Preheat the oven to 250°F (120°C) or as directed on the packaging. Using parchment paper, cover a pizza stone or baking sheet.
- Follow the package directions for making the gluten-free bread mix, then spoon it onto the parchment paper. Spread the dough into a big circle (approximately 12 inches/30 cm in diameter) with the back of a metal spoon soaked in water if needed. Brush the olive oil on the pizza crust and bake for 15 minutes, or until it is gently browned.
- Preheat the oven to 350 degrees Fahrenheit (180 degrees Celsius). Cook for 15 minutes, or until the toppings are warmed through and the cheese (if used) has melted, after topping the crust with your preferred Ingredients.

38. Smoked Salmon

Prep time: 30 min | Serves: 4 | Difficulty: Moderate
Nutrition: Calories: 373 kcal | Fat: 12 g | Protein: 44 g | Carbohydrates: 24 g

Ingredients
- 1/4 cup (60 ml) tomato sauce
- 2 teaspoons garlic-infused olive oil
- 3/4 cup (2 3/4 ounces/75 g) grated mozzarella
- 4 ounces (115 g) smoked salmon, cut into strips
- 1 cup (100 g) halved cherry tomatoes
- 1/2 cup (125 g) light sour cream
- Chopped chives or dill, to garnish

Instructions
- Over the pizza crust, evenly sprinkle the tomato sauce, oil, and mozzarella. Finish with the cherry tomatoes and smoked salmon on top. Bake according to the package directions.
- Serve with a sprinkling of chives or dill and tiny dollops of sour cream.

39. Autumn Veggie

Prep time: 30 min | Serves: 4 | Difficulty: Moderate
Nutrition: Calories: 277 kcal | Fat:11 g | Protein:16 g | Carbohydrates: 30.3 g

Ingredients
- 1/4 cup (60 ml) tomato sauce
- 2 heaping tablespoons Basil Pesto
- 1/2 cup (1 3/4 ounces/50 g) grated mozzarella
- 1 small (3 1/2-ounce/100 g) sweet potato, cut into 1/8-inch (3 mm) slices and grilled or broiled
- Handful of baby spinach leaves, rinsed and dried
- 1 heaping tablespoon roasted, unsalted shelled sunflower seeds
- 2 teaspoons roasted, unsalted shelled pumpkin seeds
- 1/3 cup (1 3/4 ounces/50 g) crumbled blue cheese

Instructions
- Evenly spread the tomato sauce and pesto over the pizza crust. Top with half of the mozzarella. Arrange the sweet potato and spinach over the cheese and sprinkle with the sunflower seeds, pumpkin seeds, blue cheese, and remaining mozzarella. Bake as directed.

40. Pesto Margherita

Prep time: 30 min | Serves: 4 | Difficulty: Moderate
Nutrition: Calories: 311 kcal | Fat: 7.1 g | Protein: 44 g | Carbohydrates: 16 g

Ingredients
- 2 heaping tablespoons Basil Pesto
- 1/2 cup (1 3/4 ounces/50 g) grated mozzarella
- 3 to 4 mozzarella bocconcini, thinly sliced
- 2 medium tomatoes, sliced
- Torn basil leaves, to garnish

Instructions
- Spread the pesto evenly over the pizza crust and sprinkle the shredded mozzarella on top.
- Place a layer of bocconcini on top, followed by a layer of tomatoes. Bake according to the package directions. Serve with basil leaves as a garnish.

41. Potato and Rosemary

Prep time: 30 min | Serves: 4 | Difficulty: Moderate
Nutrition: Calories: 374 kcal | Fat:10 g | Protein:14 g | Carbohydrates:54 g

Ingredients
- 2 small red-skin potatoes, peeled (if desired)
- 2 teaspoons garlic-infused olive oil
- 2 teaspoons olive oil
- 2 heaping tablespoons roughly chopped rosemary
- 1/4 cup (60 ml) tomato sauce
- 1/2 cup (50 g) grated mozzarella (optional)
- 1/4 cup (40 g) roughly chopped thinly sliced prosciutto, or 1/4 cup (35 g) roughly chopped grilled
- zucchini or eggplant

Instructions
- Fill a medium saucepan halfway with cold water and add the entire potatoes.
- Bring to a boil over high heat, then lower to medium-high heat and continue to cook for 10 to 12 minutes, or until just tender. Drain. Allow it

cool for a few minutes before slicing as thinly as possible.

- In a large frying pan, heat the garlic-infused oil and olive oil, then add the potato slices and rosemary and cook until golden brown on both sides.
- Spread the tomato sauce evenly over the pizza dough and, if using, sprinkle the mozzarella on top. On top, arrange the potatoes and prosciutto.
- Bake according to the package directions.

42. Grilled Fish with Coconut-Lime Rice

Prep time: 2hr -15 min | Serves: 4 | Difficulty: Moderate
Nutrition: Calories: 399 kcal | Fat:13 g | Protein: 44 g | Carbohydrates:43 g

Ingredients

Marinade
- 1 tablespoon plus 1 teaspoon fresh lemon juice
- 1 tablespoon plus 1 teaspoon sesame oil
- 1 teaspoon garlic-infused olive oil
- 1/4 small red chile pepper, seeded and finely chopped (optional)
- Freshly ground black pepper
- 4 large boneless, skinless firm white fish fillets (such as snapper or cod; 51/2 ounces/160 g each)
- 1 1/2 cups (300 g) jasmine rice
- 3 kaffir lime leaves, very thinly sliced
- 1/2 cup (125 ml) coconut milk
- Garlic-infused olive oil

Instructions

- In a large glass or ceramic dish, add all of the marinade Ingredients and swirl well to incorporate.
- Toss in the fish fillets carefully to coat. Cover and marinate for 2 to 3 hours in the refrigerator, rotating every hour to achieve uniform marinating.
- Over high heat, bring a large saucepan of water to a boil. Reduce the heat to medium, add the rice and one-third of the lime leaves, and simmer for 10 minutes, or until the rice is cooked, stirring periodically.
- Drain and rinse well with hot water. In a mixing dish, combine the washed rice, coconut milk, and remaining lime leaves.
- Keep warm by covering. Heat the garlic-infused oil in a ridged grill pan or cast-iron skillet over medium-high heat.
- Drain the fish fillets and fry for 2 to 3 minutes per side, or until done to your liking. Serve over rice made with coconut and lime.

43. Baked Atlantic Salmon on Soft Blue Cheese Polenta

Prep time: 30 min | Serves: 4 | Difficulty: Moderate
Nutrition: Calories: 547 kcal | Fat: 38 g | Protein: 33.7 g | Carbohydrates: 19.8 g

Ingredients

- Olive oil
- Four 51/2-ounce (160 g) Atlantic salmon fillets, skin on, pin bones removed
- 3 cups (750 ml) low-fat milk, lactose-free milk, or suitable plant-based milk
- 2 garlic cloves, peeled and halved
- 2/3 cup (110 g) coarse cornmeal (instant polenta)
- 2/3 cup (90 g) strong blue cheese (or to taste)
- Salt and freshly ground black pepper
- Green salad or vegetables, for serving

Instructions

- Preheat the oven to 350 degrees Fahrenheit (180 degrees Celsius).
- Using a pastry brush, gently coat a baking sheet in olive oil. Brush the salmon fillets with olive oil and bake for 10 to 12 minutes, or until done to your liking. Meanwhile, in a medium saucepan over medium heat, add the milk and garlic and bring to just below a boil. Remove and discard the garlic cloves using a slotted spoon.
- Stir in the cornmeal and milk until the polenta comes to a boil. Reduce the heat to low and simmer for another 3 to 5 minutes, stirring regularly.
- The polenta should have a smooth mashed potato texture.
- Allow the blue cheese to melt in the mixture.
- Season with salt and pepper to taste. Serve the polenta on warmed plates with the salmon fillets on top and a salad or vegetables on the side.

44. Chicken with Olives, Sun-Dried Tomato, and Basil with Mediterranean Vegetables

Prep time: 40 min | Serves: 4 | Difficulty: Moderate
Ingredients

- 2 heaping tablespoons pitted black or kalamata olives
- 1/2 cup (75 g) sun-dried tomatoes, drained (if packed in oil)
- Small handful of basil leaves
- 2 tablespoons olive oil
- Salt and freshly ground black pepper
- Four 6-ounce (170 g) boneless, skinless chicken breasts

Mediterranean Vegetables
- Nonstick cooking spray
- 2 small zucchinis, thinly sliced lengthwise
- 1 small (80 g) eggplant, thinly sliced lengthwise
- 1/2 cup (80 g) kalamata olives, pitted

- 2 tablespoons plus 2 teaspoons balsamic vinegar

Instructions
- Preheat the oven to 325 degrees Fahrenheit (170 degrees Celsius). Using parchment paper, line a baking sheet.
- Crush the black olives, sun-dried tomatoes, basil, 1 tablespoon olive oil, and salt & pepper to taste in a mortar and pestle until a smooth paste forms (it can be as smooth or chunky as you like). Use a blender or a tiny food processor if you don't have a mortar and pestle.
- In a large frying pan, heat the remaining 1 tablespoon of olive oil over medium-low heat. Cook for 5 minutes on each side, until the chicken breasts are gently browned and cooked through.
- Place the chicken on the prepared baking sheet and drizzle with the olive paste.
- Bake for 10 to 15 minutes, covered with foil. Meanwhile, oil a ridged grill pan or cast-iron skillet with cooking spray and heat over medium heat to prepare the Mediterranean vegetables.
- Cook for 3 to 4 minutes on each side, until the zucchini and eggplant are soft (in batches if required).
- Warm the kalamata olives in the pan. Serve the chicken and veggies together with a little sprinkling of balsamic vinegar.

45. Pan-Fried Chicken with Brown Butter–Sage Sauce

Prep time: 3hr-20 min| Serves: 4| Difficulty: Moderate
Nutrition: Calories: 338 kcal| Fat: 11 g| Protein:35 g| Carbohydrates:24g

Ingredients
- 2 teaspoons garlic-infused olive oil
- 2 teaspoons olive oil
- 1 tablespoon plus 1 teaspoon fresh lemon juice
- Salt and freshly ground black pepper
- Four 6-ounce (170 g) boneless, skinless chicken breasts
- 5 tablespoons (75 g) salted butter
- 2 garlic cloves, peeled and halved
- 20 sage leaves
- Shaved pecorino, for garnish
- Green salad or vegetables, for serving

Instructions
- In a mixing bowl, combine the garlic-infused oil, olive oil, lemon juice, salt, and pepper. Toss in the chicken breasts to coat. Refrigerate for 3 to 4 hours or overnight, covered.
- In a large frying pan over medium-low heat, melt 1 tablespoon of butter. Cook for 4 to 5 minutes on each side, until the chicken breasts are just done and golden brown.
- Meanwhile, in a small frying pan, heat the remaining 4 tablespoons butter and sauté the

garlic until golden brown. Remove and discard the garlic cloves from the pan. Cook until the butter is golden brown before adding the sage leaves.
- Serve the chicken with the brown butter sauce and shaved pecorino cheese on top. Serve with a salad or vegetables of your choice.

46. Chile Chicken Stir-Fry

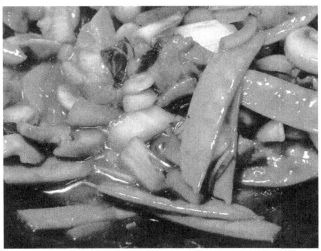

Prep time: 30 min| Serves: 4| Difficulty: Moderate
Nutrition: Calories: 373 kcal| Fat: 12 g| Protein: 44 g| Carbohydrates: 24 g

Ingredients
- 2 tablespoons plus 2 teaspoons sesame oil
- 1 pound 5 ounces (600 g) boneless, skinless chicken breasts or thighs, cut into thin strips
- 1 small red chile pepper, seeded and finely chopped, or 1/2 teaspoon cayenne pepper
- 1 bunch bok choy, leaves separated, cut if large, rinsed, and drained
- 5 ounces (125 g) green beans, trimmed and halved (1 heaping cup)
- 1 heaping cup (150 g) baby corn (about two thirds of a 15-ounce/425 g can, drained)
- 1 cup (80 g) bean sprouts
- One 8-ounce (225 g) can bamboo shoots, drained
- 1 heaping tablespoon cornstarch
- 2 tablespoons plus 2 teaspoons gluten-free soy sauce
- 1 cup (250 ml) gluten-free, onion-free chicken or vegetable stock*
- Steamed rice or prepared rice noodles, for serving

Instructions
- In a wok, heat the sesame oil over medium heat.
- Stir-fry the chicken with the chile pepper for 4 to 5 minutes, or until the chicken is well browned. Increase the heat to medium-high and stir-fry the bok choy, green beans, baby corn, bean

sprouts, and bamboo shoots for 2 to 3 minutes, or until the veggies are soft.

- In a small dish, make a paste with the cornstarch, soy sauce, and 2 tablespoons of the stock.
- Slowly pour in the remaining stock, stirring constantly to avoid lumps. Toss the chicken and veggies in the sauce until it is cooked through and thickened.
- Serve over rice or rice noodles right away.

47. Spanish Chicken with Creamy Herbed Rice

Prep time: 2hr | Serves: 4 | Difficulty: Moderate
Nutrition: Calories: 456 kcal | Fat: 12 g | Protein:28 g | Carbohydrates:43 g

Ingredients

- 2 tablespoons plus 2 teaspoons garlic-infused olive oil
- 1 heaping tablespoon smoked paprika
- 1 heaping tablespoon ground cumin
- 1/2 teaspoon ground turmeric
- Salt and freshly ground black pepper
- Four 6-ounce (170 g) boneless, skinless chicken breasts

Creamy Herbed Rice

- 2 cups (300 g) cooked basmati rice, at room temperature (made from
- 2/3 cup/130 g uncooked rice)
- 2 teaspoons garlic-infused olive oil
- 3 tablespoons olive oil
- 1/4 cup (60 ml) red wine vinegar
- 3/4 cup (200 g) gluten-free low-fat plain yogurt
- 1/3 cup (90 g) Basil Pesto
- 1/4 cup (15 g) flat-leaf parsley leaves
- 2 heaping tablespoons finely chopped mint
- Mint or flat-leaf parsley leaves, for garnish

Instructions

- Preheat the oven to 350 degrees Fahrenheit (180 degrees Celsius). In a small bowl, combine the garlic-infused oil, paprika, cumin, turmeric, salt, and pepper.
- Rub about three-quarters of the spice mixture over the chicken in a large baking dish. Cook the chicken for 20 minutes, or until it is fully done.
- Remove from the oven and put aside for 1 to 2 hours, reserving any cooking fluids separately. To prepare the creamy herbed rice, whisk together all of the Ingredients in a large mixing basin.
- In a small frying pan over medium heat, combine the remaining spice mix, cooking juices, and a little water. Simmer until well warmed.
- Cut the chicken into thick slices and serve over rice, a drizzle of spicy sauce, and a sprinkle of mint or parsley leaves at room temperature.
- Serve at room temperature or chilled.

48. Chicken and Vegetable Curry

Prep time: 30 min | Serves: 4 | Difficulty: Moderate
Nutrition: Calories: 229 kcal | Fat: 7.7 g | Protein: 32.2 g | Carbohydrates: 8.3 g

Ingredients

- 2 teaspoons garlic-infused olive oil
- 2 tablespoons olive oil
- 1 heaping tablespoon garam masala
- 1 heaping tablespoon ground cumin
- 2 teaspoons ground turmeric
- 1/2 teaspoon cayenne pepper (or to taste)
- 1 tablespoon sesame oil
- Four 7-ounce (200 g) boneless, skinless chicken thighs, trimmed of fat
- 3 Roma (plum) tomatoes, chopped
- 1 zucchini, halved lengthwise and sliced
- 13/4 cups (180 g) trimmed and halved green beans
- 9 ounces (250 g) kabocha or other suitable winter squash, peeled, seeded, and cut into 3/4-inch (2 cm)
- pieces
- 1/4 cup (55 g) packed light brown sugar
- Steamed rice, for serving

Instructions

- In a large heavy-bottomed pot or Dutch oven, heat the garlic-infused oil and olive oil over medium heat.
- Cook for 1 to 2 minutes, until aromatic, with the garam masala, cumin, turmeric, cayenne, and sesame oil.
- Add 1/2 cup (125 ml) water, chicken, tomatoes, zucchini, green beans, squash, brown sugar
- Reduce the heat to medium-low, cover, and simmer until the chicken and veggies are cooked and the sauce has thickened, about 20 minutes. Serve with steamed rice as a side dish.

49. Chicken Parmigiana

Prep time: 45 min | Serves: 4 | Difficulty: Moderate
Nutrition: Calories: 407 kcal | Fat: 35 g | Protein: 7 g | Carbohydrates: 6 g

Ingredients

Tomato Sauce

- One 14.5-ounce (425 g) can crush tomatoes
- 2 heaping tablespoons chopped flat-leaf parsley
- 1 teaspoon sweet paprika
- 2 teaspoons sugar
- 1/2 cup (80 g) sliced black olives
- 1/2 cup (75 g) cornstarch
- 2 large eggs
- 1 cup (120 g) dried gluten-free, soy-free bread crumbs*
- Salt and freshly ground black pepper
- Four 6-ounce (170 g) boneless, skinless chicken breasts
- 1 tablespoon olive oil

- 2/3 cup (80 g) grated reduced-fat Parmesan or cheddar
- Green salad or vegetables, for serving

Instructions

- Preheat the oven to 350 degrees Fahrenheit (180 degrees Celsius). To create the sauce, in a small frying pan, mix the tomatoes, parsley, paprika, sugar, and olives and simmer for 15 minutes, stirring regularly.
- Fill three small dishes halfway with cornstarch, halfway with eggs, and halfway with bread crumbs mixed with salt and pepper.
- Lightly whisk the eggs. Coat the chicken breasts with cornstarch, brushing off any excess, then dunk them in the egg, then throw them in the bread crumbs until well coated.
- In a large frying pan, heat the olive oil over medium-low heat.
- Cook for 3 to 4 minutes each side on each side, until golden brown and cooked through.
- Place the chicken breasts in a baking dish with the sauce and the cheddar cheese on top. Bake for 15 minutes, or until the cheese has melted and become brown.
- Serve with a salad or vegetables of your choice.

---

50. Baked Chicken and Mozzarella Croquettes

Prep time: 45 min | Serves: 4 | Difficulty: Moderate
Nutrition: Calories: 311 kcal | Fat: 7.1 g | Protein: 44 g | Carbohydrates: 16 g

Ingredients

- Nonstick cooking spray
- 5 large boneless, skinless chicken thighs, excess fat removed, cut into chunks
- 2/3 cup (80 g) dried gluten-free, soy-free bread crumbs*
- 1 large egg
- 1/4 cup (60 ml) Basil Pesto
- 4 ounces (115 g) mozzarella, cut into 8 cubes
- 8 basil leaves
- 8 prosciutto slices (optional)

Garlic-Infused Cream Sauce

- 1/4 cup (60 ml) light cream
- 1 teaspoon garlic-infused olive oil
- Salt and freshly ground black pepper
- Green salad or vegetables, for serving

Instructions

- Preheat the oven to 350 degrees Fahrenheit (180 degrees Celsius). Using nonstick cooking spray, grease a baking sheet.
- In a food processor or blender, add the chicken, bread crumbs, egg, and pesto and process until barely combined—do not puree. Form the mixture into 8 balls by dividing it into 8 halves.
- Flatten each ball gently and insert a slice of mozzarella and a basil leaf in the centre. Re-form the balls to surround the cheese and basil,

then cut into 2-inch (5-cm) long and 1-inch (3-cm) broad croquettes.

- Wrap each croquette in a piece of prosciutto and attach with a toothpick if using prosciutto. Place the croquettes on a baking sheet and set aside. Bake for 20 minutes, or until chicken is well done (and the prosciutto, if using, is crisp).
- Cut a croquette into a test to see if it's opaque. In a small saucepan over medium-low heat, mix the cream and garlic-infused oil and season well with salt and pepper to prepare the sauce.
- Cook, stirring constantly, until well warmed.
- Serve two chicken croquettes per person with the sauce and salad or vegetables of your choice.

---

51. Tarragon Chicken Terrine

Prep time: 3hr | Serves: 8 | Difficulty: Moderate
Nutrition: Calories: 547 kcal | Fat: 38 g | Protein: 33.7 g | Carbohydrates: 19.8 g

Ingredients

- 2 teaspoons garlic-infused olive oil
- 2 tablespoons olive oil
- 2 tablespoons (30 g) salted butter
- 1/4 cup (60 ml) dry white wine
- 14 ounces (400 g) boneless, skinless chicken thighs, excess fat removed, finely chopped
- 12 ounces (340 g) ground white meat chicken
- Nine 1-ounce (28 g) slices gluten-free, soy-free bread, crusts removed, crumbled into coarse crumbs
- 1 large egg, lightly beaten
- 1/2 cup (125 ml) light cream
- Small handful of flat-leaf parsley leaves, chopped
- Small handful of tarragon leaves, chopped
- Salt and freshly ground black pepper
- 14 long, thin prosciutto slices (about 12 ounces/340 g total)
- Boiling water
- Green salad, for serving

Instructions

- Preheat the oven to 350 degrees Fahrenheit (180 degrees Celsius). In a small heavy-bottomed frying pan, heat the garlic-infused oil, olive oil, and butter over medium heat until the butter has melted.
- Set aside after adding the wine. In a large mixing bowl, combine the chicken thigh flesh, ground chicken, bread crumbs, egg, cream, parsley, and tarragon. Pour in the wine mixture and stir thoroughly.
- Season with salt and pepper to taste. Using overlapping slices of prosciutto, line a deep 8 x 4-inch (20 x 10-cm) loaf pan, allowing a little overhang on both long sides.

- Smooth the surface of the chicken mixture in the pan. To surround the filling, fold in the excess prosciutto.
- Place the pan in a large baking dish and cover with foil. Fill the dish with boiling water until it reaches two-thirds of the way up the side of the pan. Bake for 1 hour, or until a toothpick inserted in the center of the terrine comes out clean.
- Allow to cool to room temperature before serving. To drain the juices, remove the foil and invert the pan onto a wire rack over the baking dish.
- Turn the pan upright and cover with foil after the fluids have stopped flowing. To compress the terrine, top with another loaf pan containing two or three heavy cans.
- Refrigerate for a couple of hours or overnight.
- Remove the weights, additional pan, and foil before serving, and turn out the terrine onto a cutting board to dry.
- Serve with your favorite salad after cutting into thick pieces.

52. Soy-Infused Roast Chicken

Prep time: 1hr-30 min | Serves: 6 | Difficulty: Moderate
Nutrition: Calories: 311 kcal | Fat: 7.1 g | Protein: 44 g | Carbohydrates: 16 g
Ingredients
- 1/2 cup (125 ml) gluten-free soy sauce
- 2 tablespoons plus 2 teaspoons sesame oil
- 2 heaping tablespoons light brown sugar
- 2 teaspoons grated ginger
- 3-star anise (or 2 teaspoons ground star anise)
- 1/2 teaspoon ground cinnamon
- One 4-pound (1.8 kg) whole chicken, excess fat removed
- 2 cups (500 ml) gluten-free, onion-free chicken stock*
- Vegetables, for serving
Instructions
- In a bowl, whisk together the soy sauce, sesame oil, brown sugar, ginger, star anise, and cinnamon until the sugar has dissolved.
- Place the chicken on a baking dish, breast side up. Pour the marinade over the chicken and use a pastry brush to coat it completely.
- Refrigerate the chicken for 3 to 4 hours, coating it with the marinade every 1 to 2 hours. Preheat the oven to 350 degrees Fahrenheit (180 degrees Celsius).
- Roast for 30 minutes after uncovering the chicken and pouring the liquid into the baking dish.
- Cover loosely with foil and continue roasting for another 20 to 30 minutes, or until the juices flow clear when a toothpick is inserted into the thickest portion of the thigh.

- Allow for a few minutes to rest before cutting.
- Serve with pan juices and veggies of your choice.

53. Swiss Chicken with Mustard Sauce

Prep time: 30 min | Serves: 4 | Difficulty: Moderate
Nutrition: Calories: 305 kcal | Fat: 27 g | Protein: 15 g | Carbohydrates: 2 g
Ingredients
- Four 6-ounce (170 g) boneless, skinless chicken breasts
- 2 slices Swiss cheese, halved
- 2 slices gluten-free smoked or double-smoked ham, halved
- 1/4 cup (35 g) cornstarch
- 2 large eggs
- 1 cup (120 g) dried gluten-free, soy-free bread crumbs*
- 1/4 cup (60 ml) canola oil
- MUSTARD SAUCE
- 1/4 cup (60 ml) light cream
- 1/4 cup (75 g) gluten-free mayonnaise
- 2 to 3 teaspoons gluten-free smooth mild mustard
- Green salad or vegetables, for serving
Instructions
- Without cutting all the way through, cut each chicken breast roughly in half horizontally. As if it were a book, open it up.
- Fold the top over the filling and fasten with a toothpick. Place a slice of cheese and a piece of ham on each.
- 3 shallow bowls should be placed on the table. Fill one with cornstarch, another with eggs, and yet another with bread crumbs. Lightly whisk the eggs.
- Coat the chicken breasts with cornstarch, brushing off any excess, then dip them in the egg, then bread crumbs.
- Assemble the chicken breasts so that the stuffing is completely enclosed. In a large nonstick skillet, heat the canola oil over medium-low heat. Cook for 4 to 5 minutes on each side, until the chicken is golden brown and cooked through.
- In a small saucepan, mix the cream, mayonnaise, and mustard to make the mustard sauce. Stir for 3 to 5 minutes over medium heat, until the sauce has thickened somewhat.
- Serve the chicken on four dishes, drizzled with the sauce, and accompanied by a salad or vegetables of your choosing.

54. Chicken Pockets

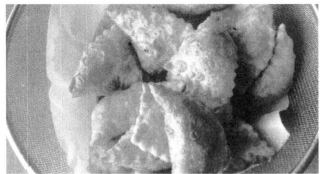

Prep time: 45 min | Serves: 4 | Difficulty: Moderate
Nutrition: Calories: 396 kcal | Fat: 13 g | Protein:31 g | Carbohydrates:32 g
Ingredients
Four 6-ounce (170 g) boneless, skinless chicken breasts
Sun-Dried Tomato and Feta
- 2/3 cup (100 g) sun-dried tomatoes, drained (if packed in oil) and finely chopped
- 1 cup (150 g) cooked white rice
- 3 1/2 ounces (100 g) feta, finely diced (about 2/3 cup)
- 1 heaping tablespoon finely grated lemon zest
- 1 large egg white
- 2 heaping tablespoons fresh oregano
- Salt and freshly ground black pepper
- Basting liquid
- 2 teaspoons garlic-infused olive oil
- 3 tablespoons olive oil
- 1 teaspoon fresh oregano
- 1 teaspoon finely grated lemon zest
Middle Eastern
- 6 ounces (170 g) mashed sweet potato (from about 1 small sweet potato)
- 1 cup (150 g) cooked white rice
- 1 teaspoon ground cumin
- 1 large egg white
- Salt and freshly ground black pepper
- Basting liquid
- 2 teaspoons garlic-infused olive oil
- 3 tablespoons olive oil
- 1 teaspoon ground cumin
Pesto
- 2 heaping tablespoons Basil Pesto
- 1 cup (150 g) cooked white rice
- 1 large egg white
- Salt and freshly ground black pepper
Basting liquid
- 2 teaspoons garlic-infused olive oil
- 3 tablespoons olive oil
- 1 teaspoon Basil Pesto
- Small basil leaves, for garnish (optional)
- Green salad or vegetables, for serving
Instructions
1. Preheat the oven to 350 degrees Fahrenheit (180 degrees Celsius).

- Insert the blade into the center of the chicken breast using a tiny sharp knife and work to produce a pocket (cut to approximately 13 inch/1 cm from the interior edge).
- In a medium mixing bowl, combine all of the Ingredients for your filling of choice and stir thoroughly.
- Fill the chicken pockets with the filling, pushing it firmly into place and spreading it evenly.
- Using a toothpick, secure the ends. On a baking pan, arrange the chicken breasts. To make your basting liquid, whisk together all of the Ingredients and spread it over the chicken.
- Bake for 15 minutes, or until golden brown, then cover with foil and continue baking for another 5 to 10 minutes, or until well done (no longer pink inside).
- Allow for a 5- to 10-minute recovery period. Serve with your choice of salad or vegetables, cut into thick slices and garnished with basil leaves (if preferred).

---

55. Pork and Vegetable Fricassee with Buttered Quinoa

Prep time: 1hr-30 min | Serves: 6 | Difficulty: Moderate
Nutrition: Calories: 397 kcal | Fat:16 g | Protein:36 g | Carbohydrates: 30 g
Ingredients
- 1/4 cup (35 g) cornstarch
- Salt and freshly ground black pepper
- 2 pounds (900 g) lean pork, diced
- 2 teaspoons garlic-infused olive oil
- 2 teaspoons olive oil
- One 14.5-ounce (400 g) can crush tomatoes
- 1/2 cup (125 ml) tomato puree
- 2 carrots, sliced
- 1 1/2 cups (375 ml) gluten-free, onion-free beef or vegetable stock*
- 1 large rosemary sprig
- 4 ounces (120 g) baby spinach leaves (4 cups)
- 7 ounces (200 g) green beans, trimmed and halved (2 cups)

Buttered Quinoa
- 2/3 cup (70 g) quinoa
- 1 tablespoon (15 g) salted butter
- Salt and freshly ground black pepper
Instructions
- In a small dish, combine the cornstarch, salt, and pepper.
- Shake off any excess cornstarch before coating the meat. In a large heavy-bottomed saucepan or stockpot, heat the garlic-infused oil and olive oil over medium-high heat.
- Cook for 2 to 3 minutes, tossing occasionally, until the meat is browned. With a slotted spoon, transfer to a platter and cover to keep warm.

- Rep with the rest of the pork. Return the leftover pork and any liquids to the pot after adding the tomatoes, tomato puree, carrots, stock, and rosemary to the last batch of pork.
- Bring to a boil, then turn down to a low heat. Cover and simmer for 1 hour, or until the meat is very tender, stirring periodically.
- Remove the rosemary stem from the pan and turn it off (the leaves should have cooked off). Season with salt and pepper to taste after adding the spinach and green beans.
- Cook, stirring occasionally, for 5 minutes, or until the beans have softened. Bring a medium pot of water to a boil in the meantime.
- Boil for 10 to 12 minutes, or until the quinoa is barely soft. Drain and rinse under hot water before draining once more. Season with salt and pepper to taste after stirring in the butter until it has melted.
- Serve the quinoa in shallow bowls with a liberal dollop of fricassee on top.

56. Pork Tenderloin on Creamy Garlic Polenta with Cranberry Sauce

Prep time: 3hr | Serves: 4 | Difficulty: Moderate
Nutrition: Calories: 381 kcal | Fat: 14 g | Protein: 26 g | Carbohydrates: 19 g

Ingredients
- 1 teaspoon garlic-infused olive oil
- 1 tablespoon plus 1 teaspoon olive oil
- 1 tablespoon plus 1 teaspoon fresh lemon juice
- Salt and freshly ground black pepper
- 1-pound (450 g) pork tenderloin
- 1/3 cup (80 g) whole berry cranberry sauce

Creamy Garlic Polenta
- 3 cups (750 ml) low-fat milk, lactose-free milk, or suitable plant-based milk
- 2 garlic cloves, peeled and halved
- 2/3 cup (135 g) coarse cornmeal (instant polenta)
- Salt and freshly ground black pepper
- Green salad or vegetables, for serving

Instructions
- In a baking dish, combine the garlic-infused oil, olive oil, lemon juice, salt, and pepper. Brush the meat all over with the marinade. Refrigerate for at least 3 hours after covering.
- Preheat the oven to 350 degrees Fahrenheit (180 degrees Celsius). Remove the pork from the fridge and bake for 30 minutes, uncovered, or until done to your liking.
- In a medium saucepan over medium heat, mix the milk and garlic for the polenta and bring to just below a boil.
- Remove and discard the garlic cloves using a slotted spoon. Stir in the cornmeal until the Polenta reaches a boil. Reduce the heat to low and cook for another 3 to 5 minutes, stirring

regularly, until the polenta has the consistency of smooth mashed potatoes.
- Season with salt and pepper to taste. Remove the pork from the baking dish and transfer the cooking juices into a small frying pan with caution.
- Return the pork to the dish and keep it warm in the oven while you make the sauce.
- Cook, stirring constantly, until the cranberry sauce is warmed through and fully blended in the frying pan with the cooking juices.
- Pork should be cut into thick pieces. Top the polenta with the pork and a generous tablespoon of cranberry sauce on warmed plates.
- Finish with a pinch of black pepper and a salad or vegetables of your choosing.

57. Pork Sausages with Cheesy Potato Rösti

Prep time: 45 min | Serves: 4 | Difficulty: Moderate
Nutrition: Calories:612 kcal | Fat: 24.7 g | Protein: 41.1 g | Carbohydrates:59g

Ingredients
- 3 or 4 medium russet potatoes (1 pound 10 ounces/750 g), peeled
- 3 tablespoons (45 g) salted butter, melted
- Salt and freshly ground black pepper
- Nonstick cooking spray
- Four 2½-ounce (70 g) gluten-free, onion-free pork sausages
- Four 1-ounce (28 g) Jarlsberg cheese slices
- Gluten-free mustard (optional)
- Green salad or vegetables, for serving

Instructions
- Fill a medium saucepan halfway with cold water and add the potatoes.
- Over high heat, bring to a boil. Reduce to medium-high heat and continue to boil for 12 to 15 minutes. Insert a toothpick into the center of a potato to check for doneness; there should be no resistance.
- Drain and allow to cool fully before serving. Preheat the oven to 250°F (120°C) for creating individual rösti.
- In a large mixing bowl, grate the potatoes and add the butter, salt, and pepper to taste. Toss everything together well. Cook over medium heat in a small frying pan coated with cooking spray.
- Place one-quarter of the potatoes on top and firmly push down. Cook for 15 minutes, or until golden brown and crisp on the bottom. Slide the rösti out of the pan onto a cutting board or big plate using a spatula.
- Return it to the pan after flipping it over. Cook for another 10 minutes, or until golden brown and cooked through.

- Place on a baking sheet in the oven to keep warm while you finish the rest of the rösti. (Alternatively, in a big frying pan, create one huge rösti and cut into wedges to serve.) Preheat a ridged grill pan, cast-iron skillet, frying pan, or grill to medium-high and cook the sausages until done to your liking.
- Place a piece of Jarlsberg cheese on top of each rösti and broil until the cheese has melted.
- Serve with the sausages and your choice of salad or veggies, as well as a teaspoon of mustard (if preferred).

58. Lime Pork Stir-Fry with Rice Noodles

Prep time: 3hr | Serves: 4 | Difficulty: Moderate
Nutrition: Calories: 311 kcal | Fat: 7.1 g | Protein: 44 g | Carbohydrates: 16 g
Ingredients
- 1 heaping tablespoon finely grated ginger
- 6 kaffir lime leaves, shredded, or 11⁄2 heaping tablespoons grated lime zest
- 1 small red chile pepper, seeded and thinly sliced
- 2 tablespoons plus 2 teaspoons fresh lime juice
- 1⁄4 cup (55 g) brown sugar
- 1⁄3 cup (80 ml) gluten-free soy sauce
- 3 tablespoons sesame oil
- 1 pound 5 ounces (600 g) lean pork, cut into 1⁄8-inch (3 to 4 mm) strips
- 8 ounces (225 g) rice noodles
- 1 bunch bok choy, leaves separated, cut if large, rinsed, and drained
- 1 red bell pepper, seeded and cut into thin strips
- 11⁄2 cups (150 g) broccoli florets
- 1⁄4 cup (5 g) roughly chopped cilantro

Instructions
- In a large mixing bowl, combine the ginger, lime leaves, chile pepper, lime juice, brown sugar, 1 tablespoon soy sauce, and 1 tablespoon sesame oil.
- Cover and chill for 3 to 4 hours or overnight after adding the pork and tossing to coat. Soak the noodles in boiling water for 5 minutes or until soft, just before you're ready to eat.
- Drain the water and set it away until you're ready to use it. In a wok, heat the remaining 2 tablespoons sesame oil and stir-fry the pork strips until barely done.
- Cook until the veggies are just soft, then add the bok choy, bell pepper, and broccoli, along with the remaining soy sauce.
- Toss in the noodles to blend. Serve with a garnish of cilantro.

59. Beef Stir-Fry with Chinese Broccoli and Green Beans

Prep time: 2hr-15 min | Serves: 4 | Difficulty: Moderate
Nutrition: Calories: 407 kcal | Fat: 35 g | Protein: 7 g | Carbohydrates: 6 g
Ingredients
- 1 heaping tablespoon grated ginger
- 2 teaspoons garlic-infused olive oil
- 2 teaspoons olive oil
- 1⁄4 cup (60 ml) sesame oil
- 1-pound (450 g) beef sirloin or top round steak, very thinly sliced
- 1 bunch Chinese broccoli, cut into 1-inch (3 cm) lengths
- 7 ounces (200 g) green beans, trimmed (13⁄4 cups)
- 1 cup (80 g) bean sprouts
- 1 tablespoon gluten-free, onion-free, garlic-free oyster sauce
- 1⁄4 teaspoon cayenne pepper
- Steamed rice or prepared rice noodles, for serving

Instructions
- In a mixing bowl, combine the ginger, garlic-infused oil, olive oil, and 2 tablespoons sesame oil. Toss in the meat to coat it.
- Refrigerate for 2 to 3 hours, covered. In a wok over medium-high heat, heat the remaining 2 tablespoons sesame oil.
- Cook for 2 minutes, or until the meat is lightly browned. Stir in the Chinese broccoli, green beans, and bean sprouts for 2 to 4 minutes, or until the vegetables are soft.
- Stir in the oyster sauce and cayenne pepper for 1 to 2 minutes, or until the sauce has warmed up and the meat and veggies have been coated.
- Serve with rice or rice noodles as a side dish.

60. Spanish Meatloaf with Garlic Mashed Potatoes

Prep time: 1hr | Serves: 6 | Difficulty: Moderate
Nutrition: Calories: 547 kcal | Fat: 38 g | Protein: 33.7 g | Carbohydrates: 19.8 g
Ingredients
- Nonstick cooking spray
- 11⁄2 pounds (700 g) extra-lean ground beef
- 1⁄2 cup (125 ml) tomato paste
- 3⁄4 cup (90 g) dried gluten-free, soy-free bread crumbs*
- 2 large eggs, lightly beaten
- 2 teaspoons garlic-infused olive oil
- 2 teaspoons olive oil
- Small handful of flat-leaf parsley leaves, roughly chopped
- 3⁄4 teaspoon ground ginger
- 1 teaspoon chili powder
- 11⁄2 teaspoons cayenne pepper

- 1 1/2 teaspoons sweet paprika
- Salt and freshly ground black pepper

Garlic Mashed Potatoes
- 4 potatoes, peeled (if desired) and quartered
- 1 tablespoon garlic-infused olive oil
- 2 tablespoons (30 g) salted butter
- 1/3 cup (80 ml) low-fat milk, lactose-free milk, or suitable plant-based milk
- Salt and freshly ground black pepper
- Green salad or vegetables, for serving

Instructions
- Preheat the oven to 350 degrees Fahrenheit (180 degrees Celsius). Spray an 812 x 412 inch (21.5 x 11.5 cm) loaf pan with cooking spray before lining it with foil.
- In a large mixing bowl, mix together the meat, tomato paste, bread crumbs, eggs, garlic-infused oil, olive oil, parsley, ginger, chilli powder, cayenne, paprika, salt, and pepper. Using your hands, thoroughly combine the Ingredients. Place the dough in the loaf pan and press it down.
- Bake for 40 to 45 minutes, or until well done. (When you pierce the center with a little knife, the fluids will stream clean.) Allow for at least 5 minutes of resting time before serving.
- Meanwhile, prepare the potatoes in a saucepan of boiling water until very soft, about 10 minutes, to produce the garlic mashed potatoes. Drain. Using a potato masher, mash the potatoes.
- Season with salt and pepper after adding the garlic-infused oil, butter, and milk.
- If necessary, adjust the Ingredients for taste or texture.
- Serve with a heaping spoonful (or two) of mashed potatoes and your choice of salad or veggies after cutting the meatloaf into thick pieces.

61. Grilled Steak with Pesto and Potato Wedges

Prep time: 45 min | Serves: 4 | Difficulty: Moderate
Nutrition: Calories: 653 kcal | Fat:18 g | Protein: 44 g | Carbohydrates:54 g

Ingredients
- 8 skin-on new potatoes, scrubbed
- 2 heaping tablespoons cornstarch
- 1 heaping tablespoon minced herbs (such as rosemary and/or oregano)
- 1/2 teaspoon salt
- 2 tablespoons olive oil
- 2 pounds (900 g) beef sirloin or top round steaks, or beef fillet
- Basil Pesto

Instructions
- Preheat the oven to 400 degrees Fahrenheit (200 degrees Celsius). Using parchment paper, line a baking sheet. Potatoes should be cut in half and then into 12-inch (1.5 cm) wedges.

- In a resalable plastic bag, combine the cornstarch, herbs, and salt. Seal the bag and toss in the potato wedges to coat.
- Shake off any excess coating in a sieve; the potatoes should only be lightly covered. Brush the wedges with the oil and bake for 10 minutes in a single layer on the baking sheet.
- Reduce the oven temperature to 350°F (180°C) and bake for another 20 minutes, or until crisp and golden brown, flipping the wedges halfway through.
- Preheat the broiler or grill to medium-high, or heat the steaks in a ridged grill pan or cast-iron skillet over medium-high heat until done to your liking.
- Allow to rest for a few minutes after covering. With a dollop of pesto on top, serve the steaks and potato wedges.

62. Beef Satay Stir-Fry with Peanut Sauce

Prep time: 20 min | Serves: 6-8 | Difficulty: Moderate
Nutrition: Calories: 453 kcal | Fat: 16 g | Protein:56 g | Carbohydrates:33 g

Ingredients

Peanut Sauce
- 1 heaping tablespoon cornstarch
- 3/4 cup (210 g) creamy peanut butter
- 2 cups (500 ml) gluten-free, onion-free beef stock*
- 2 teaspoons garlic-infused olive oil
- 2 tablespoons rice bran oil or peanut oil
- 1/4 cup (60 ml) gluten-free soy sauce
- 1/4 cup (55 g) packed light brown sugar
- Salt and freshly ground black pepper
- 2 tablespoons peanut oil, plus more if needed
- 1 1/2 pounds (700 g) lean beef, sliced 1/8-inch (3 mm) thick
- 5 ounces (150 g) green beans, trimmed (1-1/3 cups)
- 1 red bell pepper, seeded and cut into strips
- 1 1/2 cups (150 g) broccoli florets
- 2 carrots, diced
- Steamed rice, for serving

Instructions
- To prepare the peanut sauce, whisk together the cornstarch, peanut butter, and 2 tablespoons of the stock until smooth.
- Season with salt and pepper after adding the garlic-infused oil, rice bran oil, soy sauce, brown sugar, and the remaining stock.
- In a wok, heat the peanut oil over medium heat. Stir-fry one-third of the meat until it is just done (it should still be pink on the inside).
- Remove the wok from the heat and set it aside. Set aside the leftover meat, which was cooked in two batches.

- Add the veggies to the pan and stir-fry for 2 to 5 minutes, or until just tender, over high heat, adding a little more oil if necessary.
- Return the steak to the pan, along with any juices. Stir in the sauce until it has thickened and cooked thoroughly. Serve with a side of rice.

63. Beef Rolls with Horseradish Cream

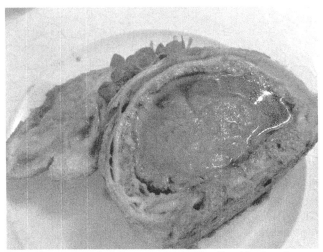

Prep time: 45 min | Serves: 4 | Difficulty: Moderate
Nutrition: Calories: 407 kcal | Fat: 35 g | Protein: 7 g | Carbohydrates: 6 g
Ingredients
- 11/2 pounds (675 g) flank, sirloin, or top round steak, trimmed of fat and cut into 4 pieces
- 2 ounces (60 g) baby spinach leaves (2 cups), rinsed, dried, and finely chopped
- 2 heaping tablespoons finely chopped pitted black olives
- 1/4 cup plus 1 tablespoon (75 g) reduced-fat cream cheese, at room temperature
- Salt and freshly ground black pepper

Horseradish Cream
- 1 heaping tablespoon freshly grated horseradish
- Squeeze of fresh lemon juice
- 1/4 cup (60 ml) light cream
- 2 heaping tablespoons finely chopped flat-leaf parsley
- Salt and freshly ground black pepper
- Green salad or vegetables, for serving

Instructions
- Preheat the oven to 350°F (180°C). Grease a baking dish with nonstick cooking spray.
- Place each steak between two sheets of parchment or waxed paper and flatten with a meat tenderizer or rolling pin until the steak is about a third of its original thickness.
- Cut each steak in half to make 8 thin steaks. Set aside. Mix together the spinach, olives, and cream cheese and season with salt and pepper.
- Place about 1 tablespoon of the cream cheese filling across the center of each steak portion

and roll up to enclose the filling. Secure with a toothpick.
- Place the rolls in the baking dish and bake for 10 minutes. Cover with foil and bake for 5 minutes more or until cooked through. Meanwhile, to make the horseradish cream, combine all the Ingredients in a small saucepan and simmer gently over medium-low heat for 5 to 8 minutes, until thickened slightly.
- (Don't let it boil.) 6. Serve 2 beef rolls per person with the horseradish cream and your choice of salad or vegetables.

64. Stuffed Rolled Roast Beef with Popovers and Gravy

Prep time: 2hr | Serves: 8 | Difficulty: Moderate
Nutrition: Calories: 547 kcal | Fat: 38 g | Protein: 33.7 g | Carbohydrates: 19.8 g
Ingredients
Popovers
- 1/2 cup (65 g) superfine white rice flour
- 1/3 cup (50 g) cornstarch
- 1 teaspoon salt
- 2 large eggs
- 1/2 cup (125 ml) skim milk, lactose-free milk, or suitable plant-based milk

Herb and Mustard Stuffing
- 2/3 cup (80 g) dried gluten-free, soy-free bread crumbs*
- 1 large egg
- 1/4 cup (60 ml) gluten-free whole grain mustard
- 3 to 4 heaping tablespoons roughly chopped flat-leaf parsley
- 1 heaping tablespoon tomato paste or puree
- 1/4 teaspoon salt
- 1/4 teaspoon freshly ground black pepper
- 2 teaspoons paprika
- 2 pounds 10 ounces (1.2 kg) beef tenderloin
- 1 tablespoon olive oil
- 2 teaspoons salt
- 2 tablespoons vegetable oil

Gravy
- About 1 cup (250 ml) boiling water
- 1/4 cup (85 g) gluten-free, onion-free gravy mix*
- Roasted vegetables, for serving

Instructions
- Preheat the oven to 400 degrees Fahrenheit (200 degrees Celsius). Sift the rice flour, cornstarch, and salt three times into a large mixing basin to create the popovers (or whisk in the bowl until well combined).
- In the centre, make a well and pour in the eggs and one-third of the milk. Mix the mixture with a wooden spoon from the centre out, starting with the eggs and milk and gradually adding the flour from the edges. The batter should be smooth and glossy.

- Stir in the rest of the milk and let aside for an hour. In a mixing dish, combine all of the Ingredients for the filling. Remove from the equation.
- Place the beef on a chopping board and cut horizontally across the thickest area, like a book, to open it out. Stuff the middle with stuffing. Roll the meat carefully around the filling, securing it with kitchen twine at 34-inch (2 cm) intervals.
- Place the rolled beef, seam-side down, in a metal baking dish, drizzle with olive oil, and season with salt. For medium-rare, roast for 40 to 45 minutes, or until done to your liking.
- Remove the baking sheet from the oven and raise the temperature to 425°F (220°C). While making the popovers, transfer the beef to a cutting board and cover loosely with foil to rest. Fill each cup of a 12-cup muffin tray with 12 teaspoon vegetable oil to produce the popovers.
- Heat the oil for 5 minutes on the highest level of the oven. Pour the batter into each cup with care. Reduce the heat to 375°F (190°C) and bake the popovers for 6 to 8 minutes, or until golden brown.
- To prepare the gravy, whisk together the pan contents and enough hot water to produce 1 cup (250 ml) liquid. Return the baking dish to the oven and stir in the gravy mix. Cook, whisking continually, over medium heat until thickened and well mixed.
- Remove the thread from the meat and slice it gently so that the filling is not disturbed.
- Serve with popovers, gravy, and roasted veggies of your choice.

65. Rib-Eye Steak with Creamy Shrimp Sauce

Prep time: 3hr | Serves: 6 | Difficulty: Moderate
Nutrition: Calories: 311 kcal | Fat: 7.1 g | Protein: 44 g | Carbohydrates: 16 g
Ingredients
- 2 teaspoons garlic-infused olive oil
- 2 teaspoons olive oil
- 1 tablespoon plus 1 teaspoon fresh lemon juice
- Salt and freshly ground black pepper
- Six 6-to 7-ounce (190 g) rib-eye steaks (21/2 pounds/1.125 kg total), trimmed of excess fat
- Creamy Shrimp Sauce
- 1/2 cup (125 ml) light cream
- 1 teaspoon cornstarch
- 1 teaspoon garlic-infused olive oil
- 1 pound (450 g) raw jumbo shrimp, peeled and deveined, tails intact
- 2 teaspoons roughly chopped flat-leaf parsley
- Salt and freshly ground black pepper
- Green salad or vegetables, for serving

Instructions
- In a baking dish, combine the garlic-infused oil, olive oil, lemon juice, salt, and pepper. Turn the steaks to cover them with the sauce.
- Refrigerate for at least 3 hours after covering. To prepare the sauce, whisk together the cream and cornstarch in a small mixing basin, making sure there are no lumps.
- In a medium frying pan, heat the garlic-infused oil. Cook until the shrimp are barely pink and the sauce has thickened, then add the cream mixture, shrimp, and parsley.
- Season with salt and pepper to taste. Preheat the grill, a ridged grill pan, or a cast-iron skillet to medium-high.
- Cook the steaks until they're done to your liking. Remove the pan from the heat, cover, and set aside for a few minutes to cool. Serve the steaks with the shrimp sauce and a salad or vegetables of your choice.

66. Lamb and Vegetable Pilaf

Prep time: 20 min | Serves: 4-6 | Difficulty: Moderate
Nutrition: Calories: 407 kcal | Fat: 35 g | Protein: 7 g | Carbohydrates: 6 g
Ingredients
- 2 tablespoons olive oil
- 2 teaspoons garlic-infused olive oil
- 21/2 teaspoons grated ginger
- 2 teaspoons ground cinnamon
- 6 whole cloves
- 1/2 teaspoon cayenne pepper
- 2 teaspoons ground cumin
- 11/4 pounds (500 g) boneless lamb loin, sliced
- 11/2 cups (300 g) white basmati rice
- 1 small sweet potato, chopped
- 21/2 cups (625 ml) gluten-free, onion-free beef or vegetable stock*
- 2/3 cup (65 g) slivered almonds
- 1 large eggplant, trimmed and sliced
- 2 medium zucchinis, halved lengthwise and thickly sliced
- Salt and freshly ground black pepper
- 1/4 cup (5 g) roughly chopped cilantro
- 3 tablespoons roughly chopped flat-leaf parsley

Instructions
- In a large skillet or Dutch oven, heat 1 tablespoon plus 2 teaspoons olive oil and 2 teaspoons garlic-infused oil over medium heat.
- Cook for 1 to 2 minutes, until aromatic, with the ginger, cinnamon, cloves, cayenne, and cumin. Toss in the lamb and cook until it is browned.
- Add the rice, sweet potato, and eggplant to the pan and simmer for 2 to 3 minutes, stirring constantly, until the rice is well coated in the seasoned oil.
- Bring the stock to a boil, then lower to a low heat and cover and simmer for 10 minutes. In a

small frying pan, heat the remaining 1 teaspoon of olive oil over medium heat.

- Cook, stirring constantly, until the almonds are golden. Using paper towels, absorb any excess liquid. Cook for 5 minutes more after adding the zucchini to the rice mixture, or until all of the liquid has been absorbed and the rice is soft.
- Remove the entire cloves and toss them out. Stir in the almonds, cilantro, and parsley after seasoning with salt and pepper. Serve immediately.

67. Mild Lamb Curry

Prep time: 2hr-40 min| Serves: 6-8| Difficulty: Moderate
Nutrition: Calories: 229 kcal| Fat: 7.7 g| Protein: 32.2 g| Carbohydrates: 8.3 g
Ingredients
- 1⁄2 cup (75 g) cornstarch
- 2 pounds 10 ounces (1.2 kg) lean lamb steaks, cut into 3⁄4-inch (2 cm) pieces
- 2 teaspoons garlic-infused olive oil
- 2 tablespoons rice bran oil or sunflower oil
- 2 teaspoons ground cinnamon
- 2 heaping tablespoons ground cumin
- 2 teaspoons ground ginger
- 1 heaping tablespoon ground turmeric
- 2 teaspoons paprika
- 1 teaspoon cayenne pepper
- 1 teaspoon salt
- 1 teaspoon freshly ground black pepper
- 4 cups (1 liter) gluten-free, onion-free beef stock*
- 2 heaping tablespoons light brown sugar
- One 14.5-ounce (425 g) can crush tomatoes
- Steamed rice and cilantro leaves, for serving

Instructions
- In a small basin, combine the cornstarch and the water. Toss in the lamb parts to thoroughly coat them.
- Remove any excess by shaking it off. In a large heavy-bottomed saucepan or Dutch oven, heat the garlic-infused oil and rice bran oil over medium heat.
- Cook for 1 to 2 minutes, until aromatic, with the cinnamon, cumin, ginger, turmeric, paprika, cayenne, salt, and pepper.
- Cook, tossing periodically, for 5 to 7 minutes, or until the lamb is beautifully browned. Bring the stock and brown sugar to a boil, then reduce to a low heat and cook, stirring regularly, for 112 hours.
- Cook for another hour or until the meat is very soft, stirring in the crushed tomatoes. Make sure the heat is kept low to prevent the lamb from drying out. (If required, add a splash of water.) Season with salt and pepper to taste and serve with steamed rice and cilantro on top.

68. Roasted Lamb Racks on Buttered Mashed Rutabaga

Prep time: 50 min| Serves: 4-8| Difficulty: Moderate
Nutrition: Calories: 280 kcal| Fat: 15 g| Protein: 54 g| Carbohydrates:17 g
Ingredients
- 2 tablespoons (30 g) salted butter, at room temperature
- 1 teaspoon ground cumin
- Salt and freshly ground black pepper
- 2 lamb racks (8 chops each, about 3 pounds/1360 g total), trimmed of fat

Buttered Mashed Rutabaga
- 2 large rutabagas (13⁄4 pounds/800 g total), peeled and cut into 2-inch (5 cm) chunks
- 1 tablespoon (15 g) salted butter, at room temperature
- Salt and freshly ground black pepper

Intrusions:
- Preheat the oven to 350 degrees Fahrenheit (180 degrees Celsius). In a small bowl, combine the butter, cumin, salt, and pepper. Rub all over the racks of lamb.
- Place the lamb in a baking dish and roast for 30 minutes, or until cooked through but still pink in the center.
- Allow to cool for a few minutes after removing from the oven. Meanwhile, boil the rutabagas for 8 to 10 minutes, or until soft, to produce the mashed rutabagas.
- Drain the potatoes and mash them with a potato masher. While the butter is still hot, stir it in and season with salt and pepper.
- Serve atop a bed of mashed rutabagas with each rack of lamb cut in half or quarters.

69. Spinach- Salmon

Prep time: 50 min| Serves: 4-8| Difficulty: Moderate
Nutrition: Calories: 285 kcal| Fat: 8.7 g| Protein: 13 g| Carbohydrates: 20 g
Ingredients
- 1 bag (16 ounces, or 455 g) frozen spinach, thawed and stems removed, or fresh spinach, stems removed
- 1 large squash, peeled and cut lengthwise into '/2-inch (1.25-cm) thick slices
- 1 can (7 ounces, or 200 g) wild salmon or 6 ounces (170 g) wild salmon, cooked medium-rare (see note)
- 2 cups (520 g) Omega 3 Pesto

Instructions
- Preheat the oven to 300 degrees F (180 degrees C, gas mark 2) Using cooking spray, coat a 9-inch (22-cm) oval baking dish. To drain all liquid, press the spinach against the base of a sieve. Heat a sauté pan over medium heat with cooking spray. Arrange the squash on the pan, flat against the pan and not overlapping.

- Sauté the squash until it becomes transparent and the edges begin to brown. To ensure consistent cooking, turn the pan once or twice. Remove the squash from the heat and let it to cool on a flat platter. (Don't stack the pieces on top of one another.) In the prepared baking dish, arrange the squash in a vertical row along the center, filling the full length of the pan. (There will be space on the sides if the pieces overlap.)
- Unfold half of the spinach leaves and stack them on top of the squash in a layer. On top, layer the salmon. Place the remaining half of the spinach on top of the salmon. Bake for about S minutes, or until the lasagna is warmed through but the top layer of spinach isn't dried out or scorched. Take the lasagna out of the oven. Place the pesto on top of the spinach and spread it out evenly. To make 12 servings, cut once lengthwise and six times width-wise. Warm the dish before serving.

70. Stir-Fried Scallops and Sweet Potatoes

Prep time: 50 min | Serves: 4-8 | Difficulty: Moderate
Nutrition: Calories: 277 kcal | Fat: 7.5 g | Protein: 21 g | Carbohydrates: 22 g
Ingredients
- 2 tablespoons (28 ml) grapeseed oil, divided
- 1 large or 3 small sweet potatoes, peeled and cut into '/2 -inch (1.25-cm) slices
- 1 medium red pepper, seeded and cut into squares
- 5 shitake mushrooms, cleaned and halved (see note)
- 1/2 teaspoon peeled, minced fresh ginger
- 10 snow pea pods, washed, dried, and trimmed
- 1 pound (455 g) sea scallops, halved if very large
- 1/2 cup (120 ml) low-sodium vegetable broth, heated
- 1/2 cup (120 ml) light coconut milk
- 2 tablespoons (28 ml) dark agave nectar
Instructions
- Boil the sweet potatoes first.
- Then mix all the ingredients, add in the boiled sweet potatoes and stir fry them for 7 minutes.
- Serve with fried scallops.

71. Beef in a Pillow

Prep time: 50 min | Serves: 4-8 | Difficulty: Moderate
Nutrition: Calories: 311 kcal | Fat: 7.1 g | Protein: 44 g | Carbohydrates: 16 g
Ingredients
- 2 tablespoons coconut oil
- 1/4 pound free-range lean ground beef
- 4 eggs
- 1/2 teaspoon salt

Instructions
- 1 tablespoon coconut oil, heated in a medium pan over medium heat Cook the ground beef until it is well cooked and broken up into tiny bits. Remove the meat from the skillet and place it on paper towels to drain the fat.
- In a mixing dish, whisk together the eggs and salt.
- Heat the remaining coconut oil in a clean, hot pan before adding the eggs. Sprinkle the cooked beef into the center of the omelet as the eggs begin to set (approximately 3 minutes). Flip the omelet in half, slide it halfway down the pan, and cook for an additional minute.
- Remove the pan from the heat and cover it for a few minutes to allow the omelet to finish cooking in the middle. Serve immediately after cutting into four portions.

72. Eggs in a Basket

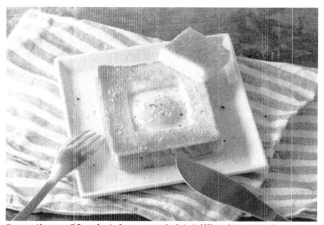

Prep time: 50 min | Serves: 4-8 | Difficulty: Moderate
Nutrition: Calories: 311 kcal | Fat: 7.1 g | Protein: 44 g | Carbohydrates: 16 g
Ingredients
- 2 eggs
- 2 slices of sourdough bread
- 2 teaspoons butter or ghee
- Dash of paprika (optional)
Instructions
- In a deep skillet (with a cover), add 3 to 4 inches of water and cook on high. When the water in the skillet boils, crack each egg into a separate tiny cup; carefully put the egg into the water and cover immediately.
- Turn off the heat and cook for 3 minutes, or until the eggs are just little runny. Toast the bread (if preferred), put butter or ghee on each slice, and then make a hole in the centre of each piece while the eggs are frying. After the eggs have finished cooking, place each egg in the hole of one piece of bread with a slotted spoon. Add a pinch of paprika as a finishing touch (if desired).

73. Sheila's Tea Biscuits

Prep time: 50 min | Serves: 4 | Difficulty: Moderate
Nutrition: Calories: 256 kcal | Fat: 15 g | Protein: 13 g | Carbohydrates: 28 g

Ingredients
- 2 1/3 cups almond flour
- 1/2 cup creamy peanut butter
- 3 eggs
- 1/4 cup plain yogurt (or water)
- 1/2 teaspoon salt
- 1 teaspoon honey (optional)
- 1/2 teaspoon baking soda

Instructions
- Preheat oven to 325 degrees Fahrenheit. Set aside the almond flour and peanut butter after thoroughly mixing them together.
- After beating the eggs, add the yoghurt or water, salt, honey (if using), and baking soda. Mix the egg mixture into the flour mixture until it is stiff.
- Roll heaping portions between barely moist palms, rewetting your hands as needed with a basin of water. Flatten biscuits to approximately a third of an inch in height on a prepared baking sheet. Preheat oven to 350°F and bake for 15 minutes, or until gently browned. Keep it cool and have fun.

74. Pita Pizza

Prep time: 55 min | Serves: 4 | Difficulty: Moderate
Nutrition: Calories: 373 kcal | Fat: 12 g | Protein: 44 g | Carbohydrates: 24 g

Ingredients
- 1 piece of non-wheat pita bread
- 1 tablespoon tomato sauce
- 4 medium mushrooms, sliced
- 1/4 cup SCD-safe medium cheddar cheese
- 1 /8 teaspoon each dried basil and dried oregano

Instructions
- Preheat the oven to 350 degrees (for a softer crust) or turn on the broiler (for a crispier crust). Spread the pita with a small amount of tomato sauce. Sprinkle on the mushrooms, a bit of cheese as a highlight rather than a blanket, and the dried basil and oregano.
- Put the pizza on a cookie sheet and bake or broil until the mushrooms are a little wilted and any cheese is melted/browned to your liking.

75. Colorful Kids Pasta Salad

Prep time: 55 min | Serves: 4 | Difficulty: Moderate
Nutrition: Calories: 298 kcal | Fat: 9 g | Protein: 24 g | Carbohydrates: 44 g

Ingredients
- One 8.8-ounce package dried pasta, cooked and drained
- 1 cup frozen peas, thawed under running water
- One 12-ounce can of tuna packed in water, drained
- 1 tablespoon lemon juice
- 1/2 tablespoon olive oil
- ¼ teaspoon each salt and pepper, or to taste

Instructions
- Place the cooked pasta in a big bowl; have the kid(s) add in the peas and tuna and stir.
- Put the lemon juice and olive oil in a small jar and let the kid(s) shake it and pour it over the pasta mixture. Add salt and pepper to taste.

76. Fried-Free Fish for Four

Prep time: 55 min | Serves: 4 | Difficulty: Moderate
Nutrition: Calories: 295 kcal | Fat: 8 g | Protein:22 g | Carbohydrates: 30 g

Ingredients
- Four 8-ounce tilapia fillets
- 1 egg white, beaten
- 1 /2 to 1 cup dry breadcrumbs or panko breadcrumbs
- 1 teaspoon dried parsley
- 1/2 teaspoon dried sage or basil

Instructions
- Using cold running water, rinse the fish and wipe dry with a paper towel. Preheat oven to 350 degrees Fahrenheit.
- Combine the breadcrumbs or panko and herbs in a basin large enough to hold the fish pieces. Turn the fish to cover it with the egg white and then the bread crumbs.
- Place the coated fish on a parchment-lined baking sheet that has been sprayed with cooking spray. Bake for 20 to 25 minutes, or until the surface is a rich golden brown and the inside flakes when pierced with a fork, flipping after approximately 10 minutes to ensure crispy edges on both sides.

77. Happy Mac 'n' Cheese

Prep time: 55 min | Serves: 4 | Difficulty: Moderate
Nutrition: Calories: 257 kcal | Fat:11 g | Protein:15 g | Carbohydrates:28 g

Ingredients
- 8 ounces dry short rice or wheat pasta (such as elbow macaroni, penne, shells, or fusilli)
- 1/2 tablespoon butter
- 1 1/2 tablespoons flour

- 1 teaspoon powdered mustard
- 2 1/2 cups plain soymilk
- 1 teaspoon paprika
- 8 ounces grated cheddar cheese
- 1 teaspoon dry parsley, or 1 tablespoon fresh
- 1 /2 cup breadcrumbs or panko crumbs (optional)
- 1/2 teaspoon salt

Instructions
- A big pot of water should be brought to a boil. Cook the pasta according to the package guidelines, but add 1 minute to the cooking time to account for the time spent in the oven afterwards. To stop the pasta from cooking, drain and rinse it with cold water.
- Turn on the broiler and position the oven rack approximately a third of the way up.
- Melt 12 tbsp. butter in a large saucepan over medium heat. Whisk or fork-mix in the flour and powdered mustard for approximately a minute to cook the flour and prevent it from tasting pasty in the sauce. Slowly pour in the soymilk, stirring constantly to ensure that the flour mixture is uniformly distributed and does not get lumpy. Add a quarter teaspoon of paprika to the mixture.
- Bring the sauce mixture to a boil over high heat, then reduce to a low heat until the sauce is barely bubbling. Simmer for 3 to 5 minutes to thicken, stirring often.
- Add the cheese in handfuls, stirring after each addition, until the cheese melts and the sauce is smooth and gooey. Turn the heat to medium-low and toss in the cooked pasta for a few minutes to heat it up and make sure it's properly coated. Spray an 8- or 9-inch baking dish with cooking spray and pour in the cheesy spaghetti. If preferred, sprinkle the breadcrumbs on top, followed by the remaining paprika and parsley.
- Broil the pan under a hot broiler until the crumbs are golden brown or the spaghetti is toasty brown, keeping the oven door open to prevent overheating. Remove it from the oven and put it aside for 5 minutes to enable the flavors to meld.

78. Smashed Potatoes with Rosemary
Prep time: 55 min| Serves: 4| Difficulty: Moderate
Nutrition: Calories: 311 kcal |Fat: 7.1 g| Protein: 44 g| Carbohydrates: 16 g
Ingredients
- 2 pounds white, red, or purple baby potatoes
- 2 sprigs fresh rosemary, needles stripped and chopped
- 2 cloves garlic, peeled and chopped
- 6 tablespoons olive oil
- 1 /8 teaspoon each salt and pepper

Instructions
- Preheat the oven to 350 degrees Fahrenheit. Boil the potatoes for about 15 minutes in salted water, or until a fork can be put into one with minor resistance.
- Combine the rosemary, garlic, olive oil, salt, and pepper in a mixing bowl. Transfer the potatoes to a chopping board with a slotted spoon and ask the kids to smash them with the back of a big spoon to make a disc. It's a good idea to aim for an inch of thickness, but your kids might not be about symmetry.
- Brush the flavored olive oil on top of the discs on a rimmed baking sheet lined with parchment paper. Roast in the oven for 15 to 20 minutes, or until golden and crispy.

79. Paprika Calamari with Garden Salad
Prep time: 4hr-15 min| Serves: 4| Difficulty: Moderate
Nutrition: Calories: 229 kcal| Fat: 7.7 g| Protein: 32.2 g| Carbohydrates: 8.3 g
Ingredients:
- 4 large or 8 regular squid bodies, cleaned
- 1/2 teaspoon salt
- 1/2 teaspoon finely ground black pepper
- 1 teaspoon paprika
- 1/3 cup (50 g) cornstarch
- Olive oil

Garden Salad
- 1 small head romaine lettuce, roughly chopped
- 1/2 large cucumber, halved lengthwise and sliced 2 stalks celery, thinly sliced
- 1/2 green bell pepper, seeded and sliced 1 cup (50 g) snow pea shoots

Dressing
- 2 tablespoons garlic-infused olive oil
- 1 1/2 tablespoons lemon juice
- 1/2 teaspoon brown sugar
- Salt

Instructions:
- To produce two huge pieces, cut the squid bodies down the long sides (if using large squid, cut them into quarters). Cut the squid pieces in a 12-inch (1 cm) crisscross pattern with a sharp knife, being careful not to cut all the way through. Using paper towels, pat dry.
- In a large mixing basin, combine the salt, pepper, paprika, and cornstarch; add the squid pieces and toss to coat. Refrigerate for 3 to 4 hours, covered.
- In a large salad bowl, toss together the lettuce, cucumber, celery, bell pepper, and snow pea shoots.
- To create the dressing, whisk together the oil, lemon juice, and brown sugar in a small screw-top container. Season with salt to taste.

- Preheat the grill to high heat, or heat a skillet or ridged grill pan. Oil the grill or frying pan. Cook for 2 to 3 minutes with the squid, scored-side down. Cook for 1 to 2 minutes more on the opposite side, until the squid is opaque white throughout.
- Drizzle the dressing over the salad and divide it among four bowls or plates. Place the calamari on top and serve immediately.

80. Chili Salmon with Cilantro Salad

Prep time: 30 min | Serves: 4 | Difficulty: Moderate
Nutrition: Calories: 357 kcal | Fat:12 g | Protein:19 g | Carbohydrates:27 g
Ingredients:
- Four 5½-ounce (160 g) salmon fillets, skin on, pin bones removed
- 1 tablespoon garlic-free sweet chili sauce
- Salt and freshly ground black pepper

Cilantro Salad
- 5 cups (150 g) roughly chopped lettuce leaves
- ½ large cucumber, halved lengthwise and sliced
- 2 stalks celery, thinly sliced on the diagonal
- ½ green bell pepper, thinly sliced
- ½ cup (25 g) firmly packed chopped cilantro
- ½ small red chile, finely chopped
- 2 tablespoons lime juice
- 1 tablespoon rice vinegar
- 2 tablespoons fish sauce
- 2 tablespoons brown sugar

Instruction
- Set an oven rack 5 inches from the broiler element and line a broiler pan with foil. Place the salmon fillets skin-side up on the pan and broil for 1 to 2 minutes, or until the skin crisps up.
- Turn the fillets over and brush each with a quarter teaspoon of sweet chilli sauce. Salt & pepper to taste. Broil for another 3 to 4 minutes, or until the chicken is cooked to your taste.
- In a large mixing basin, combine the lettuce, cucumber, celery, bell pepper, and cilantro to form the salad. In a small bowl, combine the chile, lime juice, rice vinegar, fish sauce, and brown sugar; pour over the salad. With the salmon, serve.

81. Dukkah

Prep time: 35 min | Serves: 4 | Difficulty: Moderate
Nutrition: Calories: 487 kcal | Fat:19 g | Protein:29 g | Carbohydrates:31 g
Ingredients:
- ½ cup (75 g) blanched almonds
- ¼ cup (30 g) pine nuts
- 1 teaspoon ground coriander
- 1 teaspoon cumin seeds
- 1 teaspoon sesame seeds
- ½ teaspoon chili powder
- Four 7-ounce (200 g) snapper fillets (ideally about 1-inch/3 cm thick), or other lean fish
- 2 tablespoons canola oil
- Cilantro leaves
- Cooked basmati rice
- Lemon wedges

Instructions:
- Preheat the oven to 350°F (180°C) and prepare a baking sheet with parchment paper to create the dukkah. On a baking sheet, spread out the almonds and pine nuts and bake for 5 minutes, or until brown.
- Bring to room temperature before serving. In a food processor, pulse all of the nuts and spices until fine crumbs form. 4 tablespoons will be reserved for serving, and the remainder will be transferred to a platter.
- Brush the oil all over the fish fillets before pressing them into the dukkah to cover both sides. Over medium-high heat, heat a ridged grill pan or a cast-iron skillet.
- Cook for 3 to 4 minutes on each side, until the salmon is just done. Garnish with the cilantro and dukkah that was set aside. Serve with lemon wedges and basmati rice.

82. Swordfish steaks

Prep time: 4hr-20 min | Serves: 4 | Difficulty: Moderate
Nutrition: Calories: 457 kcal | Fat:19 g | Protein:14 g | Carbohydrates:23 g
Ingredients:
- 3 tablespoons balsamic vinegar
- 2 tablespoons soy sauce (gluten-free if following a gluten-free diet)
- 2 tablespoons brown sugar
- 4 large swordfish steaks
- 1½ tablespoons sesame seeds
- Steamed Asian greens

Instructions:
- Combine the balsamic vinegar, soy sauce, and brown sugar in a nonmetallic bowl. Add the swordfish steaks and turn to coat in the marinade.
- Cover and refrigerate for 3 to 4 hours, turning regularly. 2. Preheat the oven to 450°F (230°C). Line a large baking sheet with parchment paper.
- Place the swordfish steaks on the baking sheet, reserving the marinade, and bake for 10 minutes. Turn the steaks over and baste with the marinade.
- Sprinkle with sesame seeds and bake for an additional 5 to 10 minutes, until cooked through. Serve with the steamed Asian greens.

83. Lemon-Oregano Chicken Drumsticks

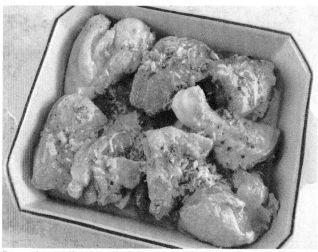

Prep time: 4hr 15 min | Serves: 6 | Difficulty: Moderate
Nutrition: Calories: 407 kcal | Fat: 35 g | Protein: 7 g | Carbohydrates: 6 g
Ingredients:
- 18 skinless chicken drumsticks
- 1/4 cup (15 g) finely chopped oregano, plus additional for garnish
- 1 tablespoon finely grated lemon zest
- 2 tablespoons extra virgin olive oil
- Salt and freshly ground black pepper

Greek Salad
- 2 cups (120 g) shredded iceberg lettuce
- 12 cherry tomatoes, cut in half
- 1/2 cup (75 g) pitted kalamata olives
- 4 ounces (125 g) feta, cut into 1/2-inch (1 cm) cubes
- 2 tablespoons olive oil
- 2 teaspoons balsamic vinegar

Instructions:
- Using a tiny knife, equally puncture the chicken all over.
- In a large mixing bowl, combine the oregano, lemon zest, and oil. Toss in the chicken, seasoning it with salt and pepper. Cover and chill for 3 to 4 hours, rotating occasionally.
- Preheat the oven to 450 degrees Fahrenheit (230 degrees Celsius). Preheat oven to 350°F. Line two baking pans with parchment paper.
- Bake the drumsticks for 10 to 15 minutes, until golden brown and cooked through, on the baking pans.
- In a large mixing basin, gently toss the lettuce, tomatoes, olives, and feta to form the salad. In a small screw-top jar, add the oil and vinegar and shake vigorously to incorporate.
- Toss the salad quickly with the dressing. Serve with the chicken and a sprinkle of oregano on top.

84. Garlic Chicken Steak

Prep time: 35 min | Serves: 4 | Difficulty: Moderate
Nutrition: Calories: 387 kcal | Fat:19 g | Protein:24 g | Carbohydrates:28 g
Ingredients:
- 2 tablespoons garlic-infused canola oil
- Four 6-ounce (170 g) boneless skinless chicken breasts

Maple-Mustard Sauce
- 1 tablespoon cornstarch
- 1 cup (250 ml) onion-free chicken stock (gluten-free if following a gluten-free diet)
- 3 tablespoons pure maple syrup
- 1 tablespoon whole grain mustard
- 1 tablespoon chopped thyme
- 1/2 teaspoon freshly ground black pepper
- 2 tablespoons light whipping cream
- Salt

Instructions:
- In a large skillet, heat the oil over medium-low heat. Cook for 3 to 5 minutes on each side, until the chicken is just done and golden brown. Remove the pan from the heat. Cover and set aside while preparing the sauce.
- To make the sauce, make a paste with the cornstarch and a little chicken stock. Pour in the remaining stock slowly, stirring constantly to avoid lumps. Combine the maple syrup, mustard, thyme, pepper, and cream in a mixing bowl.
- Pour the sauce into the skillet and cook, stirring constantly, for 3 to 5 minutes, until it thickens.
- Return the chicken to the pan and stir in the sauce for 1 to 2 minutes, or until well cooked. Season with salt and pepper to taste, then serve right away.

85. Tarragon Chicken Steak

Prep time: 45 min | Serves: 6 | Difficulty: Moderate
Nutrition: Calories: 466 kcal | Fat:17 g | Protein:29 g | Carbohydrates:31 g
Ingredients:
- 1 tablespoon finely chopped tarragon
- 1 tablespoon olive oil
- 2 tablespoons freshly ground black pepper
- 2 teaspoons cornstarch
- Six 6-ounce (170 g) boneless skinless chicken breasts

Herb Rösti
- 4 large red-skin potatoes, such as Pontiac
- 2 tablespoons chopped flat-leaf parsley
- 6 sage leaves, chopped
- 8 tablespoons (115 g) butter, melted
- Salt and freshly ground black pepper
- 2 tablespoons vegetable oil
- 1/2 cup (125 ml) onion-free beef stock (gluten-free if following a gluten-free diet)

- 1/3 cup (80 ml) red wine, or additional onion-free beef stock Steamed baby carrots
- Whole grain mustard

Instructions:
- In a small screw-top jar, add the tarragon, olive oil, pepper, and cornstarch and shake vigorously to incorporate. Brush the chicken breasts all over with the mixture. Refrigerate for 1 to 2 hours, covered.
- Place the potatoes in a big saucepan, cover with cold water, and bring to a boil to make the rösti. Reduce the heat to low and continue to cook for another 10 minutes. Drain. Allow to cool fully before serving.
- Peel and grate the flesh of the potatoes into a large mixing basin. Season to taste with the herbs and melted butter. Make six equal amounts of the mixture. To make a flat patty, roll each part into a ball and gently press flat with your palm.
- In a large nonstick skillet, heat the vegetable oil over medium heat. Cook for 10 to 15 minutes, until the rösti is crisp and golden on the bottom. Cook for another 10 minutes, or until golden brown and cooked through using a spatula.
- Cook the chicken for 3 to 4 minutes on each side in a large nonstick pan coated with cooking spray over high heat, until cooked through. Allow the chicken to cool for a few minutes before serving.
-
- Bring the pan back up to medium-high heat. Bring the stock and red wine to a low simmer. Heat for 2 minutes after adding the chicken. With the herb rösti, steamed carrots, and a teaspoon of mustard, serve right away.

86. Prosciutto Chicken with Sage Polenta

Prep time: 45 min| Serves: 4| Difficulty: Moderate
Nutrition: Calories: 492 kcal| Fat: 33.1 g| Protein: 7.5 g| Carbohydrates: 44.6 g
Ingredients:
- Four 6-ounce (170 g) boneless skinless chicken breasts
- 4 slices prosciutto

Sage Polenta
- 3 cups (750 ml) low-fat milk, lactose-free milk, or suitable plant-based milk
- 2 tablespoons garlic-infused olive oil
- 2/3 cup (85 g) cornmeal
- 2 tablespoons sage leaves, torn if large,
- Plus additional for garnish Salt and freshly ground black pepper

Instructions:
- Preheat oven to 350 degrees Fahrenheit (180 degrees Celsius) and line a baking sheet with parchment paper.

- Wrap a piece of prosciutto around each chicken breast and fasten with a toothpick. Bake for 20 minutes, or until the chicken is cooked through and the prosciutto is crisp, on the baking sheet.
- In a medium saucepan, heat the milk and oil until almost boiling to make the sage polenta. Stir in the cornmeal until the mixture boils.
- Reduce the heat to low and simmer for an additional 3 to 5 minutes, stirring regularly, until the polenta is done (it should be the texture of smooth mashed potatoes). Season with salt and pepper after adding the sage.
- Serve the polenta with the prosciutto chicken on four heated plates. Serve with a sprinkling of sage leaves on top.

87. Chicken Kibbeh

Prep time: 1hr-20 min| Serves: 8-10| Difficulty: Moderate
Nutrition: Calories: 141 Kcal |Fat: 18 g| Protein: 6 g| Carbohydrates: 14 g
Ingredients:
- 1 cup (170 g) quinoa

Filling
- 1/2 cup (80 g) pine nuts, toasted
- 3 small tomatoes, finely chopped
- 1 teaspoon ground cinnamon
- 1 cup (30 g) chopped flat-leaf parsley
- 1 teaspoon grated lemon zest
- 2 pounds (1 kg) ground chicken
- 2 tablespoons garlic-infused olive oil
- 3 tablespoons finely chopped tarragon, plus additional leaves for garnish
- 2 teaspoons ground allspice
- 2 tablespoons tahini
- Salt and freshly ground black pepper
- Garden Salad

Instructions:
- Preheat the oven to 350°F (180°C). Grease a 9 x 13-inch (25 x 30 cm) rimmed baking sheet and line with parchment paper.
- Bring a medium saucepan of water to a boil and add the quinoa. Stir, then bring back to a boil. Cook for 10 to 12 minutes, until just tender. Drain and rinse under cold water, then drain again.
- To make the filling, combine the pine nuts, tomatoes, cinnamon, parsley, and lemon zest in a small bowl.
- Place the cooked quinoa, chicken, oil, tarragon, allspice, and tahini in a bowl and mix until well combined. Season to taste with salt and pepper. Divide into two portions. Press half of the mixture into the prepared baking sheet and cover evenly with the filling. Top with the remaining kibbeh mixture, spreading it evenly over the filling.

- Bake for 50 to 60 minutes, until cooked through—a toothpick inserted into the center should come out clean. Remove and let rest for 5 to 10 minutes before cutting into squares. Garnish with the extra tarragon leaves and serve with the salad.

88. Roast Pork with Almond Stuffing

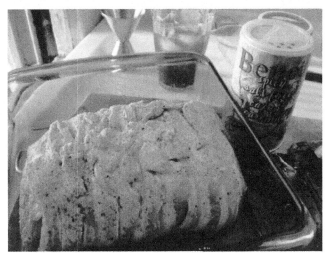

Prep time: 55 min | Serves: 8 | Difficulty: Moderate
Nutrition: Calories: 311 kcal | Fat: 7.1 g | Protein: 44 g | Carbohydrates: 16 g
Ingredients:
- Scant 3⁄4 cup (75 g) natural almond meal or chestnut flour
- 1 1⁄2 cups (110 g) fresh gluten-free bread crumbs (made from day-old bread)
- 1⁄3 cup (10 g) chopped flat-leaf parsley
- 2 tablespoons chopped sage, plus additional leaves for garnish
- 3 tablespoons brown sugar
- Salt and freshly ground black pepper
- 3 tablespoons balsamic vinegar
- 4-pound (1.8 kg) boneless center-cut pork loin, butterflied for stuffing
- Roasted vegetables, such as potatoes, carrots, and parsnips
- Steamed zucchini flowers, optional

Instructions:
- Preheat the oven to 425°F (220°C).
- Combine the almond flour, bread crumbs, herbs, and brown sugar in a bowl. Season with salt and pepper. Stir in the balsamic vinegar.
- Open up the pork on a clean surface and spoon the stuffing along the center. Roll up the pork around the filling and tie it with kitchen string at 1-inch (2 cm) intervals.
- Transfer the pork to a roasting pan and roast for 25 minutes. Reduce the temperature to 375°F (190°C) and roast for another hour. Transfer the pork to a plate and cover with foil. Let rest for 20 minutes.

- Remove the foil and cut the pork into slices. Garnish with the additional sage leaves and serve with the roasted vegetables and steamed zucchini flowers, if desired.

89. Peppered Lamb with Rosemary Cottage Potatoes

Prep time: 8hr | Serves: 8 | Difficulty: Moderate
Nutrition: Calories: 407 kcal | Fat: 35 g | Protein: 7 g | Carbohydrates: 6 g
Ingredients:
- 3-pound (1.5 kg) leg of lamb
- 2 tablespoons freshly ground black pepper

Rosemary Cottage Potatoes
- 10 new potatoes
- 5 ounces (150 g) reduced-fat Cheddar, cubed (1 cup)
- Salt and freshly ground black pepper
- 2 tablespoons (30 g) butter
- 2 tablespoons rosemary leaves
- 1⁄2 cup (125 ml) low-fat milk, lactose-free milk, or suitable plant-based milk SAUCE
- 1⁄2 cup (125 ml) dry red wine, or onion-free beef stock (gluten-free if following a gluten-free diet)
- 1 cup (250 ml) onion-free beef stock (gluten-free if following a gluten-free diet)
- 3 tablespoons light sour cream
- Salt and freshly ground black pepper
- Steamed vegetables

Instructions:
- Place the lamb in a roasting pan. Rub all over with the pepper, then cover with plastic wrap and refrigerate for 3 to 4 hours.
- Preheat the oven to 400°F (200°C). Roast the lamb for 1 hour 20 minutes, until slightly pink in the middle and an instant-read thermometer inserted into the thickest part reaches 140°F (60°C) for medium, or until desired doneness. As soon as the lamb is out of the oven, remove it from the roasting pan and transfer to a plate. Cover with foil and let rest.
- Meanwhile, place the potatoes in a large saucepan of cold water. Bring to a boil and cook for 10 to 12 minutes, until tender. Drain and cool, then peel and cut in half. Combine the potatoes and Cheddar in a large bowl and season with salt and pepper. Transfer the mixture to a medium baking dish.
- Place the butter and rosemary in a small skillet over medium heat and stir until the butter is melted and lightly golden. Pour it over the potato mixture, followed by the milk. Bake the cottage potatoes for 20 to 25 minutes.
- While the potatoes are baking, place the empty roasting pan on the stove over medium heat. Add the wine and cook for 5 minutes, or until the wine is reduced by half. Add the stock and bring to a boil. Reduce the heat and simmer, stirring regularly, for 5 minutes, or until the sauce starts to

thicken. Remove the pan from the heat and stir in the sour cream until melted and well combined. Season with salt and pepper.

- Carve the lamb and serve with the red wine sauce and cottage potatoes, with the steamed vegetables on the side.

90. Herbed Beef Meatballs with Creamy Mashed Potatoes

Prep time: 45 min | Serves: 6 | Difficulty: Moderate
Nutrition: Calories: 279 kcal | Fat: 7.7 g | Protein: 32.2 g | Carbohydrates: 18.3 g
Ingredients:
Creamy Mashed Potatoes
- 6 large russet potatoes
- 1/2 cup (125 ml) low-fat milk
- 3 tablespoons (45 g) butter
- Pinch of salt
- 1/3 cup (40 g) coarsely grated reduced-fat Cheddar Pinch of ground nutmeg

Herbed Beef Meatballs
- 11/4 pounds (600 g) extra lean ground beef
- 1/2 cup (50 g) dried gluten-free bread crumbs
- 3 eggs, lightly beaten
- 2 tablespoons chopped oregano, plus additional leaves for garnish
- 2 tablespoons chopped marjoram
- 1/3 cup (10 g) chopped flat-leaf parsley
- Salt and freshly ground black pepper
- Canola oil

Tomato Gravy
- 3 tablespoons onion-free gravy powder (gluten-free if following a gluten-free diet)
- 2 tablespoons tomato paste
- 2 tablespoons dry red wine, optional

Instructions:
- Place the potatoes in a large saucepan and cover with cold water to make the mashed potatoes. Bring to a boil, then reduce to a low heat and simmer for 15 minutes, or until the potatoes are soft when pierced with a fork. Drain and lay aside for 5 minutes to allow the juices to settle. Return the potatoes to the pan after peeling them. Add the other ingredients and mash until smooth using a potato masher. Keep warm by covering.
- In a large mixing bowl, combine the meat, bread crumbs, eggs, oregano, marjoram, and parsley. Salt & pepper to taste. Make walnut-sized balls out of the mixture.
- In a big heavy-bottomed skillet, heat a little oil over medium heat. Cook for 6 to 8 minutes, or until the meatballs are browned and cooked through.
- To prepare the gravy, in a small mixing bowl, add the gravy powder, tomato paste, and red wine, if using, and whisk to form a paste. Slowly pour in 1 cup (250 ml) boiling water (or the

quantity specified on the gravy packaging instructions), whisking regularly to avoid lumps and an even thickening of the gravy.

- Serve the meatballs on top of the mashed potatoes on six plates. Pour the sauce over the meatballs and top with more oregano, if desired.

91. Beef Pumpkin Stew

Prep time: 5 hr 20min | Serves: 4 | Difficulty: Moderate
Nutrition: Calories: 311 kcal | Fat: 7.1 g | Protein: 44 g | Carbohydrates: 16 g
Ingredients:
- 1 tablespoon olive oil
- 1 medium or 1/2 of a large onion, cut up
- 4 cloves garlic, pressed
- 31/2 cups raw pumpkin, cut into 1-inch squares
- 1/2 of a chili pepper, diced
- 1 carrot, sliced
- 6 to 7 cups water
- 2 large celery stalks
- 3 tomatoes, chopped
- 6 standard-size mushrooms, sliced
- 3 tablespoons tomato sauce (jarred, canned, or from the Marinara Sauce recipe later in this chapter)
- 1 pound stew beef (top round)
- 1/2 teaspoon each salt and pepper
- 11/2 tablespoons Italian seasoning
- 4 to 5 bay leaves

Instructions
- In a large saucepan, heat the olive oil over high heat. Sauté until the onion is transparent, then add the onion and garlic (about 8 minutes).
- One cup water, along with the pumpkin, chilli pepper, and carrots Cover with a towel and steam for 1 minute. Combine the celery, tomatoes, and mushrooms in a large mixing bowl. Steam for around 2 minutes with the lid on.
- While the vegetables are steaming, season your meat well with salt, pepper, and Italian seasoning. Cover the pot with the beef and heat for 1 to 2 minutes (the meat does not need to be fully cooked).
- 3 tablespoons tomato sauce and 5 to 6 glasses of water Cover and cook for 3 to 5 minutes with the by leaves on top.

92. Sabra Chicken

Prep time: 3 hr 5min | Serves: 6 | Difficulty: Moderate
Nutrition: Calories: 305 kcal | Fat: 27 g | Protein: 15 g | Carbohydrates: 2 g
Ingredients:
- 2 cups chicken stock
- Zest of 1/2 an orange, grated or julienned
- 1/2 cup fresh orange juice
- 1/8 teaspoon paprika

- 1/4 teaspoon each salt and freshly ground black pepper Six 5-ounce chicken breasts, with skin and bones
- 2 tablespoons olive oil
- 1 medium onion, finely chopped
- 8 green olives, pitted Chopped fresh mint to garnish

Instructions

- Combine 1 cup of the chicken stock, the zest, orange juice, and paprika in a shallow baking dish with a pinch of salt and pepper. Add the chicken and marinate for 2 hours in the refrigerator, rotating the chicken a few times to ensure it is completely submerged in the marinade.
- Remove the chicken breasts from the marinade, brush off the excess liquid, and pat dry well.
- Heat the oil in a big skillet with sides over medium-high heat until your hand feels hot 1 inch above the pan. Cook the chicken, skin side down, for about 4 minutes per side, until golden brown, adding extra oil if the pan is too dry. Remove the cooked chicken from the pan and set it aside on a platter.

93. Meatloaf (Turkey-Style)

Prep time: 1 hr 50min | Serves: 6 | Difficulty: Moderate
Nutrition: Calories: 232 kcal | Fat: 21 g | Protein: 21 g | Carbohydrates: 44.6 g
Ingredients:

- 2 pounds ground white-meat turkey
- 1 package extra-firm tofu, drained and mashed (optional)
- 1/2 cup quick-cooking rolled oats
- 1/2 cup finely chopped onions
- 1/3 cup finely chopped red bell pepper
- 1 large or 2 small eggs, gently beaten with a fork
- 1/2 teaspoon each salt, black pepper, and chili powder
- 1 teaspoon dried parsley, plus extra for the top
- 1/4 cup ketchup

Instructions

- Preheat the oven to 350 degrees Fahrenheit.
- Mix everything together gently except the ketchup and frying spray; the more you work it, the tougher the beef will become.
- Grease a loaf pan lightly and spoon the mixture into it, gently patting it down. Pour the ketchup over the top and top with a pinch of dry parsley. Preheat oven to 325°F and bake for 90 minutes.

94. Fancy Chicken Roll-Ups

Prep time: 55 min | Serves: 4 | Difficulty: Moderate
Nutrition: Calories: 392 kcal | Fat: 33.1 g | Protein: 7.5 g | Carbohydrates: 44.6 g
Ingredients:

- Four 5-ounce chicken breast fillets, butterflied
- 1/2 teaspoon butter
- 1 large clove garlic, minced
- 12 spears asparagus
- 4 slices Tofutti soy cheese
- 1 teaspoon sea salt
- 1 teaspoon sage
- 1 cup chicken broth
- 2 tablespoons flour, such as brown rice flour

Instructions

- Preheat oven to 350 degrees Fahrenheit.
- Place the chicken fillets on a cutting board, cut side up, dot with butter, and sprinkle the garlic on one side of each fillet.
- Wash the asparagus, remove the ends, and cut into pieces that are just a little longer than the chicken fillets' breasts. Arrange the asparagus evenly among the fillets, atop the garlic, with the tips dangling out a little for added visual appeal.
- Place one piece of soy cheese on top of each asparagus fillet, then roll the chicken up, closing the edges with toothpicks dipped in water for 10 minutes (to avoid burning). Season the tops of each breast with sea salt and sage, pressing the sage.

95. Sun-Dried and Wined Chicken

Prep time: 40min | Serves: 2 | Difficulty: Moderate
Nutrition: Calories: 311 kcal | Fat: 7.1 g | Protein: 44 g | Carbohydrates: 16 g
Ingredients:

- 3 teaspoons olive oil
- 2 to 3 cloves of garlic, diced
- 1 small onion, cut
- 4 to 5 sun-dried tomatoes, diced up
- 4 to 6 mushrooms, sliced
- Generous splash of white wine (about 3 tablespoons)
- 10 to 15 basil up leaves
- Three 5-ounce boneless,
- skinless chicken breasts

Instructions

- Preheat the oven to 350 degrees.
- In a small pan, heat the oil over medium heat. Add the garlic, onion, and sun-dried tomatoes and sauté for about 3 to 4 minutes.
- Add the mushrooms. When the mushrooms cook down to half their size (about 5 minutes), splash in white wine and cook for about 1 to 2 minutes. Turn off heat and sprinkle basil over the top of the wine mixture.
- Measure out 3 pieces of tinfoil big enough to fully surround one chicken breast each. 5 Place

one chicken breast onto each piece of foil and cover with 1/3 of the white wine mixture. Seal off the foil packets, place them on a cookie sheet, and bake them for about 20 to 25 minutes.

96. Spiced Honey Chicken

Prep time: 1hr30min | Serves: 2 | Difficulty: Moderate
Nutrition: Calories: 311 kcal | Fat: 7.1 g | Protein: 44 g | Carbohydrates: 16 g
Ingredients:
- 1/2 cup honey
- 2 garlic cloves, pressed
- 2 tablespoons plain yogurt
- 1 teaspoon lemon zest
- 1 tablespoon lemon juice
- 3 to 4 pounds chicken parts with bones and skin
- 1/2 teaspoon each salt and black pepper
- 1/4 teaspoon each ground nutmeg and ground cloves
- 1 cup almond slivers
- 1 cup raisins
- 6 cinnamon sticks

Instructions
- Preheat oven to 350 degrees Fahrenheit. In a 10-x-15-inch casserole dish, place the chicken with the skin side up.
- Half of the honey, garlic, yoghurt, lemon peel, and lemon juice should be drizzled over the meat in a bowl.
- Place the cinnamon sticks evenly around the casserole dish and season the meat with salt, pepper, nutmeg, cloves, almonds, and raisins. Over the chicken and spices, pour the remaining honey mixture.
- Keep for 1 hour and 20 minutes in the oven, basting every 30 minutes. Check at the one-hour mark to see if it's done.
- Before serving, remove the pan from the oven and baste it with the sauce.

97. Seared Salmon with Sautéed Summer Vegetables

Prep time: 1hr30min | Serves: 2 | Difficulty: Moderate
Nutrition: Calories: 492 kcal | Fat: 33.1 g | Protein: 7.5 g | Carbohydrates: 44.6 g
Ingredients:
- 3 cups broccoli florets
- 1 tablespoon olive oil
- 1 carrot, peeled and cut into 1/4-inch-thick rounds
- 1 yellow pepper, chopped
- 1 red pepper, chopped
- 1 cucumber, peeled, seeded, and cut into 2-inch spears
- 1 bunch of radishes (about 5 radishes), quartered and keeping some of the greens attached

- 1 teaspoon lemon juice
- 4 basil leaves, chopped
- 1/4 teaspoon salt
- 1 teaspoon coconut oil Four 5-ounce salmon fillets

Instructions
- Set aside the broccoli florets after steaming them for 3 to 6 minutes.
- Heat the olive oil in a big skillet. Cook for 1 to 3 minutes after adding the carrot. Sauté for 1 to 3 minutes with the peppers, broccoli, cucumber, and radishes. Toss with lemon juice, basil, and salt in a mixing bowl.
- In a skillet over medium-high heat, melt the coconut oil. Season the salmon with salt and pepper before searing it for 4 minutes on each side in a skillet. Check to see if the salmon is cooked through at 8 minutes. Cook for a further minute on each side if necessary.
  1. Serve the salmon on top of the vegetables that have been sautéed.

98. Herbed Tilapia with Lime

Prep time: 20min | Serves: 2 | Difficulty: Moderate
Nutrition: Calories: 342 kcal | Fat: 12g | Protein: 23 g | Carbohydrates: 22 g
Ingredients:
- 1 tablespoon olive oil
- 1/8 teaspoon each thyme and dried basil
- 1/4 teaspoon salt Two 6-ounce tilapia fillets
- Juice of 1/2 a lime (about 1/8 cup)

Instructions
- In a stovetop pan, heat the olive oil over medium heat.
- On both sides of the fillets, evenly sprinkle the thyme, basil, and salt. Cook for 5 to 7 minutes on each side, or until cooked through, in the pan with the fillets.
- Place the fillets on serving dishes and drizzle with lime juice before serving.

99. Coconut Panko Shrimp

Prep time: 20min | Serves: 2 | Difficulty: Moderate
Nutrition: Calories: 492 kcal | Fat: 16 g | Protein: 25 g | Carbohydrates: 16 g
Ingredients:
- 2 pounds large or jumbo shrimp, tail on and deveined
- 1/2 cup rough or fine panko flakes (see the following recipe or use store-bought)
- One 4-ounce bag sweetened coconut flakes
- 4 eggs, lightly beaten
- 1 cup coconut oil

Instructions
- Set aside the shrimp in a basin after butterflying them. In one bowl, combine the panko flakes

and coconut flakes; in another, separate the eggs.

- Place the shrimp on a dish after dipping them in the egg and then the panko/coconut mixture. Heat the coconut oil in a skillet over medium-high heat once all of the shrimp are prepared and ready to go.
- Add a few shrimp to the skillet, providing enough room to flip them once one side is golden brown. Cook for 2 minutes on each side, then remove and drain on several layers of paper towels. Rep with the remaining shrimp.

100. Panko

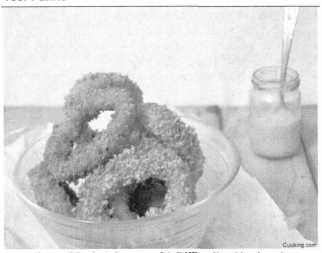

Cuuking.com

Prep time: 25min | Serves: 3 | Difficulty: Moderate
Nutrition: Calories: 142 kcal | Fat: 12 g | Protein: 3 g | Carbohydrates: 46 g
Ingredients:
- 1 loaf of day-old French or sourdough white bread

Instructions
- Preheat oven to 150 degrees Fahrenheit. Remove the crusts from the bread and crush or flake it into crumbs using your hands or a cheese grater; you should have about 3 cups of crumbs.
- Spread the crumbs out on baking trays and bake for about an hour, or until they are crunchy but not browned – check after 20 minutes. Refrigerate panko in plastic zipped bags or glass jars inside or outside the refrigerator.

101. Easy Chicken Curry

Prep time: 35min | Serves: 4 | Difficulty: Moderate
Nutrition: Calories: 407 kcal | Fat: 35 g | Protein: 7 g | Carbohydrates: 6 g
Ingredients:
- 1/2 tablespoon olive oil
- 1 to 11/2 pounds white-meat chicken breast, cut into chunks medium onion (optional) 1/4 cup golden raisins (optional)

- 1 cup cooked potatoes, chopped into about 1-inch squares
- 1/2 teaspoon each cumin, cinnamon, and cardamom
- 1 teaspoon mild yellow curry powder
- 1 cup plain yogurt
- 1/2 teaspoon salt
- 1/4 teaspoon pepper

Instructions
- In a large pot, heat the olive oil over medium-high heat. When the pot is heated, add the chicken and cook it quickly on both sides (less than one minute on each side — you don't need to worry about it being done yet). Remove the chicken and set it aside.
- Cook for about 5 minutes, stirring regularly, after adding the onions, raisins (if preferred), and potatoes to the saucepan. Reduce to medium-low heat and stir in the cumin, cinnamon, cardamom, and curry powder. Cook for approximately a minute, stirring occasionally, to bring the spices' tastes to life.
- Cook until the quick-fried chicken is cooked through (approximately 10 to 15 minutes depending on the chunk size — split a piece in half to check; if it's not pink, it's done).

102. Zucchini Lasagna

Prep time: 35min | Serves: 4 | Difficulty: Moderate
Nutrition: Calories: 256 kcal | Fat: 8 g | Protein:11 g | Carbohydrates:32 g
Ingredients:
- 2 zucchinis, peeled and trimmed
- 1 cup farmer's cheese, crumbled
- 1 cup Asiago cheese, freshly grated
- 1 cup Monterey Jack cheese, freshly grated
- 1 cup Parmesan cheese, freshly grated
- 1 cup Classic Tomato Sauce
- 1/4 cup of olive oil

Instructions
- Preheat oven to 375 degrees Fahrenheit. Slice the zucchinis lengthwise into long, thin slices with a mandoline and set aside. Make a separate bowl for each cheese and tomato sauce.
- In a casserole pan, spread 12 cup tomato sauce. Top with zucchini and a sprinkle of olive oil. Repeat the process, layering the cheeses on top of the zucchini (in whichever order you like) until all of the components are used up, finishing with the Parmesan. Add the leftover tomato sauce on top.
- Bake for 40 to 45 minutes, or until the top is bubbling. Allow 15 minutes for the melted cheese to solidify before slicing and serving.

103. Classic Tomato Sauce

Prep time: 1hr30min | Serves: 6 | Difficulty: Moderate
Nutrition: Calories: 229 kcal | Fat: 7.7 g | Protein: 32.2 g | Carbohydrates: 8.3 g
Ingredients:

- 4 tablespoons olive oil
- 1/2 cup chopped onion
- 6 cloves chopped garlic
- 1 carrot, chopped
- 1/8 teaspoon each sea salt and freshly cracked pepper
- Two 28-ounce cans or cartons Italian no-sugar-added whole tomatoes
- 1 bay leaf
- 2 tablespoons unsalted butter
- 1 big handful (about 1 cup) fresh basil

Instructions

- Heat the oil in a large saucepan over medium-high heat; add the onions and cook for 5 minutes, or until they're transparent. Cook for one minute after adding the garlic. Cook for 10 minutes, stirring regularly to avoid scorching, with the carrot, salt, and pepper.
- Cook for 1 hour, uncovered, with the tomatoes and bay leaf. Add the butter after removing the bay leaf. To avoid a saucy eruption, puree in batches in a food processor, adding basil to each batch. If you have one, you can also use a hand (immersion) blender (no pun intended).

104. Eggplant Lasagna

Prep time: 55min | Serves: 4 | Difficulty: Moderate
Nutrition: Calories: 252 kcal | Fat:12 g | Protein: 11 g | Carbohydrates: 36 g
Ingredients:

- 1large eggplant
- 1/4 of a medium pumpkin
- 1/8 teaspoon each salt and pepper
- 2 cups Marinara Sauce (see the following recipe)
- 7 ounces SCD-safe cheddar cheese

Instructions

- The eggplant should be cut into 14-inch round slices, and the pumpkin should be thinly sliced.
- Preheat oven to 425 degrees Fahrenheit.
- Roast the pumpkin for 15 minutes on a flat baking sheet wrapped in tinfoil. Season the eggplant with salt and pepper while it's cooking, then add it to the baking sheet after the pumpkin has roasted for about 5 minutes, so the eggplant roasts for about 10 minutes and finishes about the same time as the pumpkin. Alternatively, you can roast them on separate sheets. When they're done, cool them on a rack.
- After the eggplant and pumpkin have cooled, grease a baking dish and layer the lasagna with sauce, eggplant, pumpkin, and cheese in the following order: sauce, eggplant, pumpkin, and cheese. Repeat the layering process and make sure cheese end on top.

105. Home-style Marinara Sauce over Chicken balls

Prep time: 3hr10min | Serves: 4 | Difficulty: Moderate
Nutrition: Calories: 256 kcal | Fat: 8 g | Protein:11 g | Carbohydrates:32 g
Ingredients:

- 2 teaspoons olive oil
- 1 small onion, diced
- 4 cloves garlic, pressed
- 4 to 6 mushrooms, chopped
- 1 small red pepper, diced
- 1/3 to 1/2 of a chili pepper, diced
- 1/3 to 1/2 of a zucchini, diced
- 2 to 3 fresh tomatoes, diced
- 1 tablespoon mixed dried, Thyme, oregano, basil and rosemary, all herbs together
- Two 15-ounce cans skinless stewed tomatoes, juice included
- 2 tablespoons tomato paste
- 12 Chicken meat balls

Instructions

- In a large frying pan, heat the olive oil. Sauté for 5 minutes with the onion and garlic. To avoid sticking, use a tablespoon or two of water instead of extra oil throughout this process.
- Sauté for another 5 minutes with the mushrooms and red pepper.
- Cover and cook for 2 to 3 hours on low heat with the chili, zucchini, fresh tomatoes, stewed tomatoes, and tomato paste.
- Sprinkle all mixed dried herbs
- Pour over stir fried chicken meatballs and serve

106. Shannon's Gourmet Zucchini Angel-Hair "Pasta"

Prep time: 15min | Serves: 4 | Difficulty: Moderate
Nutrition: Calories: 215kcal | Fat: 21 g | Protein: 15 g | Carbohydrates: 26 g
Ingredients:

- 1 large or 2 medium green or yellow zucchinis
- 12 black olives, pitted
- 1 cup tiny broccoli florets
- 4 sun-dried tomatoes, sliced
- 1 to 2 fresh tomatoes, finely diced
- 1 tablespoon balsamic vinegar
- 1 clove of garlic, minced
- 3 oyster mushrooms, sliced
- 1/4 teaspoon each sea salt and cracked pepper, or to taste
- 1/8 teaspoon oregano, or to taste

Instructions

- Spiralize, mandolin or grate the zucchini into thin strips and place on a large serving plate.
- In a mixing dish, combine the olives, broccoli, and both types of tomatoes with the vinegar

and garlic. Add the oil mixture, salt, pepper, and oregano to the mushrooms.

- Serve the olive-mushroom combination on top of the zucchini "pasta."

107. Quinoa Casserole with Baked Sweet Potatoes

Prep time: 65min | Serves: 4 | Difficulty: Moderate
Nutrition: Calories: 327 kcal | Fat: 12 g | Protein: 7 g | Carbohydrates:26 g
Ingredients:

- 4 sweet potatoes
- 1 tablespoon of ghee, or coconut oil or butter (see recipe in Chapter 6)
- 1 small onion, diced
- 2 chopped garlic cloves
- 1 carrot, diced
- 1/2 teaspoon turmeric
- 1/2 teaspoon thyme
- 1 cup diced zucchini
- 1 cup sliced mushrooms
- 1 cup frozen peas
- 2 cups chicken stock
- 3 cups cooked quinoa

Instructions

- Preheat oven to 400 degrees Fahrenheit.
- Bake the sweet potatoes for 50 to 60 minutes. Allow to cool before removing the skins and slicing the potatoes.
- Meanwhile, in a 12-inch sauté pan over medium heat, heat the ghee or oil and sauté the onions until transparent. Cook for 1 minute after adding the garlic and carrot.
- Combine the turmeric, thyme, zucchini, mushrooms, peas, chicken stock, and cooked quinoa in a large mixing bowl. Bring to a boil, then reduce to a low heat for 10 minutes, stirring occasionally to avoid sticking.
- Serve with baked sweet potato pieces and additional herbs if you want it to be spicier.

108. Creamy Vegan Stroganoff with Caramelized Onions

Prep time: 65min | Serves: 4 | Difficulty: Moderate
Nutrition: Calories: 279 kcal | Fat: 8.9 g | Protein: 13 g | Carbohydrates:26 g
Ingredients:

- 2 tablespoons olive oil
- 1 large yellow onion, sliced from root to tip in long slices
- 1/2 cup white wine
- 7 ounces brown rice fettuccine, cooked and drained
- 1 cup tofu "Sour Cream" (see the following recipe)
- 2 cups tempeh, cubed Salt and pepper to taste (optional)
- 1/2 cup olive oil-fried gluten-free breadcrumbs

Instructions

- In a large frying pan, heat the oil over medium heat. Add the onions and cook for about 15 minutes, or until they are slightly brown. Cook until the liquid has reduced slightly, then add the wine.
- Reduce the heat to low and toss in the cooked fettuccine with the wine mixture. Toss the noodles in the sauce to coat them.
- 1 cup tofu "sour cream" is poured into the pan and stirred. Season with salt and pepper to taste, then add the tempeh and continue to reheat over low heat (if desired).
- Serve the noodles in a serving dish with fried gluten-free bread crumbs on top.

109. Vegetarian Dreamy Coconut Curry

Prep time: 1hr15min | Serves: 4 | Difficulty: Moderate
Nutrition: Calories:612 kcal | Fat: 24.7 g | Protein: 41.1 g | Carbohydrates:59g
Ingredients:

- 4 Thai young coconuts, water (62/3 cups liquid total) and meat
- 2 cloves of garlic
- 2 tablespoons Thai basil
- Juice of 1/2 a lemon (about 1/8 cup)
- 1/2 cup cilantro
- 3 green onions
- 1/4 teaspoon Celtic salt, or to taste
- 2 tablespoons yellow curry powder
- 1 hot green chili pepper
- 1 fresh lemongrass stick
- 3/4 cup julienned carrot
- 3/4 cup julienned Asian cabbage
- 1/2 cup soaked and drained wild rice

Instructions

- Everything except the lemongrass stick, julienned veggies, and rice should be blended in a blender. Place the pureed curry in a double boiler with the lemongrass stick and reheat slowly. Cook for 30 minutes with the lid on.
- Remove the lemongrass sprig and check the curry's consistency. Thin it up with water or coconut juice as needed. Toss in the julienned vegetables and rice while the curry is still warm and ready to eat.

110. Gourmet Pizza

Prep time: 30min | Serves: 4 | Difficulty: Moderate
Nutrition: Calories: 305 kcal | Fat: 27 g | Protein: 15 g | Carbohydrates: 2 g
Ingredients:

- 1/2 cup almond flour
- 1 tablespoon plus
- 1 cup grated Parmesan cheese
- 1/4 teaspoon salt
- 1/2 teaspoon dried basil

- 1/2 teaspoon dried oregano
- 1/4 teaspoon dried thyme (optional)
- 1 teaspoon olive oil, plus more for greasing the baking sheet and drizzling
- 1 large egg
- 1/4 cup tomato sauce, or to taste depending on your level of tomato sensitivity
- 1/4 to 1/2 cup each of mushrooms, red peppers, zucchini, and onions

Instructions

- Preheat oven to 325 degrees Fahrenheit. Grease a cookie sheet with olive oil and line it with parchment paper.
- In a mixing dish, combine the almond flour, 1 tablespoon Parmesan, salt, basil, oregano, thyme (if preferred), olive oil, and egg until the dough resembles cookie batter.
- On the cookie sheet, spread the dough thinly into a 6- to 8-inch circle. Spread tomato paste or sauce on top, then top with your pizza toppings and a good amount of parmesan cheese. 4 Drizzle the pizza with olive oil and bake for 18 to 20 minutes.

110. Black 'n' White Chicken Nuggets

Prep time: 55 min | Serves: 4 | Difficulty: Moderate
Nutrition: Calories: 256 kcal | Fat: 8 g | Protein:11 g | Carbohydrates:32 g

Ingredients

- 1/2 cup black sesame seeds
- 1/2 cup white sesame seeds
- 1/4 cup honey
- 2 egg whites, beaten
- 1 tablespoon tamari or low-sodium soy sauce
- 1 teaspoon water
- 1/4 teaspoon each salt and pepper
- 4 boneless, skinless
- 6-ounce chicken breasts, cut into nugget-sized chunks
- 2 teaspoons olive oil

Instructions

- Preheat oven to 400 degrees Fahrenheit. Fill a big plastic zipper bag halfway with black sesame seeds and a second bag halfway with white sesame seeds.
- Whisk together the honey, egg whites, tamari or soy sauce, water, salt, and pepper in a medium mixing bowl using a fork. With a slotted spoon, mix in the chicken until all of the pieces are uniformly coated. With the slotted spoon, remove the chicken and let the excess liquid to drop out.
- Half of the chicken should be placed in the black sesame seed bag, and the other half should be placed in the white sesame seed bag. Seal the bags and shake, shake, shake until the seeds are evenly distributed throughout the chicken, adding additional seeds as needed.

- Apply a thin layer of olive oil or parchment paper on two cookie sheets. Remove the chicken chunks from the bags with a clean slotted spoon and place them on the cookie sheets, ensuring sure they don't contact to ensure speedier cooking. Bake for 20 to 25 minutes, or until no pink remains in the middle of a piece sliced open.

112. Pesto without the Pain

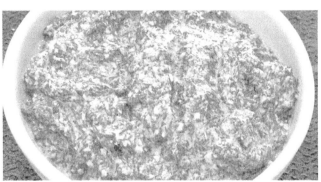

Prep time: 10min | Serves: 2 | Difficulty: Moderate
Nutrition: Calories: 229 kcal | Fat: 7.7 g | Protein: 32.2 g | Carbohydrates: 8.3 g

Ingredients:

- 2 cloves of garlic
- 1/2 cup almonds
- 1 cup fresh basil leaves, lightly packed
- 1 cup fresh parsley, lightly packed
- 1/3 cup lemon juice
- 1/4 cup olive oil
- 1/3 cup chicken broth

Instructions

- Combine the garlic and almonds in a food processor or blender and process until a thick paste forms. Blend in the basil and parsley one more. Blend in the lemon juice once more.
- Slowly drizzle in the olive oil until you have a smooth purée. Blend in the chicken broth until it's completely smooth.

113. Smoked Chicken Pasta

Prep time: 30 min | Serves: 4-6 | Difficulty: Moderate
Nutrition: Calories: 427 kcal | Fat: 15 g | Protein: 28 g | Carbohydrates: 31 g

Ingredients

- 1-pound (450 g) gluten-free pasta
- 1/4 cup (60 ml) extra virgin olive oil
- 2 teaspoons garlic-infused olive oil, plus more for serving (optional)
- 10 ounces (285 g) boneless, skinless smoked chicken breast or plain roast chicken breast sliced
- 2 large handfuls of baby spinach leaves, rinsed and dried
- 1/3 cup (50 g) pine nuts

- 1/2 cup (40 g) grated Parmesan
- Salt and freshly ground black pepper

Instructions

- A big pot of water should be brought to a boil. Cook until the pasta is barely soft, according to the package guidelines.
- Return to the pot after draining. 2 tablespoons olive oil, stirred in, covered and kept heated. In a large frying pan, heat the garlic-infused oil and the remaining 2 tablespoons olive oil.
- Stir in the chicken, spinach, and pine nuts until the spinach has wilted and the chicken and pine nuts are golden brown, about 5 minutes.
- Toss in the drained pasta and Parmesan until the cheese has melted over medium heat.
- Season with salt and pepper to taste, then sprinkle with more garlic-infused oil if preferred.

Chapter 7: Soups, Stews and Salads

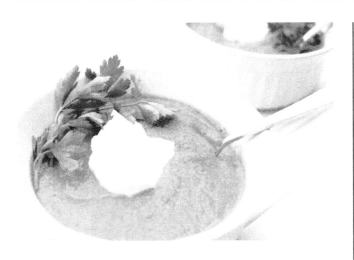

1. Spinach and Bell Pepper Salad with Fried Tofu Puffs

Prep time: 15 min | Serves: 4 | Difficulty: Moderate
Nutrition: Calories: 143 kcal | Fat: 3.2 g | Protein:11 g | Carbohydrates: 16 g

Ingredients
- 1/4 cup gluten-free soy sauce
- 1/4 cup fresh lemon juice
- 1 tablespoon plus 1 teaspoon seasoned rice vinegar
- 1/4 cup packed light brown sugar
- 1/4 cup sesame oil
- 10 cups baby spinach leaves, rinsed and dried
- 1 1/2 cups snow pea shoots or bean sprouts
- 1 green bell pepper, seeded and sliced
- 14 ounces fried tofu puffs, cut into cubes
- 1/3 cup pine nuts
- Salt and freshly ground black pepper

Instructions
- In a small bowl, mix together the soy sauce, lemon juice, vinegar, brown sugar, and sesame oil.
- In a large mixing bowl, combine the spinach, snow pea shoots, bell pepper, tofu, and pine nuts.
- Drizzle the dressing over the salad and stir briefly. Season with salt and pepper to taste and serve.

2. Peppered Beef and Citrus Salad

Prep time: 20 min | Serves: 1 | Difficulty: Moderate
Nutrition: Calories: 305 kcal | Fat: 27 g | Protein: 15 g | Carbohydrates: 2 g

Ingredients
- 2 teaspoons olive oil
- 1-pound beef sirloin or top round steak
- 2 teaspoons garlic-infused olive oil
- 1 heaping tablespoon freshly ground black pepper, plus more for serving

- 1/4 cup fresh lemon juice
- 1 heaping tablespoon light brown sugar
- Salt
- 1 orange, peeled and cut into segments
- 1 head butter lettuce (Boston or Bibb), leaves separated
- One 8-ounce can water chestnuts, drained and roughly chopped

Instructions
- In a frying pan, heat the olive oil over medium heat.
- Cook the beef for 4 minutes on each side for medium-rare, or until done to your liking. Allow 10 minutes for the steak to rest before slicing thinly.
- In a medium bowl, mix together the garlic-infused oil, pepper, lemon juice, brown sugar, and seasoning to taste. Toss in the steak until it is well covered in the marinade. Refrigerate for 3 hours, covered.
- In a large mixing bowl, combine the orange segments, lettuce, water chestnuts, meat, and any residual marinade. Serve immediately with a few grinds of black pepper on top.

3. Roasted Sweet Potato Salad with Spiced Lamb and Spinach

Prep time: 45 min | Serves: 4 | Difficulty: Moderate
Nutrition: Calories: 287 kcal | Fat: 12 g | Protein: 7 g | Carbohydrates:26 g

Ingredients
- 4 small sweet potatoes, peeled (if desired) and cut into 3/4-inch cubes
- 1 red bell pepper, seeded and cut into quarters
- Olive oil
- 1 heaping tablespoon ground cumin
- 2 teaspoons ground coriander
- 1/2 teaspoon ground cardamom
- 2 teaspoons ground turmeric
- 1/2 teaspoon ground sumac, or 1/2 teaspoon paprika plus 1/2 teaspoon lemon zest
- 1 pound lean lamb steak, cut into thin strips
- 8 ounces baby spinach leaves (8 cups), rinsed and dried

Instructions
- Preheat the oven to 350 degrees Fahrenheit (180 degrees Celsius). Brush the sweet potato and bell pepper with olive oil on a large baking sheet.
- Cook for 30 minutes, or until the vegetables are soft and browned. Allow to cool before serving. Remove the skin off the bell pepper once it has cooled enough to handle.

- In a medium frying pan, heat a little olive oil over medium-low heat. Heat for 1 minute or until aromatic, then add the cumin, coriander, cardamom, turmeric, and sumac.
- Stir in the lamb to coat it in the spice mixture. Cook, stirring occasionally, for 3 to 5 minutes, or until lightly browned.
- Turn off the heat. In a large mixing basin, combine the spinach, sweet potato, and bell pepper.
- Finish with a sprinkle of olive oil and the lamb and any pan juices.

4. Caramelized Squash Salad with Sun- Dried Tomatoes and Basil

Prep time: 2h-25 min | Serves: 4 | Difficulty: Moderate
Nutrition: Calories: 226 kcal | Fat: 13 g | Protein: 16 g | Carbohydrates: 18 g
Ingredients
- 1.2 kg kabocha or other suitable winter squash, peeled, seeded, and cut into 3⁄4- inch cubes
- 1 eggplant, cut into 1⁄4-inch slices
- 1⁄4 cup olive oil
- 12 or 13 pieces sun-dried tomatoes in oil, drained and sliced
- 1⁄2 cup thawed frozen corn kernels
- Small handful of basil leaves, roughly chopped
Instructions
- Preheat the oven to 350 degrees Fahrenheit (180 degrees Celsius). Brush 2 tablespoons of olive oil over the squash and eggplant on two separate baking sheets.
- Bake for 25 minutes, or until golden brown and soft. Allow it cool to room temperature before chopping the eggplant.
- In a large mixing bowl, combine the squash, eggplant, sun-dried tomatoes, corn, basil, and the remaining 2 tablespoons olive oil. Allow for flavor development by refrigerating for 2 to 3 hours.
- Before serving, allow it cool to room temperature.

5. Blue Cheese and Arugula Salad with Red Wine Dressing

Prep time: 15 min | Serves: 4 | Difficulty: Moderate
Nutrition: Calories: 274 Kcal | Fat: 18 g | Protein: 23 g | Carbohydrates: 6 g
Ingredients
- 4 handfuls of arugulas
- 1 cup snow pea shoots or bean sprouts
- 7 ounces blue cheese, cut into small chunks
- 1⁄2 English cucumber, sliced
- 1 avocado, pitted, peeled, and sliced (optional)
- 1⁄2 green bell pepper, seeded and thinly sliced
Red Wine Dressing
- 1⁄4 cup (60 ml) olive oil

- 2 tablespoons plus 2 teaspoons fresh lemon juice
- 1 tablespoon red wine vinegar
- 1 teaspoon gluten-free whole grain mustard
- 1 teaspoon sugar
- 2 heaping tablespoons chopped tarragon or flat-leaf parsley

Instructions
- In a large mixing bowl, combine the arugula, snow pea shoots, blue cheese, cucumber, avocado (if using), and bell pepper.
- To prepare the dressing, whisk together all of the Ingredients in a small screw-top jar until thoroughly combined. Pour the dressing over the salad just before serving and gently toss to incorporate.

6. Vietnamese Beef Noodle Salad

Prep time: 3h-10 min | Serves: 4 | Difficulty: Moderate
Nutrition: Calories: 286 kcal | Fat:14 g | Protein: 26 g | Carbohydrates: 18 g
Ingredients
- 2 teaspoons garlic-infused olive oil
- 2 teaspoons olive oil
- 1 heaping tablespoon Chinese five-spice powder
- 1⁄4 cup fish sauce, or 3 tablespoons soy sauce and 1 tablespoon fresh lime juice
- 1⁄4 cup seasoned rice vinegar
- 2 teaspoons grated ginger
- 1 heaping tablespoon light brown sugar
- 1-pound beef sirloin or top round steak, cut into thin strips
- 8 ounces gluten-free rice vermicelli
- 2 tablespoons sesame oil
- 1 cup snow pea shoots or bean sprouts
- 1⁄4 cup roughly chopped Vietnamese mint, or a combination of mint and cilantro
Instructions
- In a medium glass or ceramic bowl, mix the garlic-infused oil, olive oil, five-spice powder, fish sauce, vinegar, ginger, and brown sugar to prepare the marinade.
- Toss in the beef strips, making sure they are fully coated in the marinade. Refrigerate for 3 hours, covered.
- Fill a large mixing basin halfway with boiling water. Soak the vermicelli for 4 to 5 minutes, or until it softens. Drain and rinse under cold water before draining one more.
- In a nonstick frying pan or wok, heat the sesame oil over medium heat. Toss the beef strips with any residual marinade for 2 to 4 minutes, or until just cooked through.
- You want the meat to be lovely and soft, so don't overcook it. In a mixing dish, combine the meat, any liquids, vermicelli, snow pea shoots, and mint. Serve immediately.

7. Smoked Chicken and Walnut Salad

Prep time: 45 min | Serves: 4 | Difficulty: Moderate
Nutrition: Calories: 236 kcal | Fat: 7 g | Protein: 13 g | Carbohydrates: 16 g

Ingredients

- 1/2 cup gluten-free mayonnaise
- 1/2 teaspoon gluten-free soy sauce
- 3 tablespoons fresh lemon juice
- 2 heads baby romaine lettuce, leaves separated
- 1/2 cup alfalfa sprouts
- 4 large hard-boiled eggs, halved
- 1 avocado, pitted, peeled, and sliced (optional)
- 14 ounces smoked chicken or plain roast chicken, thinly sliced
- 1/4 cup toasted walnuts
- Salt and freshly ground black pepper

Instructions

- In a separate bowl, mix together the mayonnaise, soy sauce, and lemon juice to make the dressing.
- In a large salad bowl, combine the lettuce, sprouts, eggs, and avocado (if using). Drizzle the dressing on top and gently stir to coat.
- Add the chicken and walnuts just before serving, season to taste, and serve.

8. Vermicelli Salad with Chicken, Cilantro, and Mint

Prep time: 2-3h | Serves: 4-6 | Difficulty: Moderate
Nutrition: Calories: 256 kcal | Fat: 8 g | Protein:11 g | Carbohydrates:32 g

Ingredients

- 101/2 ounces gluten-free rice vermicelli

Dressing
- 2 tablespoons fresh lime juice
- 1 tablespoon fish sauce, or 2 teaspoons soy sauce and 1 extra teaspoon fresh lime juice
- 2 tablespoons light brown sugar
- 1/2 red chile pepper, seeded and finely chopped
- 1 tablespoon sesame oil
- 4-1/3 cups shredded cooked chicken breasts
- Small handful of cilantro leaves, roughly chopped
- Small handful of mint leaves, roughly chopped
- Salt and freshly ground black pepper

Instructions

- Fill a large mixing basin halfway with boiling water. Soak the vermicelli for 4 to 5 minutes, or until it softens.
- Drain and rinse under cold water before draining one more. To prepare the dressing, whisk together all of the Ingredients in a small screw-top jar until thoroughly combined.
- In a large mixing dish, combine the noodles, chicken, cilantro, and mint. Toss in the dressing, season with salt and pepper to taste, and toss to incorporate.

- Allow for flavor melding by refrigerating for 2 to 3 hours before serving.

9. Vegetable Soup

Prep time: 15 min | Serves: 4-6 | Difficulty: Moderate
Nutrition: Calories: 286 kcal | Fat: 12g | Protein: 21 g | Carbohydrates: 21 g

Ingredients

- 2 tablespoons garlic-infused olive oil
- 2 celery stalks, tough strings removed, halved lengthwise and cut into 1/4-inch (5 mm) slices
- 1 head broccoli, cut into chunks (including stalks)
- 3 rutabagas, peeled and cut into chunks
- 2 large carrots, cut into chunks
- 14 ounces kabocha or other suitable winter squash, peeled, seeded, and cut into chunks
- 3 potatoes, cut into chunks
- 4 cups gluten-free, onion-free vegetable stock*
- 11/2 cups low-fat milk, lactose-free milk, or suitable plant-based milk
- Salt and freshly ground black pepper

Instructions

- In a large heavy-bottomed stockpot, heat the oil over medium heat.
- Cook, stirring constantly, until the celery is golden brown.
- Combine the broccoli, rutabagas, carrots, squash, and potatoes in a large mixing bowl.
- Pour the stock in. Bring to a boil, then lower to a low heat and cover and simmer for 1 hour, or until the veggies are soft.
- Allow to cool to room temperature after removing from the heat. To get a smooth purée of the veggies, use an immersion blender. (Alternatively, place the veggies in a food processor and blend until smooth.) Stir in the milk, season with salt and pepper to taste, and gently reheat.

10. Spicy Clear Soup

Prep time: 15 min | Serves: 4 | Difficulty: Moderate
Nutrition: Calories: 241 kcal | Fat: 18 g | Protein: 17 g | Carbohydrates: 4 g

Ingredients

- 1 tablespoon sesame oil
- 2 teaspoons garlic-infused olive oil
- 2 teaspoons rice bran oil or sunflower oil
- 2 heaping tablespoons finely chopped lemongrass (white portion only)
- 1/2 to 1 red chile pepper, seeded and finely chopped
- 6 pieces dried galangal root (optional)
- 61/2 cups gluten-free, onion-free chicken or vegetable stock*

- 2 tablespoons plus 2 teaspoons fish sauce, or 4 teaspoons soy sauce and 2 teaspoons fresh lime juice
- 1 tablespoon plus 1 teaspoon fresh lime juice
- 3 bunches baby bok choy, quartered, rinsed, and drained
- 2 heaping tablespoons chopped cilantro
- One 8-ounce can bamboo shoots, drained
- One 14-to 15-ounce can baby corn, drained, or 7½ ounces fresh baby corn, cut on the
- diagonal
- 2 cups gluten-free rice vermicelli

Instructions
- In a large saucepan, heat the sesame oil, garlic-infused oil, and rice bran oil over medium heat.
- Cook for 2 minutes, or until the lemongrass and chile are aromatic.
- Bring the stock, fish sauce, and lime juice to a boil, along with the galangal (if using). Combine the bok choy, cilantro, bamboo shoots, baby corn, and vermicelli in a large mixing bowl. Reduce the heat to low and cook the veggies and noodles for 3 minutes, or until they are soft. (Take away the galangal.) Serve right away.

11. Chicken Noodle Soup with Bok Choy

Prep time: 15 min | Serves: 4 | Difficulty: Moderate
Nutrition: Calories: 317 kcal | Fat: 5.7 g | Protein:7 g | Carbohydrates: 16g
Ingredients
- 8 cups gluten-free, onion-free chicken or vegetable stock*
- 1 heaping tablespoon grated ginger
- 4 kaffir lime leaves
- 1 pound boneless, skinless chicken breasts, very thinly sliced
- 8 ounces gluten-free rice vermicelli, broken into 2-inch (5 cm) pieces
- 3 bunches baby bok choy, leaves separated, rinsed and drained
- ½ cup bean sprouts
- 2 teaspoons gluten-free soy sauce

Instructions
- Bring the stock, ginger, and lime leaves to a boil in a big heavy-bottomed pot.
- Reduce the heat to low and cook the chicken for 5 minutes.
- Simmer for a further 5 minutes, or until the rice noodles, bok choy, and bean sprouts are soft.
- Remove the lime leaves and mix in the soy sauce before serving.

12. Curried Potato and Parsnip Soup

Prep time: 40 min | Serves: 4 | Difficulty: Moderate
Nutrition: Calories: 218 kcal | Fat: 7 g | Protein:8 g | Carbohydrates: 36g
Ingredients

- 1 tablespoon canola oil
- 2 parsnips peeled and cut into ¾-inch pieces
- 4 potatoes peeled and cut into ¾-inch pieces
- 6½ cups gluten-free, onion-free chicken or vegetable stock*
- 1 teaspoon gluten-free curry powder, or to taste
- 1 cup (250 ml) low-fat milk, lactose-free milk, or suitable plant-based milk
- Salt and freshly ground black pepper
- Chopped flat-leaf parsley, to garnish

Instructions
- In a large heavy-bottomed saucepan, heat the canola oil over medium heat.
- Cook, turning often, for 3 to 5 minutes, until the parsnips and potatoes are gently browned.
- Bring the stock to a boil, then remove from the heat. Reduce the heat to low and cook, stirring occasionally, for 15 to 20 minutes, or until the veggies are tender.
- Remove from the fire and set aside for 10 minutes to cool. Blend until smooth with an immersion blender (or in batches with a normal blender).
- Blend in the curry powder and milk until thoroughly mixed.
- Season with salt and pepper to taste. Gently reheat without boiling. Serve with a dusting of parsley as a garnish.

13. Carrot and Ginger Soup

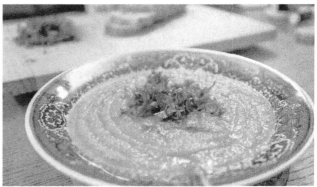

Prep time: 40 min | Serves: 4 | Difficulty: Moderate
Nutrition: Calories: 255 kcal | Fat: 7 g | Protein: 12g | Carbohydrates: 22g
Ingredients
- 1 tablespoon olive oil
- 1 small celery root, peeled, halved, and cut into ¼-inch slices
- 4 pounds carrots, cut into ¾-inch (2 cm) chunks
- 2 large potatoes,npeeled and cut into quarters
- 6½ cups gluten-free, onion-free chicken or vegetable stock*
- 1 heaping tablespoon ground ginger
- 1 cup low-fat milk, lactose-free milk, or suitable plant-based milk

- Salt and freshly ground black pepper

Instructions

- In a large heavy-bottomed skillet, heat the olive oil over medium heat, then add the celery root and sauté until golden. Combine the carrots, potatoes, and stock in a large mixing bowl. Bring to a boil, then lower to a low heat, cover, and cook for 20 minutes, or until the veggies are soft.
- Allow it cool for 10 minutes before blending until smooth with an immersion blender (or in stages in a conventional blender). Combine the ginger and milk in a large mixing bowl.
- Depending on how thick you prefer your soup, you may vary the amount of milk.
- Season with salt and pepper to taste. Serve after a gentle reheating without boiling.

14. Roasted Squash and Chestnut Soup

Prep time: 1h-10min | Serves: 4 | Difficulty: Moderate
Nutrition: Calories: 437 kcal | Fat: 12 g | Protein: 21g | Carbohydrates:31 g

Ingredients.

- 2 kg peeled, seeded, and cubed kabocha or other suitable winter squash
- 2 tablespoons olive oil
- 2 cups unsweetened chestnut puree
- 8 cups gluten-free, onion-free chicken or vegetable stock*
- 2 teaspoons ground ginger
- 1 cup low-fat milk, lactose-free milk, or suitable plant-based milk, warmed, plus more for serving (optional)
- Salt and freshly ground black pepper

Instructions

- Preheat the oven to 350 degrees Fahrenheit (180 degrees Celsius).
- Drizzle the olive oil over the squash and spread it out on a baking pan. Bake for 30 to 40 minutes, flipping regularly, until brown and cooked through. In a large saucepan or stockpot, place the squash. Bring the stock, chestnut purée, and ginger to a boil. Reduce the heat to medium-low and cook, stirring occasionally, for 15 to 20 minutes, or until the squash is soft. Allow for a 10-minute cooling period.
- Puree the soup with an immersion blender (or in batches in a conventional blender) until completely smooth.
- Season with salt and pepper to taste. Serve with a swirl of additional milk over top (if preferred).

15. Creamy Seafood Soup

Prep time: 45 min | Serves: 6 | Difficulty: Moderate
Nutrition: Calories: 241 kcal | Fat: 18 g | Protein: 17 g | Carbohydrates: 4 g

Ingredients

- 3 tablespoons salted butter
- 2 large carrots, diced
- 1/2 cup of long-grain white rice
- 5 cups gluten-free, onion-free chicken stock*
- 2 tablespoons plus 2 teaspoons fish sauce, or 4 teaspoons soy sauce plus 2 teaspoons fresh lime juice
- 1/2 cup tomato pure
- 1/2 fennel bulb, finely chopped
- 1/2 cup white wine (optional)
- 1 pound raw medium shrimp, peeled and deveined
- 2 large or 5 small squid bodies, cleaned and sliced
- 5 ounces boneless, skinless firm fish fillets, cut into cubes
- 6 cooked jumbo shrimp
- 1 cup low-fat milk, lactose-free milk, or suitable plant-based milk
- Salt and freshly ground black pepper
- Extra virgin olive oil, to garnish (optional)

Instructions

- In a large heavy-bottomed saucepan, melt the butter over medium heat.
- Cook, stirring often, for 5 minutes after adding the carrots and rice. Stir together the stock, fish sauce, tomato puree, fennel, and wine (if using).
- Bring to a boil, then lower to a low heat and continue to cook for another 20 minutes, or until the rice is tender. Allow 10 minutes for cooling. Blend until smooth with an immersion blender (or in batches with a normal blender).
- Return the pan to the burner and bring the soup to a simmer over medium heat. Add the uncooked shrimp, squid, and fish to the pot and cook for 4 to 5 minutes, or until the seafood is just done.
- Stir in the jumbo shrimp and milk until thoroughly cooked and mixed.
- Season with salt and pepper to taste, drizzle with olive oil (if wanted), and serve right away.

16. Mussels in Chili, Bacon, and Tomato Broth

Prep time: 50 min | Serves: 4 | Difficulty: Moderate
Nutrition: Calories: 427 kcal | Fat:14 g | Protein:32 g | Carbohydrates:26g

Ingredients

- 4 ounces lean bacon slices, cut crosswise into thin strips
- 2 tablespoons olive oil
- 3 cups (750 ml) tomato puree
- 1/2 teaspoon cayenne pepper (or to taste)

- 6 1/2 cups reduced sodium gluten-free, onion-free chicken stock*
- 5 1/2 pounds mussels, scrubbed and debearded
- Salt and freshly ground black pepper
- Gluten-free bread, for serving

Instructions
- Cook the bacon in a big heavy-bottomed saucepan over medium heat until it is barely brown. Remove and discard any extra fat before adding the olive oil, tomato puree, cayenne pepper, and 2 cups (500 ml) stock. To create the smokey bacon taste, bring to a boil, then lower to a low heat and simmer for 30 to 40 minutes. Add the last of the stock.
- Bring the mixture to a boil over medium-high heat. Cook the mussels, covered, for 5 to 8 minutes, or until all of them have opened.
- Cook for a further minute after shaking the pan to disseminate the mussels. Shake once more. Any mussels that haven't opened should be discarded.
- Season with salt and pepper to taste, then serve right away with lots of gluten-free bread to lap up the wonderful soup.

17. Potato and Corn Chowder

Prep time: 20 min | Serves: 6 | Difficulty: Moderate
Nutrition: Calories: 284 kcal | Fat: 7.3 g | Protein: 12 g | Carbohydrates: 46g

Ingredients
- 8 ounces lean bacon slices, diced (optional)
- Nonstick cooking spray
- 3 large potatoes, peeled (if desired) and diced
- 8 cups (2 liters) reduced sodium gluten-free, onion-free chicken or vegetable stock
- 114.7-ounce can no-salt-add, gluten-free cream-style corn
- 1 teaspoon ground mustard
- 1 teaspoon fresh thyme leaves
- 1 heaping tablespoon roughly chopped flat-leaf parsley
- Salt and freshly ground black pepper

Instructions
- If using bacon, sauté until crisp in a large heavy-bottomed pot over medium heat, stirring occasionally.
- Remove to a plate lined with paper towels to drain. Spray the same saucepan with cooking spray, then add the potatoes and cook, turning often, over medium heat.
- Bring the stock to a boil, then remove from the heat. Reduce the heat to a low level and cook, turning periodically, for 15 minutes, or until the potatoes are soft.
- Blend until smooth with an immersion blender (or in batches with a normal blender). Season with salt and pepper after adding the corn, mustard, thyme, parsley, and reserved bacon.

- Serve after a gentle reheating without boiling.

18. Hearty Lamb Shank and Vegetable Soup

Prep time: 1h-10 min | Serves: 4 | Difficulty: Moderate
Nutrition: Calories: 381 kcal | Fat: 18 g | Protein: 37 g | Carbohydrates: 14 g

Ingredients
- 3 tablespoons olive oil
- 1 tablespoon garlic-infused olive oil
- 2 lamb shanks
- 1 1/2 pounds kabocha or other suitable winter squash, peeled, seeded, and cut into 3/4-inch pieces
- 3 large carrots, cut into 1/3-inch pieces
- 3 celery stalks, cut into 1/3-inch slices
- 6 1/2 cups gluten-free, onion-free beef stock*
- 2/3 cup long-grain white rice

Instructions
- In a large heavy-bottomed saucepan, heat the olive oil and garlic-infused oil over medium heat.
- Cook until the lamb shanks are lightly browned on both sides, about 5 to 10 minutes total, searing for 2 to 3 minutes on each side before rotating.
- Remove the shanks from the pan and place them on a platter. Cook for 2 to 3 minutes, until the squash, carrots, and celery are gently browned in the remaining oil and meat juices.
- Return the shanks to the pan and raise the heat to medium-high. Bring the stock and rice to a boil, then lower to a low heat and cook for 50 to 60 minutes, stirring regularly, until the meat is very soft.
- Remove the lamb shanks from the bones, then shred or chop the meat into big pieces. Bones and fat should be discarded.
- Return the lamb to the pan and stir thoroughly, breaking up the squash chunks as you do so.
- Season to taste with salt and pepper before serving.

19. Egg and Spinach Salad

Prep time: 15min | Serves: 4 | Difficulty: Moderate
Nutrition: Calories: 317 kcal | Fat: 8 g | Protein:22 g | Carbohydrates:26g

Ingredients:
- 1 tablespoon sesame oil
- 4 eggs, beaten

For Dressing
- 1 1/2 tablespoons soy sauce (gluten-free if following a gluten-free diet)
- 2 tablespoons lemon juice
- 2 tablespoons sesame oil
- 1 1/2 tablespoons brown sugar
- 7 cups baby spinach leaves
- 2 cups snow pea shoots
- 1 green bell pepper, sliced into 1-inch lengths

Instructions:

- In a medium nonstick pan, heat 2 tablespoons sesame oil over medium-high heat.
- Half of the beaten eggs should be added now. Cook for approximately 1 minute, or until barely cooked through, tilting the pan to produce a thin omelette.
- Remove the pan from the heat. Continue with the remaining oil and beaten eggs. Allow the omelets to cool completely before cutting them into big diamond slices.
- In a small bowl, mix the soy sauce, lemon juice, sesame oil, and brown sugar to make the dressing.
- Toss the spinach, snow pea shoots, bell pepper, and omelette strips together gently in a large mixing basin.
- Serve by dividing the salad among four bowls and drizzling the dressing on top.

20. Quinoa and Vegetable Salad

Prep time: 45min| Serves: 4| Difficulty: Moderate
Nutrition: Calories: 260 kcal |Fat: 6.7 g| Protein: 15 g| Carbohydrates: 28g
Ingredients:

- 8 ounces winter squash, peeled, cut into 1-inch cubes
- 1/4 cup plus 1tablespoon lemon-infused olive oil 1/2 cup quinoa
- 2 cups baby spinach leaves
- 1 cup cherry tomatoes, halved
- 1 small red bell pepper, seeded and finely chopped
- 1 small green bell pepper, seeded and finely chopped 2 medium carrots, peeled and cut into small cubes
- 3 tablespoons fresh thyme leaves
- 1 teaspoon lemon zest
- Salt and freshly ground black pepper

Instructions:

- Preheat the oven to 400 degrees Fahrenheit (200 degrees Celsius). Place the squash slices on a baking sheet and sprinkle with 1 tablespoon lemon-infused olive oil.
- Toss thoroughly to coat, then bake for 30–35 minutes, or until golden brown and softened. Remove from the oven and allow to cool to room temperature before serving.
- In a small saucepan, bring 2 cups (500 ml) water to a boil over medium-high heat. Reduce to medium-low heat and add the quinoa. Cook, stirring often, for 10 to 15 minutes, or until the quinoa is soft and all the water has been absorbed.
- Allow to cool to room temperature before serving. In a large mixing bowl, combine the cooked quinoa, squash, and all other ingredients, including the remaining 14 cup of

oil. Season with salt and pepper to taste. Serve right away, or cover and chill until ready to use.

21. Crab and Arugula Quinoa Salad

Prep time: 50min| Serves: 4| Difficulty: Moderate
Nutrition: Calories: 316 kcal| Fat: 13 g| Protein: 18 g| Carbohydrates: 28 g
Ingredients:

- 1/2 cup quinoa

Herb Dressing

- 3 tablespoons extra virgin olive oil
- 1 tablespoon lemon juice
- 1 teaspoon grated lemon zest
- 1/2 teaspoon finely chopped red chile pepper
- 1 tablespoon capers, drained
- 2 tablespoons roughly chopped flat-leaf parsley
- 2 tablespoons chopped chives
- 2 tomatoes, chopped
- 12 ounces canned crab meat (two 6-ounce cans)
- 2 cups arugula leaves

Instructions:

- In a small saucepan, bring 2 cups (500 ml) water to a boil over medium-high heat. Reduce to medium-low heat and add the quinoa.
- Cook, stirring often, for 10 to 15 minutes, or until the quinoa is soft and all the water has been absorbed. Allow to cool to room temperature before serving.
- To create the herb dressing, whisk together all of the dressing ingredients in a small screw-top container.
- In a large mixing bowl, combine the quinoa, tomato, crab meat, arugula, and dressing.
- To enable the flavors to merge, cover and chill for 20 to 30 minutes.

22. Mixed Potato Salad with Bacon-and-Herb Dressing

Prep time: 50min| Serves: 4-6| Difficulty: Moderate
Nutrition: Calories: 432 kcal |Fat: 9 g| Protein:15 g| Carbohydrates: 46g
Ingredients:

- 2 small sweet potatoes, washed and cut into 3/4- to 1-inch (2 to 3 cm) cubes
- 1 tablespoon canola oil
- 6 red-skin potatoes, washed and cut into 3/4- to 1-inch (2 to 3 cm) cubes
- 6 slices bacon, trimmed of fat and chopped
- 1/2 cup mayonnaise (gluten-free if following a gluten-free diet) 1/3 cup (100 g) light sour cream
- 3/4 cup drained and finely chopped dill pickles
- 1 1/2 tablespoons chopped dill
- 3 tablespoons chopped flat-leaf parsley
- 1 1/2 tablespoons capers Salt and freshly ground black pepper

- 2 eggs, hard-boiled, peeled, and cut into quarters

Instructions:
- Bake the sweet potato cubes for 30 minutes, or until soft and golden.
- Remove from the oven, wrap in foil, and set aside to cool. Meanwhile, cover the red-skin potatoes with cold water in a big saucepan.
- Bring to a boil, then reduce heat to low and simmer for 10 to 12 minutes, or until potatoes are cooked when pierced with a fork. Drain the water and set aside to cool to room temperature.
- In a small nonstick pan, cook the bacon for 3 to 4 minutes, or until barely crisp, turning often.
- Turn off the heat. Combine the mayonnaise, sour cream, pickles, herbs, capers, and bacon in a small bowl.
- In a large mixing basin, combine the cooled potatoes and sweet potatoes. Pour the mayonnaise over the top and whisk gently.
- Salt & pepper to taste. Toss gently to mix, then top with the eggs and serve.

23. Roasted Vegetable Salad

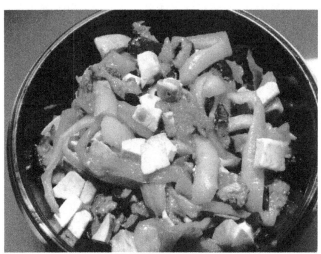

Prep time: 30min | Serves: 6 | Difficulty: Moderate
Nutrition: Calories: 367 kcal | Fat: 5.8 g | Protein: 2 g | Carbohydrates:36g
Ingredients:
- 1 eggplant, cut into 1-inch cubes
- 2 zucchinis, cut into thick slices
- 1 red bell pepper, cut into 1½-inch cubes
- 1 yellow bell pepper, cut into 1½-inch cubes
- 2 small sweet potatoes, cut into ½-inch slices
- 10 ounces winter squash, cut into ¾-inch cubes
- Garlic-infused olive oil

Balsamic Dressing
- 2 teaspoons balsamic vinegar
- 3 tablespoons garlic-infused olive oil
- 3 cups baby spinach leaves
- Salt and freshly ground black pepper

- 2 tablespoons roasted pumpkin seeds

Instructions:
- Preheat oven to 400 degrees Fahrenheit and line two baking sheets with parchment paper.
- In a large mixing bowl, combine the veggies, sprinkle with a little garlic-infused oil, and toss to coat.
- Place the veggies in a single layer on the oven trays and roast for 20 minutes, or until golden brown, rotating once or twice to achieve uniform browning. Remove the baking sheet from the oven.
- Cover with foil and set aside to chill. To create the dressing, mix the balsamic vinegar and olive oil in a small screw-top container and shake well to incorporate.
- In a large mixing basin, combine the cooled veggies and spinach. Toss in the dressing, then season with salt and pepper to taste.
- Serve with roasted pumpkin seeds on top.

24. Five-Spice Asian Pork Salad

Prep time: 3hr | Serves: 4 | Difficulty: Moderate
Nutrition: Calories: 328 kcal | Fat: 5.3g | Protein: 18 g | Carbohydrates: 32g
Ingredients:
- 1 tablespoon garlic-infused canola oil
- 3 teaspoons Chinese five-spice powder
- 3 tablespoons fish sauce
- 3 tablespoons seasoned rice vinegar
- 2 teaspoons grated ginger
- 1 tablespoon brown sugar
- 1 pound boneless pork chops, cut into thin strips
- 2 tablespoons sesame oil
- 5 cups roughly chopped iceberg lettuce
- 1 cup snow pea shoots
- ½ large cucumber, diced
- 2 stalks celery, thinly sliced
- ½ green bell pepper, diced
- ½ cup chopped cilantro or Vietnamese mint 4 ounces
- Fried rice noodles, optional.

Instructions:
- In a nonmetallic bowl, combine the canola oil, five-spice powder, fish sauce, vinegar, ginger, and brown sugar.
- Toss in the pork strips until thoroughly combined. In a wok, heat the sesame oil over medium heat. Cook, 3 to 4 minutes, until the pork is barely cooked through but still soft, adding any remaining marinade.
- Combine the lettuce, additional ingredients, pork strips, and cooking liquids in a large mixing basin.
- Serve immediately by dividing the mixture among four bowls.

25. Gluten-Free Fatoush Salad with Chicken

Prep time: 45min | Serves: 4 | Difficulty: Moderate
Nutrition: Calories: 309 kcal | Fat: 7.9 g | Protein:19 g | Carbohydrates: 22g

Ingredients:
- 1 tablespoon ground cumin
- 1 1/2 tablespoons canola oil
- 2 6-ounce boneless skinless chicken breasts
- 3 8-inch round gluten-free flatbreads
- 2 small cucumbers, cut in half lengthwise and sliced
- 2 tomatoes, chopped
- 1/2 red bell pepper, chopped
- 1/2 green bell pepper, chopped
- 1/2 cup chopped flat-leaf parsley
- 3 tablespoons chopped mint

Spiced Lemon Dressing
- 3 tablespoons olive oil
- 2 tablespoons lemon juice
- 1 tablespoon garlic-infused canola oil
- 1 teaspoon ground cinnamon
- 1 tablespoon ground cumin
- 1 teaspoon ground cilantro
- Salt and freshly ground black pepper

Instructions:
- In a small dish, combine the cumin and 1 tablespoon of canola oil. Brush the chicken on all sides.
- Cover with plastic wrap and marinate for 30 minutes in the refrigerator.
- Preheat the oven to 320 degrees Fahrenheit (160 degrees Celsius) or the broiler to high. Place the flatbreads on a baking sheet and bake for 5 minutes, or until light brown and crisp.
- Cook for only 2 to 3 minutes if broiling, keeping an eye on them to ensure they don't burn. Break them up into bite-size pieces and set them aside after they've cooled enough to handle.
- Toss the cucumbers, tomatoes, bell peppers, and chopped herbs together in a large mixing basin. To create the dressing, whisk together all of the dressing ingredients in a small screw-top container.
- In a medium pan, heat the remaining 12 tbsp. of canola oil over medium heat. Cook for 3 to 4 minutes on each side, until the chicken is just cooked through.
- Remove the chicken from the fire and set it aside to cool for 5 minutes before chopping it into rough cubes. Toss the salad gently with the toasted flatbread, chicken, and dressing before serving.

26. Chicken Salad with Herb Dressing

Prep time: 15min | Serves: 4 | Difficulty: Moderate
Nutrition: Calories: 310 kcal | Fat: 13 g | Protein: 11 g | Carbohydrates: 38 g

Ingredients:
- 2 tablespoons extra virgin olive oil
- Four 6-ounce boneless skinless chicken breasts
- 3 tablespoons mayonnaise (gluten-free if following a gluten-free diet)
- 3 tablespoons plain yogurt (gluten-free if following a gluten-free diet)
- 1 tablespoon finely chopped cilantro
- 2 tablespoons chopped flat-leaf parsley
- Grated zest and juice of 1 lemon
- 2 cups (40 g) baby spinach leaves
- Toasted sliced almonds

Instructions:
- In a large skillet, heat 1 tablespoon of the oil over medium heat.
- Cook for 4 minutes on each side, or until golden brown and cooked through, before adding the chicken breasts. Cool to room temperature after removing from the heat.
- In a small mixing bowl, whisk together the mayonnaise, yoghurt, cilantro, parsley, and 1 tablespoon lemon juice. Mix the chilled chicken into the mayonnaise dressing by shredding it into bite-size pieces.
- Shake vigorously to incorporate the lemon zest, remaining 1 tablespoon of oil, and remaining lemon juice in a small screw-top container.
- Toss the spinach leaves with the lemon oil dressing in a large mixing basin.
- Top the spinach with the chicken mixture in four separate dishes. Just before serving, top with toasted sliced almonds.

27. Chicken Noodle and Vegetable Soup

Prep time: 1hr-30min | Serves: 4 | Difficulty: Moderate
Nutrition: Calories: 347 kcal | Fat: 0 g | Protein: 29 g | Carbohydrates: 36 g

Ingredients:
- 2 tablespoons canola oil
- 3 carrots, peeled and finely chopped
- 2 large stalks celery, finely chopped
- 1 bay leaf
- 1/2 teaspoon turmeric
- 2 pounds chicken carcasses
- 5 thyme sprigs, plus 1 tablespoon finely chopped
- 3 marjoram sprigs, plus 2 teaspoons chopped, or 1 to 2 teaspoons dried
- 10 ounces boneless skinless chicken thighs
- 1 cup canned corn kernels, drained
- 1 cup rice vermicelli, broken into short lengths
- Salt and freshly ground black pepper
- 2 tablespoons finely chopped flat-leaf parsley

Instructions:

- In a large saucepan, heat the oil over medium-high heat.
- Cook, stirring occasionally, for 10 minutes, or until the vegetables have softened, adding the carrot, celery, bay leaf, and turmeric.
- 10 cups (2.5 litres) water, chicken carcasses, and thyme and marjoram sprigs Bring to a boil, then lower to a low heat and cook for 1 hour, partially covered.
- Remove the chicken carcasses and lay them aside to cool for ten minutes. Discard the bones and shred the meat into tiny pieces. Remove the bay leaf and herb sprigs from the mixture.
- Bring the soup to a low boil, then add the shredded chicken, sliced chicken thigh, and corn and cook for another 8 minutes.
- Meanwhile, cover the vermicelli noodles with boiling water and soak until softened. Drain.
- Cook for a further 2 minutes after adding the noodles to the soup. Season with salt and pepper and a sprinkle of parsley, then stir in the chopped thyme and marjoram.

28. Lemon Chicken and Rice Soup

Prep time: 50min | Serves: 4 | Difficulty: Moderate
Nutrition: Calories: 315 kcal | Fat: 8 g | Protein: 19 g | Carbohydrates: 38 g
Ingredients:

- 1 tablespoon olive oil
- 2 pounds boneless skinless chicken thighs, visible fat removed, sliced Grated zest and
- juice of 2 lemons, plus 1/2 cup additional lemon juice
- 1 tablespoon superfine sugar
- 1 cup white rice
- 3 stalks celery, finely sliced
- 1 tablespoon chopped flat-leaf parsley
- Salt and freshly ground black pepper

Instructions:

- In a large heavy-bottomed saucepan, heat the oil over medium-high heat.
- Cook, tossing often until the chicken is golden brown on both sides.
- Bring 8 cups (2 liters) of water to a boil. Reduce the heat to a low setting. Simmer, covered, for 20 to 30 minutes with the lemon zest and juice (including the excess liquid).
- Cook for 10 minutes after adding the rice to the pan.
- Cook for a further 5 minutes, or until the rice is soft, after adding the celery. Serve immediately after adding the parsley and seasoning to taste.

29. Cream of Potato and Parsnip Soup

Prep time: 50min | Serves: 4 | Difficulty: Moderate
Nutrition: Calories: 278 kcal | Fat: 8 g | Protein: 8 g | Carbohydrates: 29 g
Ingredients:

- 1 tablespoon canola oil
- 1 stalk celery, very thinly sliced
- 6 parsnips, peeled and finely diced
- 2 potatoes, peeled and finely diced
- 3 cups (750 ml) onion-free vegetable stock (gluten-free if following a gluten-free diet)
- 1/2 cup low-fat milk, lactose-free milk, or suitable plant-based milk
- 1/3 cup (80 g) crumbled feta
- Salt and freshly ground black pepper
- 2 tablespoons chopped chives

Instructions:

- In a medium saucepan over medium-low heat, heat the oil.
- Cook for 5 to 6 minutes, until the celery, is cooked and golden brown.
- Cook, occasionally stirring, for 1 to 2 minutes after adding the parsnips and potatoes. Bring the stock to a boil, then lower to low heat and cover and cook for 15 to 20 minutes, until the veggies are soft.
- Remove from the heat and leave aside to cool for 10 minutes. Combine the veggies and stock in a food processor, working in batches if required.
- Blend in the milk and feta cheese until smooth. Return the soup to the saucepan and heat over medium heat, constantly stirring, until it barely comes to a boil. (Alternatively, use an immersion blender to purée the milk and feta in the pot until smooth.)
- Season with salt and pepper after removing from the fire. Pour the soup into four bowls and top with chopped chives.

30. Pork Ragout

Prep time: 2hr | Serves: 8 | Difficulty: Moderate
Nutrition: Calories: 466 kcal | Fat: 16 g | Protein: 38 g | Carbohydrates: 18 g
Ingredients:

- 3 tablespoons garlic-infused canola oil
- 3-to 4-pound bone-in pork leg or center-cut pork loin, trimmed of fat 2 carrots, peeled and diced
- 2 stalks celery, diced
- 2 bay leaves
- 2 tablespoons chopped sage leaves
- 2 cups (onion-free chicken stock (gluten-free if following a gluten-free diet)
- 1 28-ounce can tomato puree
- 4 Yukon Gold potatoes, diced
- Salt and freshly ground black pepper
- Polenta, rice, gluten-free pasta, or mashed potatoes

Instructions:

- In a large flameproof casserole or Dutch oven, heat 2 tablespoons of the oil over medium-high heat.
- Cook for 2 to 3 minutes on each side until the pork is browned all over. Remove the pork from the pan and place it on a platter.
- In the same saucepan, heat the remaining oil, then add the carrots, celery, bay leaves, and sage and simmer, often stirring, for 5 minutes, or until the veggies soften.
- Combine the stock, tomato puree, potatoes, and meat in a large mixing bowl. Bring to a boil, then lower to a low heat setting and cover. Simmer for 11/2 hours, or until the pork is cooked, regularly tossing and basting the pig with the liquid.
- Remove Bring the sauce to a boil by increasing the heat to medium-high. Simmer for 20 minutes or until the sauce has thickened.
- Remove the meat off the bone and cut it into big chunks to add to the sauce.
- Serve over polenta, rice, gluten-free spaghetti, or mashed potatoes, and season with salt and pepper.

---

31. Lamb and Sweet Potato Curry

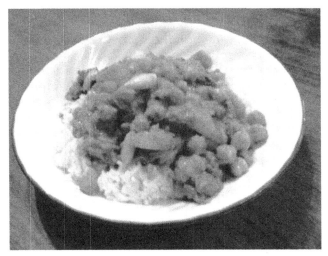

Prep time: 1hr-10min| Serves: 8| Difficulty: Moderate
Nutrition: Calories: 498 kcal |Fat: 18 g |Protein: 27 g |Carbohydrates:43 g
Ingredients:
- 1 tablespoon cornstarch
- 1/2 teaspoon paprika
- 1/2 teaspoon garam masala
- Salt and freshly ground black pepper
- 11/2 pounds boneless lamb loin chops, cut into 1-inch cubes
- 1/2 cup garlic-infused canola oil

- 1 to 2 tablespoons curry powder (gluten-free if following a gluten-free diet)
- 4 stalks celery, sliced
- 2 teaspoons tomato paste
- 2 cups (500 ml) onion-free beef stock (gluten-free if following a gluten-free diet
- 1 bay leaf
- One 14.5-ounce (425 g) can of crushed tomatoes
- 2 sweet potatoes, cut into 1/2-inch (1 cm) cubes
- 2 cups (40 g) baby spinach leaves
- Cooked basmati rice

Instructions:
- In a large mixing basin, combine the cornstarch, paprika, garam masala, salt, and pepper. Add the lamb and toss to coat.
- In a large nonstick skillet, heat little over half of the oil over medium heat. Heat for 1 to 2 minutes until the curry powder is aromatic.
- Toss the remaining oil, lamb, and celery in the pan until both sides of the meat are browned. Combine the tomato paste, stock, and bay leaf in a mixing bowl.
- Raise the heat to be high and bring the mixture to a boil, stirring often. Reduce to medium-low heat, add the crushed tomatoes, and cook for 50 to 60 minutes until the meat is cooked.
- Meanwhile, cook the sweet potatoes until just soft in a small saucepan of boiling water. Drain. Stir in the sweet potatoes and spinach until the spinach is completely wilted. Serve with a side of rice.

---

32. Warming Winter Beef Soup

Prep time: 1hr-10min| Serves: 4| Difficulty: Moderate
Nutrition: Calories: 378 kcal |Fat: 12 g |Protein:29 g |Carbohydrates:22 g
Ingredients:
- 1/3 cup cornstarch
- Salt and freshly ground black pepper
- 2 pounds chuck beef or beef stew meat, cut into 1/2-inch (1 cm) cubes
- 3 tablespoons vegetable oil
- 2 large carrots, peeled and diced
- 2 large stalks celery, diced
- 3 cups onion-free beef stock (gluten-free if following a gluten-free diet)
- 1 cup dry red wine, or additional onion-free beef stock
- 11/2 cupsTomato puree
- 2 teaspoons finely grated orange zest
- 1/4 teaspoon ground allspice
- 1/4 teaspoon crushed red pepper
- 1 cup pitted kalamata olives, sliced
- 1/3 cup chopped flat-leaf parsley

Instructions:

- In a large heavy-bottomed saucepan or stockpot, heat 1 tablespoon of the oil over medium-low heat.
- Cook for 6 to 8 minutes, until the carrots and celery are cooked and golden.
- Remove from the pan and place on a dish to cool. In the same pan, heat 1 tablespoon of oil and add half of the meat.
- Cook and stir until both sides are golden brown, then transfer to a dish with the veggies. Continue with the remaining meat and oil.
- Return the meat and veggies to the pan. Bring the stock, wine, and tomato puree to a boil over medium-high heat.
- Scrape up any browned chunks of meat from the bottom of the pan as you stir. Combine the orange zest, allspice, and crushed red pepper in a mixing bowl.
- Bring to a boil, then lower to medium-low heat and cook for 1 hour, stirring occasionally.
- Serve with the olives and parsley, seasoning to suit.

33. Beef Korma

Prep time: 3hr | Serves: 4-6 | Difficulty: Moderate
Nutrition: Calories: 332 kcal | Fat: 14 g | Protein: 29 g | Carbohydrates: 18 g
Ingredients:

- 1/4 cup garlic-infused canola oil
- 3 tablespoons ground almonds
- 2 teaspoons grated ginger
- 1 1/2 teaspoons paprika
- 1 teaspoon ground coriander
- 1 teaspoon turmeric
- 1/2 teaspoon ground cinnamon
- 1/2 teaspoon ground cardamom
- 1/2 teaspoon chili powder
- 1/2 teaspoon ground mace, optional
- 1/4 teaspoon ground cloves
- 2 pounds beef tenderloin, cut into 1/2-inch cubes
- 1 cup low-fat plain yogurt (gluten-free if following a gluten-free diet)
- 1/2 cup light sour cream Cilantro leaves
- Cooked rice

Instructions:

- In a large heavy-bottomed saucepan or stockpot, heat the oil over medium-high heat.
- Stir in the almonds, ginger, paprika, coriander, turmeric, cinnamon, cardamom, chili powder, mace (if wanted), and cloves until aromatic, about 30 to 60 seconds.
- Toss in the meat to cover it with the seasonings. Cook, occasionally stirring, for a few minutes, or until golden brown on both sides. Reduce the heat to low and continue to cook for another 5 minutes.

- Add half of the yoghurt and half of the sour cream, cover, and cook over low heat for 2 hours, or until the meat is cooked, occasionally stirring to avoid sticking.
- Cook, constantly stirring, until the remaining yogurt and sour cream are cooked through. Serve with rice and garnished with cilantro.

34. Chicken Stock

Prep time: 12min | Serves: 4 | Difficulty: Moderate
Nutrition: Calories: 310 kcal | Fat: 13 g | Protein: 11 g | Carbohydrates: 38 g
Ingredients:

- 2 onions, peeled and coarsely chopped
- 1 cleaned and sliced leek
- 1 peeled and roughly chopped turnip
- 4 sliced carrots
- 4 celery stalks, chopped
- 2 chicken carcasses, cooked
- 1 marjoram sprig
- 1 thyme sprig
- 1 rosemary sprig
- 4 bay leaves (fresh) ten black peppercorns
- 10 cups cold water (enough to cover the bones)

Instructions

- In a large pot, combine all of the ingredients and enough water to cover the chicken bones.
- Bring the pot of water to a boil. Reduce the heat to low and cook for 2 to 3 hours, adding more water as needed if the water level falls below the bones. Remove the froth that forms on the surface of the stock using a spoon while it is simmering.
- Using a sieve, strain the stock one more. The stock should then be strained again using a finer mesh sieve, kitchen towel, or muslin cloth.
- Remove the fat that rises to the top of the stock and pour it into containers to chill.

35. Beef Stock

Prep time: 3hr15min | Serves: 8 | Difficulty: Moderate
Nutrition: Calories: 281 kcal | Fat: 12 g | Protein: 31 g | Carbohydrates: 28 g
Ingredients:

- 2 onions, skin on, roughly chopped
- 1 leek, washed and chopped
- 1 turnip, peeled and chopped
- 4 carrots, peeled and chopped
- 1 cup mushroom stems, chopped
- 4 stalks celery, chopped 1-pound mix of veal, beef, or pork bones
- 2 tablespoons tomato paste
- 4 cloves garlic, peeled
- 8 stems parsley
- 8 black peppercorns
- Coldwater (enough to cover the bones — about 10 to 12 cups

Instructions

- In a large pot, combine all of the ingredients and enough water to cover the bones. Bring to a boil, then reduce to a low heat and cook for 2 to 3 hours, adding more water if the liquid level falls below the bones. Remove the froth that forms on the surface of the stock using a spoon while it is simmering.
- Using a sieve, strain the stock one more. Using a finer mesh sieve, kitchen towel, or muslin cloth, strain it a second time.
- Pour the soup into cooling containers, skimming off any fat that rises to the top before covering and storing.

36. Shellfish Stock

Prep time: 25min | Serves: 8 | Difficulty: Moderate
Nutrition: Calories: 291 kcal | Fat: 8 g | Protein: 22 g | Carbohydrates: 12 g
Ingredients:
- 2 pounds mixed seafood shells, such as shrimp and lobster
- 1 onion, peel on, quartered
- 10 whole black peppercorns
- 1 lemon, halved
- 1 bay leaf
- Cold water (enough to cover the ingredients by at least 1 inch — at least 10 cups)

Instructions
- Combine the shrimp and or lobster shells, onion, black peppercorns, lemon, and bay leaf in a large stockpot. Bring the ingredients to a boil by covering them with cold water by at least 1 inch.
- Reduce to a low heat and cook for about 20 minutes. Using a fine mesh strainer or a tea towel, strain the stock. Cool the stock in 1 cup containers before covering and storing them.

37. Vegetable Stock

Prep time: 1hr15min | Serves: 8 | Difficulty: Moderate
Nutrition: Calories: 274 Kcal | Fat: 18 g | Protein: 23 g | Carbohydrates: 6 g
Ingredients:
- 2 /3 pound each chopped mushrooms, chopped asparagus, and chopped broccoli stems
- 1 onion
- 10 black peppercorns
- 1 bay leaf
- Cold water (enough to cover the vegetables — about 10 cups)

Instructions
- Combine the shrimp and or lobster shells, onion, black peppercorns, lemon, and bay leaf in a large stockpot. Bring the ingredients to a boil by

covering them with cold water by at least 1 inch.
- Reduce to a low heat and cook for about 20 minutes. Using a fine mesh strainer or a tea towel, strain the stock. Cool the stock in 1 cup containers before covering and storing them.

38. Quinoa Soup with Miso

Prep time: 35min | Serves: 8 | Difficulty: Moderate
Nutrition: Calories: 245 kcal | Fat: 8 g | Protein:11 g | Carbohydrates:32 g
Ingredients:
- 2 tablespoons olive oil
- 1 /2 cup diced onion
- 2 garlic cloves, finely diced
- 2 carrots, sliced and cut in half moons
- 2 celery stalks, sliced
- 2 medium red potatoes, cut in quarter moons with skin
- 1 zucchini, cut in quarter moons
- 1 teaspoon salt
- 3 cups chicken stock
- 2 cups water
- 1 cup cooked quinoa
- 1 /2 teaspoon dry basil
- 1 /4 teaspoon dry oregano
- 3 tablespoons white miso paste

Instructions
- Heat the olive oil in a medium-sized pot and sauté the onion until transparent. Cook everything together for 5 minutes, including the garlic, carrots, and celery.
- Combine the potatoes, zucchini, salt, chicken stock, and water in a large mixing bowl. Bring to a boil, then reduce to a low heat for 15 minutes. Meanwhile, prepare the quinoa according to the package recommendations.
- Cook for 5 minutes with the cooked quinoa, basil, and oregano in a medium-sized pot. Turn the heat off. Stir in the white miso paste until it has completely dissolved.

39. Red Lentil and Coconut Soup

Prep time: 50min | Serves: 6 | Difficulty: Moderate
Nutrition: Calories: 401 kcal | Fat: 15 g | Protein: 21 g | Carbohydrates: 29 g
Ingredients:
- 2 tablespoons olive oil
- 1 onion, chopped
- 2 carrots, chopped
- 13/4 cups red lentils, rinsed
- 4 cups vegetable stock One 14-ounce can coconut milk
- 4 cloves garlic
- 1 /2 teaspoon salt
- 2 teaspoons lemon juice
- 11 /2 tablespoons white miso paste

Instructions

- Heat the olive oil in a large soup pot over medium-low heat. Sauté the onion and carrot for about 2 minutes, or until the onions are tender. In a large pot, combine the lentils, stock, coconut milk, garlic, and salt. Bring to a boil, stirring constantly.
- Stir the liquid again once it has reached a boil. Reduce the heat to the lowest setting, cover, and cook for 30 minutes. When the lentils are completely soft, remove the saucepan from the heat.
- Fill a blender halfway with soup and puree until smooth. Return the soup to the pot and toss in the lemon juice, white miso paste, and any other seasonings to taste. Add more vegetable stock if the soup becomes too thick.
- Pour into serving dishes.

40. Pasta e Fagioli (Yummy Italian Pasta and Bean Soup)

Prep time: 35min | Serves: 6 | Difficulty: Moderate
Nutrition: Calories: 410 kcal | Fat: 16 g | Protein: 18 g | Carbohydrates: 49 g
Ingredients:

- One 15-ounce can pinto beans, rinsed well
- 2 cups water
- 1/3 cup white rice
- 1 tablespoon olive oil
- 1/4 cup chopped celery
- 1/2 cup chopped onion
- 2 cloves garlic, minced
- 2 cups blanched tomatoes Two
- 32-ounce containers chicken broth
- 1/4 cup chopped fresh parsley
- 1 teaspoon dried basil
- 1/4 teaspoon ground black pepper
- 11/2 cups dried short pasta

Instructions

- Three fourth of a pinto bean can should be placed in a medium-sized bowl. Use a potato masher to mash the beans.
- In a medium saucepan over high heat, bring the water to a boil. Stir in the white rice. Cover the saucepan and reduce the heat to just below medium, maintaining the water at a moderate boil (the lid should not hop up and down).
- In a big pot over medium heat, heat the olive oil until a drop of water flicked from your fingers sizzles in it. Stir in the celery, onion, and garlic for 3 to 5 minutes, or until the onion is softened and translucent.
- Bring the tomatoes, pinto beans (mashed and unmashed), chicken stock, parsley, basil, and black pepper to a boil, stirring occasionally, over high heat. Reduce the heat to about midway between medium and low after a minute or so, and continue to cook for at least 10 minutes.

- Add the pasta, slightly increase the heat, and cook for 8 to 12 minutes until the pasta is done.

41. Lentil Soup from the Source

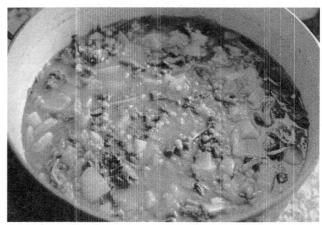

Prep time: 60min | Serves: 4 | Difficulty: Moderate
Nutrition: Calories: 276 kcal | Fat: 7.3 g | Protein: 21 g | Carbohydrates: 15.8 g
Ingredients:

- 2 teaspoons butter
- 1 carrot, chopped
- 1/2 of a medium yellow onion, chopped
- 1/2 of capsicum (a type of red pepper)
- 41/2 cups water
- 11/2 to 2 cups raw pumpkin, de-skinned and chopped into small chunks
- Two 15-ounce cans cooked lentils, drained and rinsed, or 12 ounces of dry lentils, rinsed well but not soaked
- 3 to 4 cups fresh spinach

Instructions

- Add the butter to a large pot and sauté the carrots, onion, and capsicum for a few minutes. Boil the vegetables with the water and pumpkin until they're tender. If you're using dry lentils, place them in this pot and cook for 30 minutes.
- Add the canned lentils and fresh spinach if you're using them.
- Remove one-third of the mixture from the pan and puree it in a blender, hand blender, or food processor. Return the blended-down portion to the pot, stir to combine, and serve.

42. Borscht (Beet Soup)

Prep time: 55min | Serves: 8 | Difficulty: Moderate
Nutrition: Calories: 305 kcal | Fat: 27 g | Protein: 15 g | Carbohydrates: 2 g
Ingredients:

- Two 32-ounce containers chicken broth
- 2 medium potatoes, chopped into small squares or grated
- 1 tablespoon olive oil
- 1 small onion, chopped

- 1 /3 cup red or green cabbage, grated or chopped
- 2 carrots, grated
- 5 medium beets, grated
- 1 tomato, blanched and chopped coarsely
- 1 tablespoon fresh parsley, or 1 tablespoon dried parsley
- 1 teaspoon dried dill, or 1 tablespoon fresh dill
- 1 bay leaf (optional)
- 1 teaspoon lemon juice

Instructions
- Bring the chicken stock to a boil in a big pot, then add the potatoes. If the potatoes are grated, boil for 3 minutes; if the potatoes are chunks, boil for 5 minutes.
- In a medium pot, heat the olive oil, toss in the onion, and cook, stirring periodically, until the onion is slightly translucent (approximately 2 to 5 minutes).
- Add the cabbage to the first pot after the 3 or 5 minutes from Step 1 have gone and cook for another 5 minutes.
- When the onion in the second pot is clear, add the carrots and cook for 2 to 3 minutes, stirring regularly.
- Cook for a minute with the grated beets, carrots, and onions in the pot. Then add the tomato and cook for another minute in a stir-fry. Stir in the parsley, dill, and bay leaf (if using) for one additional minute.
- Combine all of the ingredients in a pot with the chicken stock, add the lemon juice, and cook for 30 minutes.
- When the vegetables are soft, serve (making sure to remove any bay leaf).

43. Orange Chicken Soup

Prep time: 1hr20min | Serves: 16 | Difficulty: Moderate
Nutrition: Calories: 333 kcal | Fat: 9 g | Protein: 21 g | Carbohydrates: 22 g
Ingredients:
- 4 quarts chicken broth
- 1/4 cup uncooked white or brown rice
- 1 pound carrots, peeled and coarsely chopped
- 1 small butternut or acorn squash, peeled and coarsely chopped
- 2 medium yams/sweet potatoes, peeled and coarsely chopped
- 1 apple, peeled and coarsely chopped
- 1/2 teaspoon cinnamon (optional)
- 1/2 teaspoon nutmeg (optional)
- 1 teaspoon lemon juice

Instructions
- Combine the chicken stock and rice in a large pot and bring to a boil. Add the carrots, squash, yams, and apple, chopped. Combine the cinnamon and/or nutmeg in a bowl (if desired).

- Allow the soup to cook at a low boil (you should still see bubbles, but the cover shouldn't be flying up and down) for 10 to 15 minutes, stirring occasionally, until the vegetables are soft and mushy (about 20 to 60 minutes; you can start checking them with a fork after about 30 minutes).
- When the soup is still hot or lukewarm, puree it. (Don't puree the soup until it's completely cold; it'll be more difficult to purée that way.) Return the pureed soup to the pot. Juice should be stirred. Eat and enjoy.

44. Creamy Broccoli Soup in the Raw

Prep time: 2hr5min | Serves: 4 | Difficulty: Moderate
Nutrition: Calories: 287 kcal | Fat: 8 g | Protein: 13 g | Carbohydrates: 18 g
Ingredients:
- 1 1/2 cups raw cashews, soaked for 2 hours
- 2 cups chopped broccoli
- 2 cups water
- 1/8 teaspoon each salt and black pepper, or to taste
- 1 /4 teaspoon each powdered sage, dried thyme, and garlic powder

Instructions
- Drain and rinse the raw cashews after soaking them for at least 2 hours.
- In a blender, combine the soaked cashews, broccoli, water, and desired seasonings until smooth. After combining, chill the soup for about 30 minutes in the refrigerator.
- Serve with sprouted bread pieces (such as manna or Essene, which can be found in the freezer department of your local health food store), Rice Mochi (pounded rice moulded into flat cakes, which may also be found in the freezer section of your local health food store), or corn chips.

45. Raw Curry Spinach Soup

Prep time: 8min | Serves: 2 | Difficulty: Moderate
Nutrition: Calories: 256 kcal | Fat: 8 g | Protein: 11 g | Carbohydrates: 32 g
Ingredients:
- 1 bunch fresh spinach
- 1/4 cup fresh dill
- 1/2 of a red bell pepper
- 1 small ripe tomato
- 1/2 of an avocado
- 1/4 of a small onion (optional)
- 1 tablespoon Nama Shoyu (raw organic soy sauce)
- 2 tablespoons lemon juice
- 1 teaspoon curry powder
- 1/2 cup water
- 1/2 diced red or orange bell pepper

Instructions
- In a blender or food processor, combine all of the ingredients.
- Blend until smooth, then eat.

46. Carrot Ginger Soup

Prep time: 20min | Serves: 4 | Difficulty: Moderate
Nutrition: Calories: 274 Kcal | Fat: 18 g | Protein: 23 g | Carbohydrates: 6 g
Ingredients:
- 2 pounds organic carrots, or 3 cups carrot juice
- 2 ripe avocados, peeled and pitted
- 1 1/2 teaspoon salt
- 1 1/2 teaspoons lemon juice
- 1 teaspoon peeled and grated ginger
- Diced avocado or crème fraîche for serving
Instructions
- If using carrots, juice them to produce around 3 cups of carrot juice in a juicer.
- Blend the carrot juice, avocados, salt, lemon juice, and ginger until smooth in a high-powered blender.
- If preferred, season with extra lemon, ginger, or salt. Serve in bowls, topped with chopped avocado or crème fraîche.

47. French Lentil Salad

Prep time: 20min | Serves: 4 | Difficulty: Moderate
Nutrition: Calories: 355 kcal | Fat: 7 g | Protein: 19 g | Carbohydrates: 21 g
Ingredients:
- 2 tablespoons fresh thyme
- 1/2 cup (about 3 large) shallots, finely chopped Juice of one lemon (about 1/4 cup)
- Juice of 1/2 grapefruit (about 1/4 cup)
- 2 tablespoons ground cumin
- 1 tablespoon celery salt
- 2 teaspoons curry powder (no fillers or starches added)
- 1 teaspoon ground coriander
- 3 cloves garlic, minced
- 1 tablespoon freshly grated lemon zest
- 1/2 cup extra virgin olive oil
- 1/2 teaspoon cayenne pepper
- 2 cups cooked French green lentils
- 1/2 cup currants 1 fennel bulb, sliced very thinly with fronds removed
- 4 stalks of celery (about 1 cup), strings removed and finely chopped
- 1 cup fresh flat-leaf parsley, chopped
- 1/2 cup fresh cilantro, chopped
Instructions
- Thyme, shallots, lemon juice, grapefruit juice, cumin, celery salt, curry powder, coriander, garlic, lemon zest, olive oil, and cayenne pepper should all be combined in a large mixing basin. Combine all of the ingredients in a mixing bowl.

- Add the currants, fennel, celery, parsley, and cilantro to the lentils and pour the juice mixture over them. Mix thoroughly.

48. Cauliflower Salad with Dairy-Free Dill Dressing

Prep time: 25min | Serves: 4 | Difficulty: Moderate
Nutrition: Calories: 311 kcal | Fat: 8 g | Protein: 21 g | Carbohydrates: 23 g
Ingredients:
- 1 large head of cauliflower
- 1 medium red bell pepper, finely diced
- 1/4 cup red onion, minced
- 1/4 teaspoon salt, or more to taste
- 4 grinder-turns freshly ground pepper (about 1/8 teaspoon), or more to taste Dairy-Free Dill Dressing
Instructions
- Remove the cauliflower stem and discard it, then chop the head into small florets. Steam the cauliflower in a steamer basket over boiling water for 3 to 5 minutes, or until somewhat soft but still crisp and crunchy. Remove the pot from the heat and set it aside to cool.
- In the bowl of a food processor, place the cooled cauliflower. Using a food processor, coarsely chop the cauliflower. Pour into a medium mixing basin and use a knife to chop any leftover large pieces.
- Add the red bell pepper, red onion, salt, and pepper, as well as enough dressing to coat the red bell pepper and red onion. Season with salt and pepper to taste. Set aside a little amount of minced onion or bell pepper for garnish.

49. Dairy-Free Dill Dressing

Prep time: 28min | Serves: 4 | Difficulty: Moderate
Nutrition: Calories: 254 kcal | Fat:6 g | Protein: 19 g | Carbohydrates:26 g
Ingredients:
- One 12-ounce package silken tofu
- 1 medium clove of garlic
- Juice of one lemon (about 1/4 cup)
- 4 tablespoons extra-virgin olive oil
- 1 tablespoon Dijon mustard
- 2 teaspoons sea salt
- 4 tablespoons fresh dill, chopped
Instructions
- Boil some water in a small pot. Allow the water to return to a boil before adding the silken tofu and simmering for 3 minutes. Using a mesh strainer, sieve the tofu.
- In a food processor, finely chop the garlic. Combine the tofu, half of the lemon juice, olive oil, mustard, and sea salt in a mixing bowl. Blend until completely smooth. If necessary, season with extra salt and lemon juice.

- Pour into a bowl, whisk in the dill, and place in the refrigerator for 12 to 2 hours to allow the flavors to meld. Taste again, and if required, season with additional lemon juice, salt, or garlic.

50. Sprouted Salad

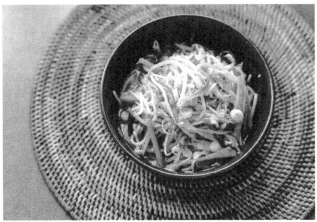

Prep time: 5min | Serves: 7 | Difficulty: Moderate
Nutrition: Calories: 202 kcal | Fat: 8 g | Protein: 17 g | Carbohydrates: 12 g
Ingredients:
- 1 cup each sunflower, broccoli, and alfalfa sprouts
- 1 head butternut lettuce
- 1 ripe avocado, halved, pitted, and peeled
Instructions
- Chop the sprouts and lettuce finely, and cut the avocado into cubes.
- Dress by combining all of the components.

51. Soba Salad

Prep time: 30min | Serves: 4 | Difficulty: Moderate
Nutrition: Calories: 305 kcal | Fat: 27 g | Protein: 15 g | Carbohydrates: 2 g
Ingredients:
- 4 quarts water, salted
- 1/2 cup broccoli florets
- 1/2 cup cauliflower florets
- 8 ounces soba noodles
- 1 tablespoon toasted sesame oil
- 1 cup thinly sliced red cabbage
- 1 head green or ruby leaf lettuce, washed, drained and thinly sliced
- 1/2 cup tahini
- 1/2 cup water
- 2 teaspoons fresh lemon juice or brown rice vinegar
- 4 medium radishes, thinly sliced into rounds
- 2 medium carrots, shredded
- 1 scallion, white and green parts, thinly sliced

Instructions
- In a large pot, bring 4 quarts of salted water to a boil. Add the broccoli and blanch until barely tender, about 3 minutes. Remove with a slotted spoon and immediately plunge into a bowl of ice water or rinse under cold water to stop the cooking. Repeat the process with the cauliflower, using the same water. When cool, drain the vegetables and set aside.
- Add the noodles to the boiling pot and cook for 6 to 8 minutes until just tender. Drain the noodles and immediately rinse under cold water. Sprinkle with the sesame oil and toss to keep the noodles from sticking.
- Combine the cabbage and lettuce in a serving bowl. Place the noodles on top and arrange the cauliflower and broccoli around the edges.
- Whisk the tahini, water, and lemon juice or vinegar in a small bowl until well combined. Pour the dressing over the salad and top with the radishes, carrots and scallions.

52. Cobb Salad with Angie's Vinaigrette

Prep time: 10min | Serves: 6 | Difficulty: Moderate
Nutrition: Calories: 167 kcal | Fat: 9 g | Protein: 12 g | Carbohydrates: 16 g
Ingredients:
- 10 ounces spinach leaves, chopped
- 3 eggs, hardboiled, peeled, and chopped into small pieces
- 1 medium tomato, chopped
- 1 to 2 avocados, stones removed and flesh scooped out of shell and sliced
- 10 ripe black olives, pitted and finely chopped
- 1/4 to 1/2 cup grated cheddar cheese
- 1 /4 cup SCD-safe bacon bits (sugar-free, smoked bacon fried very crisp)
- Angie's Vinaigrette (see the following recipe)
Instructions
- In a salad bowl, combine the spinach, egg, tomato, and avocado.
- Add the olives, cheese, and bacon bits to the top of the salad. Toss the salad with the dressing.

53. Citrus Marinated Salad

Prep time: 3hr 50min | Serves: 6 | Difficulty: Moderate
Nutrition: Calories: 274 Kcal | Fat: 18 g | Protein: 23 g | Carbohydrates: 6 g
Ingredients:
- 1/2 a medium green cabbage
- 2 large carrots
- 4 cups orange juice
- Juice of 4 lemons (about 1 cup)
- 1/4 cup umeboshi plum vinegar
- 2 tablespoons salt, divided
- 1/2 a medium red cabbage
- 1/4 cup apple cider vinegar

- 1 tablespoon salt
- 2 tablespoons toasted sesame seeds

Instructions

- Green cabbage should be thinly sliced, and carrots should be cut into 2-inch long sticks, then cut lengthwise to produce several thin wafers. Place in a big mixing basin.
- Toss the veggies with 2 cups orange juice, 12 cup lemon juice, and the umeboshi vinegar, and mix everything together with your hands.

- Allow the combination to marinade for 1 hour or until desired tenderness is reached, making sure the liquid completely covers the veggies (weighting them down with a plate if required) (anywhere between 30 minutes and 3 hours).
- Slice the red cabbage thinly and combine with the apple cider vinegar, leftover orange and lemon juice in a large mixing basin. Add the salt and stir it in with your hands. Allow the cabbage to rest.

Chapter 8: Desserts

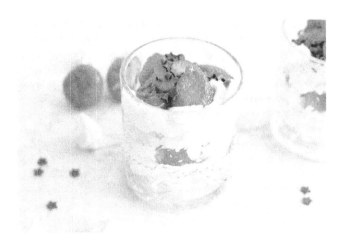

1. Macadamia–Chocolate Chip Cookies

Prep time: 30 min | Serves: 20 | Difficulty: Moderate
Nutrition: Calories: 202 Kcal | Fat: 13 g | Protein: 16 g | Carbohydrates:13 g
Ingredients
- 8 tablespoons unsalted butter, cut into cubes, at room temperature
- 1/4 cup packed light brown sugar
- 1/4 cup superfine sugar
- 1 large egg
- 1 teaspoon vanilla extract
- 2/3 cup superfine white rice flour
- 1/2 cup cornstarch
- 1/4 cup soy flour
- 1/2 teaspoon baking soda
- 1/2 cup (95 g) chocolate chips
- 1/2 cup (70 g) roasted unsalted macadamia nuts, roughly chopped

Instructions
- Preheat the oven to 325 degrees Fahrenheit (170 degrees Celsius). Preheat oven to 350°F. Line two baking pans with parchment paper.
- In a medium mixing basin, cream together the butter, brown sugar, and superfine sugar with a handheld electric mixer until thick and pale.
- In a separate bowl, whisk together the egg and vanilla extract. In a mixing bowl, sift the rice flour, cornstarch, soy flour, and baking soda three times (or whisk in the bowl until well combined).
- Toss the chocolate chips and macadamia nuts into the butter mixture and whip thoroughly. Drop spoonful of dough onto the sheets, providing enough space for them to spread.
- Preheat oven to 350°F and bake for 10 to 15 minutes, or until golden brown. Cool for 5 minutes on the sheets before transferring to a wire rack to cool fully.

2. Almond Cookies

Prep time: 40 min | Serves: 40 | Difficulty: Moderate
Nutrition: Calories: 277 kcal | Fat: 7 g | Protein: 12 g | Carbohydrates: 22 g
Ingredients
- 3/4 cup almond flour
- 1 tablespoon plus 1 teaspoon cornstarch
- 1/2 teaspoon gluten-free baking powder
- 1 large egg white
- 1/2 cup superfine sugar
- 1 teaspoon finely grated lemon zest
- 3 drops almond extract
- 1 tablespoon unsalted butter, melted

Instructions
- Preheat the oven to 275 degrees Fahrenheit (140 degrees Celsius). Preheat oven to 350°F. Line two baking pans with parchment paper.
- In a small mixing bowl, combine the almond flour, cornstarch, and baking powder. In a clean medium bowl, whisk the egg whites with a handheld electric mixer until soft peaks form.
- Gradually incorporate the sugar. Continue to beat for another 5 minutes, or until stiff peaks appear. With a big metal spoon, gradually combine the almond flour mixture, lemon zest, almond essence, and melted butter. 2 tablespoons dough rolled into a ball
- Make approximately 40 balls with the remaining dough, placing them on the baking pans with a little room for spreading.
- Slightly flatten. Bake for 25 minutes, or until a light golden color has appeared. Cool for 5 minutes on the sheets before transferring to a wire rack to cool fully.

3. Peanut Butter and Sesame Cookies

Prep time: 25 min | Serves: 20-25 | Difficulty: Moderate
Nutrition: Calories: 191 kcal | Fat: 10 g | Protein: 3 g | Carbohydrates: 23 g
Ingredients
- 2 tablespoons unsalted butter, at room temperature
- 1 cup creamy peanut butter
- 1/4 cup packed light brown sugar
- 2 heaping tablespoons superfine sugar
- 2 large eggs, lightly beaten
- 1 teaspoon vanilla extract
- 1/4 cup sesame seeds
- 2/3 cup superfine white rice flour
- 3/4 cup cornstarch
- 1/2 cup soy flour

- 1/2 teaspoon baking soda
- 1 teaspoon xanthan gum or guar gum

Instructions

- Preheat the oven to 350 degrees Fahrenheit (170 degrees Celsius). Preheat oven to 350°F. Line two baking pans with parchment paper.
- In a medium mixing basin, cream together the butter, peanut butter, brown sugar, and superfine sugar with a handheld electric mixer until smooth. Mix in the eggs, vanilla, and sesame seeds well.
- In a large mixing bowl, sift the rice flour, cornstarch, soy flour, baking soda, and xanthan gum three times (or whisk in the bowl until well combined).
- Add to the peanut butter mixture and stir until completely blended with a big metal spoon. Form the dough into walnut-sized balls and place on the baking sheets, leaving some space for spreading.
- Gently flatten to a thickness of approximately 14 inch (5 mm). Preheat oven to 350°F and bake for 10 to 12 minutes, or until golden brown. Cool for 5 minutes on the sheets before transferring to a wire rack to cool fully.

---

4. Hazelnut or Almond Crescents

Prep time: 45 min| Serves: 40| Difficulty: Moderate
Nutrition: Calories: 274 Kcal |Fat: 18 g| Protein: 23 g | Carbohydrates: 6 g

Ingredients

- 1/3 cup superfine white rice flour, plus more for the work surface
- 1/4 cup cornstarch
- 1/4 cup superfine sugar
- 11/4 cups hazelnut or almond flour
- 7 tablespoons unsalted butter, cut into cubes, at room temperature
- 1 large egg yolk, at room temperature, lightly beaten
- 1 teaspoon vanilla extract
- 1/2 cup confectioners' sugar, plus more for dusting

Instructions

- In a medium mixing bowl, sift together the rice flour and cornstarch (or whisk in the bowl until well combined). Combine the superfine sugar and hazelnut flour in a mixing bowl.
- With your fingertips, rub in the butter until the mixture resembles bread crumbs. With a big metal spoon, fold in the egg yolk and vanilla extract.
- Using rice flour, lightly dust your work surface. Form the dough into a ball and roll it out onto a floured board, kneading lightly until smooth.
- Refrigerate for 15 minutes after dividing the dough into two even halves and wrapping each

in plastic wrap. Preheat the oven to 325°F (160°C) while the dough is chilling.

- Preheat oven to 350°F. Line two baking pans with parchment paper. Remove the dough from the wrapper and roll each part into a 34-inch log (2 cm). Cut 34- to 1-inch (2- to 3-cm) slices with your hands and form them into circular crescents.
- Place on baking pans with enough space between them to allow for spreading. Bake for 15 to 20 minutes, or until golden brown. Allow to cool for 5 minutes on the sheets. In a small dish, sift the confectioners' sugar (or whisk well in the bowl).
- Roll the heated cookies in the sugar until fully covered, then set aside to cool completely on a wire rack. Just before serving, dust with more confectioners' sugar.

---

5. Amaretti

Prep time: 35 min| Serves: 20-25| Difficulty: Moderate
Nutrition: Calories: 241 kcal |Fat: 10 g| Protein: 8 g| Carbohydrates: 23 g

Ingredients

- 1 cup almond flour (preferably finely ground)
- 3/4 cup confectioners' sugar
- 1 tablespoon plus 1 teaspoon cornstarch
- 2 large egg whites
- 1/3 cup superfine sugar
- 1 teaspoon almond extract

Instructions

- Preheat the oven to 325 degrees Fahrenheit (170 degrees Celsius). Preheat oven to 350°F. Line two baking pans with parchment paper.
- In a medium mixing bowl, combine the almond flour, confectioners' sugar, and cornstarch. In a clean medium mixing basin, whisk the egg whites with a handheld electric mixer until soft peaks form. 1 tablespoon at a time, add the superfine sugar and beat until glossy and firm peaks form. Mix in the almond extract until everything is properly combined.
- With a big metal spoon, gently fold in the almond flour mixture until just combined. Place rounded tablespoons of batter on the baking sheets, providing enough area for them to spread.
- With the back of a metal spoon, smooth the tops of each biscuit. Bake for 18 to 25 minutes, or until golden brown. Allow the cookies to cool and dry in the oven after turning off the oven and leaving the door ajar.

6. Banana Friands (Mini Almond Cakes)

Prep time: 35 min | Serves: 12 | Difficulty: Moderate
Nutrition: Calories: 299 kcal | Fat: 13 g | Protein: 11 g | Carbohydrates: 28 g

Ingredients
- 9 tablespoons unsalted butter, cut into cubes
- 1 1/4 cups confectioners' sugar, plus more for dusting
- 1/4 cup cornstarch
- 1/4 cup superfine white rice flour
- 1 1/4 cups almond flour
- 5 large egg whites, lightly beaten
- 1 tablespoon plus 1 teaspoon fresh lemon juice
- 1 teaspoon vanilla extract
- 1 small ripe banana, peeled and roughly chopped

Instructions
- Preheat the oven to 350 degrees Fahrenheit (180 degrees Celsius). Using cooking spray, lightly oil a 12-cup muffin tin, fry pan, or mini loaf pan.
- In a small saucepan over low heat, melt the butter, then simmer for 3 to 4 minutes more, until brown flecks form.
- Remove from the equation. In a large mixing bowl, sift the confectioners' sugar, cornstarch, and rice flour three times (or whisk in the bowl until well combined).
- Stir in the almond flour, then combine the egg whites, lemon juice, vanilla, and melted butter using a big metal spoon. Add the banana chunks and mix well.
- Pour the batter into each cup until they are two-thirds full. Bake for 12 to 15 minutes, or until gently brown and firm (a toothpick inserted into the center should come out clean).
- Cool for 5 minutes in the pan before turning out onto a wire rack to cool fully. Before serving, dust with confectioners' sugar.

7. Berry Friands (Mini Almond Cakes)

Prep time: 35 min | Serves: 12 | Difficulty: Moderate
Nutrition: Calories: 237 kcal | Fat: 9 g | Protein: 11 g | Carbohydrates: 25 g

Ingredients
- Nonstick cooking spray
- 9 tablespoons unsalted butter, cut into cubes
- 1 1/2 cups confectioners' sugar, plus more for dusting
- 1/4 cup cornstarch
- 1/4 cup superfine white rice flour
- 1 1/4 cups almond flour
- 5 large egg whites, lightly beaten
- 1 tablespoon plus 1 teaspoon fresh lemon juice
- 2 teaspoons vanilla extract
- 1 cup blueberries or raspberries

Instructions
- Preheat the oven to 350 degrees Fahrenheit (180 degrees Celsius). Using cooking spray, lightly oil a 12-cup muffin tin, friand pan, or mini loaf pan.
- In a small saucepan over low heat, melt the butter, then simmer for 3 to 4 minutes more, until brown flecks form. Remove from the equation.
- In a large mixing bowl, sift the confectioners' sugar, cornstarch, and rice flour three times (or whisk in the bowl until well combined).
- Stir in the almond flour, then combine the egg whites, lemon juice, vanilla, and melted butter using a big metal spoon.
- Pour the batter into each cup until they are two-thirds full. 4 berries, gently pressed into the middle of each friand (without pressing all the way into the batter).
- Bake for 12 to 15 minutes, or until gently brown and firm (a toothpick inserted into the center should come out clean).
- Cool for 5 minutes in the pan before turning out onto a wire rack to cool fully. Before serving, dust with confectioners' sugar.

8. Banana Fritters with Fresh Pineapple

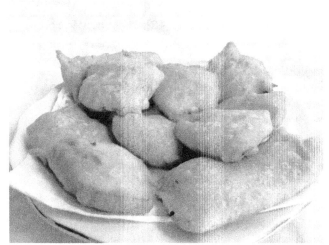

Prep time: 20 min | Serves: 4 | Difficulty: Moderate
Nutrition: Calories: 274 Kcal | Fat: 18 g | Protein: 23 g | Carbohydrates: 6 g

Ingredients
- 1 cup dried gluten-free, soy-free bread crumbs*
- 1/3 cup packed light brown sugar
- 1 tablespoon ground cinnamon
- 2 large eggs
- 1/2 teaspoon confectioners' sugar
- 4 small bananas, peeled and halved lengthwise
- 2 tablespoons unsalted butter
- Gluten-free, lactose-free vanilla ice cream, for serving
- 1/2 small pineapple, peeled, cored, and finely chopped
- Pulp of 2 passion fruits (optional)

Instructions

- Preheat the oven to 300°F. Combine the bread crumbs, brown sugar, and cinnamon on a large plate.
- Lightly beat the eggs with the confectioners' sugar in a shallow bowl. Dip the banana halves into the egg mixture, then toss in the bread crumbs until well coated.
- Melt 1 tablespoon of the butter in a large nonstick frying pan over medium- low heat. Add half of the banana pieces and cook for 3 to 4 minutes on each side, until golden brown.
- Transfer to a baking sheet and keep warm in the oven. Melt the remaining 1 tablespoon butter and cook the remaining banana halves the same way.
- Place two banana halves each on four plates. Top with ice cream, pineapple, and passion fruit pulp (if desired). Serve immediately.

9. Shortbread Fingers

Prep time: 50 min | Serves: 36 | Difficulty: Moderate
Nutrition: Calories: 122 Kcal | Fat: 13 g | Protein: 16 g | Carbohydrates:13 g

Ingredients

- 1 cup confectioners' sugar
- 1 tablespoon plus 2 teaspoons vanilla sugar, plus more for sprinkling
- 2 cups cornstarch, plus more for kneading
- 1 cup soy flour
- 1/2 cup superfine white rice flour
- 2 teaspoons xanthan gum or guar gum
- 17 tablespoons unsalted butter, cut into cubes, at room temperature

Instructions

- Preheat the oven to 275 degrees Fahrenheit (130 degrees Celsius). Preheat oven to 350°F. Line two baking pans with parchment paper. In a food processor or blender, mix the confectioners' sugar, vanilla sugar, cornstarch, soy flour, rice flour, and xanthan gum until thoroughly incorporated.
- To make a dough, add the butter and process for another 3 to 5 minutes. Using cornstarch, lightly dust your work surface.
- Turn the dough out onto the work surface and gently knead it until it comes together. Roll out the dough to a thickness of 12 inch between two pieces of parchment paper (1.25 cm).
- Place on baking sheets in 2 x 34-inch (5 x 2 cm) rectangles, giving a little room for spreading. Extra vanilla sugar can be sprinkled on top. Preheat oven to 200°F and bake for 20–25 minutes, or until golden brown. Reduce the oven temperature to 200°F (100°C) and bake for another 10 minutes, or until the cookies are golden brown.

- Cool for 10 to 12 minutes on the sheets before transferring to a wire rack to cool fully.

10. Caramel Nut Bars

Prep time: 40 min | Serves: 18-20 | Difficulty: Moderate
Nutrition: Calories: 221 kcal | Fat: 9 g | Protein: 12 g | Carbohydrates: 28 g

Ingredients

- Nonstick cooking spray
- 1/2 cup superfine white rice flour
- 1/4 cup potato flour
- 1/3 cup cornstarch
- 1/4 cup superfine sugar
- 1/4 teaspoon baking soda
- 1/4 teaspoon gluten-free baking powder
- 1 teaspoon xanthan gum or guar gum
- 4 tablespoons unsalted butter, cut into cubes, at room temperature
- 1 large egg, beaten
- 1 teaspoon vanilla extract

Nut Topping

- 1 cup packed light brown sugar
- 10 tablespoons (1 stick plus 2 tablespoons/150 g) unsalted butter, cut into cubes, at room temperature
- 1/3 cup light cream
- 3 tablespoons plus 1 teaspoon cornstarch
- 1/2 cup roasted unsalted pecans, roughly chopped
- 2/3 cup roasted unsalted Brazil nuts (skin on), roughly chopped
- 1/2 cup roasted unsalted macadamia nuts, halved

Instructions

- Preheat the oven to 350°F (180°C). Grease an 11 x 7-inch (28 x 18 cm) baking pan with cooking spray and line with parchment paper, leaving an overhang on the two long sides to help lift out the bars later.
- Sift the rice flour, potato flour, cornstarch, superfine sugar, baking soda, baking powder, and xanthan gum together three times into a bowl (or whisk in the bowl until well combined). Rub in the butter with your fingertips.
- Add the egg and vanilla and mix with a large metal spoon until well combined. As the mixture becomes more solid, use your hands to bring it together to form a ball. Roll out the dough between two sheets of parchment paper to a thickness of 1/4 inch (5 mm). Gently fit into the bottom of the pan and prick all over with a fork.
- Refrigerate for 10 minutes. Bake for 10 to 12 minutes, until the crust is firm and lightly golden. Set aside to cool, but leave the oven on. To make the topping, combine the brown sugar and butter in a large saucepan over medium heat and stir until the butter has melted and the

mixture comes to a boil. Remove from the heat and stir in the cream and cornstarch, mixing until smooth.

- Add the pecans, Brazil nuts, and macadamia nuts. Return the pan to medium heat and stir until the mixture comes to a boil.
- Reduce the heat to low and cook gently for 2 to 3 minutes more, until the mixture is thick and sticky. Spread the nut topping evenly over the crust and bake for 15 minutes, or until the topping is bubbling.
- Let cool completely in the pan, then transfer to a board, remove the parchment paper, and cut into small (or large!) pieces to serve.

11. Chocolate-Mint Bars

Prep time: 30 min | Serves: 18-20 | Difficulty: Moderate
Nutrition: Calories: 278 kcal | Fat: 11 g | Protein: 8 g | Carbohydrates: 22 g
Ingredients
- Nonstick cooking spray
- 8 tablespoons unsalted butter, cut into cubes, at room temperature
- 1/3 cup superfine sugar
- 1/2 cup superfine white rice flour
- 1/4 cup soy flour
- 1/2 cup cornstarch
- 1 teaspoon xanthan gum or guar gum
- 2 heaping tablespoons unsweetened cocoa powder

Peppermint Filling
- 1 cup confectioners' sugar
- One 8-ounce package reduced-fat cream cheese, at room temperature
- 3 to 4 teaspoons peppermint extract
- 1/2 cup plus 2 tablespoons vegetable shortening, melted

Chocolate Topping
- 4 ounces good-quality dark chocolate, broken into pieces
- 1 tablespoon plus 1 teaspoon light cream
- 3 scant tablespoons vegetable shortening
Instructions
- Preheat the oven to 325°F (170°C). Grease an 11 x 7-inch (29 × 19 cm) baking pan with nonstick cooking spray and line with parchment paper.
- Combine the butter and sugar in a medium bowl and mix with an electric beater until thick and pale.
- Sift the rice flour, soy flour, cornstarch, xanthan gum, and cocoa three times into a separate bowl (or whisk in a bowl until well combined). Add to the creamed butter and sugar and stir with a large metal spoon until well combined.
- Gently gather into a ball and knead lightly in the bowl. Press the dough into the prepared pan. Bake for 10 to 15 minutes, until lightly browned.

- Set aside to cool completely. To make the peppermint filling, combine the confectioners' sugar, cream cheese, and peppermint extract in a bowl and beat with a handheld electric mixer until well combined.
- Add the shortening and beat for 1 to 2 minutes, until smooth. Spread the filling evenly over the cookie crust and refrigerate until set. To make the chocolate topping, combine the dark chocolate, cream, and shortening in a small saucepan and stir over low heat until melted and well combined.
- Remove the pan from the refrigerator and spread the chocolate topping over the peppermint filling. Refrigerate until set, then cut into squares to serve.

12. Dark Chocolate–Macadamia Nut Brownies

Prep time: 2hr-45 min | Serves: 18-20 | Difficulty: Moderate
Nutrition: Calories: 247 kcal | Fat: 10 g | Protein: 14 g | Carbohydrates: 28 g
Ingredients
- Nonstick cooking spray
- 10 tablespoons unsalted butter, cut into cubes
- 10 1/2 ounces good-quality dark chocolate, broken into pieces
- 1 1/4 cups packed light brown sugar
- 2/3 cup superfine white rice flour
- 1/4 cup cornstarch
- 1 teaspoon xanthan gum or guar gum
- 3 large eggs
- 2 teaspoons vanilla extract
- 1/2 cup dark chocolate chips
- 1/2 cup light cream
- 3/4 cup roughly chopped macadamia nuts (optional)
Instructions
- Preheat the oven to 325 degrees Fahrenheit (160 degrees Celsius). Cooking spray an 11 x 7-inch (29 x 19-cm) baking pan and line it with parchment paper.
- In a medium saucepan, melt the butter and chocolate together over low heat, stirring constantly until smooth.
- Stir in the brown sugar until it is completely dissolved. Allow to cool to room temperature in a large mixing basin. Sift the rice flour, cornstarch, and xanthan gum into a separate bowl three times (or whisk in a bowl until well combined).
- One by one, whisk the eggs into the chocolate mixture. Combine the sifted flour, vanilla, chocolate chips, cream, and macadamia nuts in a mixing bowl (if using). Mix well, then scoop into the baking pan and level the top. Bake for 20 minutes, then cover with foil and bake for another 20 to 25 minutes, until just firm.

148

- Remove from the oven and set aside to cool to room temperature in the pan. Refrigerate for two to three hours, or overnight, until firm.
- Serve by turning out onto a cutting board, peeling away the parchment paper, and cutting into squares.

13. Chocolate Truffles

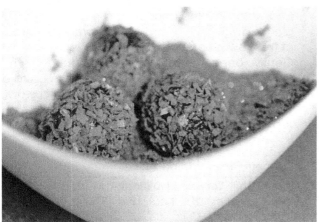

Prep time: 20 min | Serves: 25 | Difficulty: Moderate
Nutrition: Calories: 311 kcal | Fat: 7.1 g | Protein: 44 g | Carbohydrates: 16 g
Ingredients
- 7 ounces gluten-free vanilla cookies, finely crushed (about 2 cups)
- 1/3 cup unsweetened cocoa powder
- 1/3 cup sweetened condensed milk
- 2 tablespoons rum or brandy (optional)
- 11/2 cups gluten-free chocolate sprinkles
Instructions
- In a medium mixing dish, combine the crumbled cookies and cocoa. Mix in the condensed milk and rum (if using) with your hands until a firm dough forms.
- In a small dish, pour the chocolate sprinkles. With your hands, roll teaspoons of the truffle mixture into balls. To coat, toss in the chocolate sprinkles. Refrigerate until the mixture is solid.

14. Gingerbread Men

Prep time: 45 min | Serves: 20-25 | Difficulty: Moderate
Nutrition: Calories: 202 Kcal | Fat: 13 g | Protein: 16 g | Carbohydrates:13 g
Ingredients
- 1 large egg
- 1/3 cup superfine sugar
- 1/2 cup brown rice syrup
- 5 tablespoons unsalted butter, melted
- 1 cup superfine white rice flour
- 1/2 cup potato flour
- 1 cup soy flour
- 1 teaspoon xanthan gum or guar gum
- 1 teaspoon gluten-free baking powder
- 1 to 11/2 heaping tablespoons ground ginger
- Cornstarch, for rolling out dough
- Gluten-free icing (optional)
Instructions
- Preheat the oven to 300 degrees Fahrenheit (150 degrees Celsius). Preheat oven to 350°F. Line three baking pans with parchment paper (or work in batches).
- In a large mixing basin, whisk together the egg and sugar using a wooden spoon. Combine the brown rice syrup and melted butter in a mixing bowl. In a separate bowl, sift together the rice flour, potato flour, soy flour, xanthan gum, baking powder, and ginger three times (or whisk in a bowl until well combined).
- Mix thoroughly to incorporate into the syrup mixture. Refrigerate for 15 minutes to allow the mixture to thicken up somewhat. Using cornstarch, lightly dust your work surface.
- Roll out the dough to a thickness of 34 to 1 inch on a floured surface (2 to 3 mm). Cut out shapes with a cookie cutter (they don't have to be people; you could do stars, pine trees, or anything else).
- Place on baking pans with enough space between them to allow for spreading. Preheat oven to 350°F and bake for 8 to 10 minutes. Cool for 10 to 15 minutes on the sheets before transferring to a wire rack to cool fully.
- If desired, garnish with gluten-free frosting once the cake has cooled.

15. Cream Puffs with Chocolate Sauce

Prep time: 2hr | Serves: 6-8 | Difficulty: Moderate
Nutrition: Calories: 276 kcal | Fat: 12 g | Protein: 11 g | Carbohydrates: 35 g
Ingredients
Crème Filling:
- 1 cup superfine white rice flour
- 1 teaspoon xanthan gum or guar gum
- 1 heaping tablespoon sugar
- 3 large eggs
Crème Custard
- 2 cups low-fat milk, lactose-free milk, or suitable plant-based milk
- 6 large egg yolks
- 1/2 cup superfine sugar
- 1/3 cup cornstarch
- 2 teaspoons vanilla extract
Chocolate Custard
- 1/3 cup cornstarch
- 21/2 cups low-fat milk, lactose-free milk, or suitable plant-based milk
- 31/2 teaspoons sugar
- 4 ounces good-quality dark chocolate, broken into small pieces

- 2 tablespoons plus 2 teaspoons coffee liqueur or brewed strong espresso mixed with a bit of unsweetened cocoa powder
- 1/2 teaspoon vanilla extract

Chocolate Sauce
- 4 ounces good-quality dark chocolate, broken into pieces
- 1/3 cup light cream

Instructions
- Preheat the oven to 400 degrees Fahrenheit (200 degrees Celsius). Preheat oven to 350°F. Line two baking pans with parchment paper.
- In a medium saucepan, bring the butter and 34 cup (185 ml) water to a boil. In a bowl, whisk together the rice flour and xanthan gum until smooth, then add to the pan and stir quickly with a wooden spoon. The batter will pull away from the pan's sides and form a smooth ball.
- Place the dough in a medium mixing basin. Mix in the sugar using a handheld electric mixer. One at a time, beat in the eggs.
- Place rounded tablespoons of dough about 112 inches (4 cm) apart on the sheets. Preheat the oven to 350°F and bake for 7 minutes, or until the pastries puff up. Reduce the oven temperature to 350 degrees Fahrenheit (180 degrees Celsius) and bake for another 10 minutes, or until crisp and gently browned.
- Reduce the oven temperature to 275 degrees Fahrenheit (140 degrees Celsius) and remove one sheet from the oven. Cut a tiny opening in the side of each pastry quickly and gently. Replace the sheet in the oven and repeat the process with the second sheet. 5 minutes in the oven, or until the pastries are dry.
- Allow to cool to room temperature after removing from the oven. Cut the pastries open with care. Remove the soft cores from the pastry casings without crushing them.
- To create the crème custard, pour the milk into a small heavy-bottomed saucepan over medium heat and bring to just below a boil while the pastries are cooling. In a large mixing basin, whisk together the egg yolks and superfine sugar with a handheld electric mixer until thick and creamy. Add the cornstarch and mix well. Whisk together the hot milk and cream until smooth. Return the mixture to the pan and whisk gently until the custard has thickened over medium-low heat. Remove the pan from the heat and stir in the vanilla extract. Pour into a bowl, cover, and chill for 1 to 2 hours, or until completely cold.
- To prepare the chocolate custard, whisk together the cornstarch and 12 cup (125 ml) milk until smooth. In a small saucepan, combine the sugar and the remaining 2 cups (500 mL) milk and heat until just below boiling. Gradually add the cornstarch mixture to the custard, stirring

frequently until it thickens. Remove from the fire when the liquid is quite thick and whisk in the chocolate, coffee liqueur, and vanilla until creamy and the chocolate has melted. Pour into a bowl, cover, and chill for 1 to 2 hours, or until completely cold.
- In a heatproof dish or the top half of a double boiler, mix the chocolate and cream to produce the chocolate sauce. Set over a pot of boiling water or the bottom portion of a double boiler and whisk until the chocolate is melted and well blended with the cream (make sure the bottom of the bowl does not touch the water).
- Gently open each pastry and pour in the contents, half of which should be crème custard and the other half should be chocolate custard. Serve with a dollop of warm chocolate sauce on top.

---

16. Coconut Rice Pudding

Prep time: 1hr | Serves: 6 | Difficulty: Moderate
Nutrition: Calories: 202 Kcal | Fat: 13 g | Protein: 16 g | Carbohydrates:13 g

Ingredients
- 3/4 cup superfine sugar
- 3 cups milk, lactose-free milk, or suitable plant-based milk (more if needed)
- One 13.5-ounce can light coconut milk
- 2 teaspoons vanilla extract
- 11/2 cups Arborio rice
- Heaping 1/4 cup shredded sweetened or unsweetened coconut
- Maple syrup, for serving (optional)

Instructions
- In a medium saucepan over medium-high heat, combine the sugar, milk, coconut milk, and vanilla and bring to a boil, stirring often.
- Toss in the rice. Reduce the heat to low and cook for about 50 minutes, stirring occasionally, until the liquid has been absorbed and the rice is soft.
- If necessary, add more milk. Preheat the oven to 325°F (170°C) and prepare a baking sheet with foil in the meanwhile.
- Sprinkle the coconut evenly over the baking sheet and bake for 10 to 12 minutes, or until golden brown.
- Warm or at room temperature, top the rice pudding with toasted coconut and a drizzle of maple syrup, if preferred.

17. Chocolate Soufflés

Prep time: 40 min | Serves: 6 | Difficulty: Moderate
Nutrition: Calories: 241 Kcal | Fat: 18 g | Protein: 6 g | Carbohydrates: 14 g

Ingredients

- Nonstick cooking spray
- 1 1/4 cups superfine sugar
- 8 ounces good-quality dark chocolate, broken into pieces
- 1/2 cup light cream
- 6 large eggs, separated
- 2/3 cup cornstarch
- 1/4 cup packed light brown sugar
- 1/2 cup low-fat milk, lactose-free milk, or suitable plant-based milk
- Confectioners' sugar, sifted (optional)

Instructions

- Preheat the oven to 350 degrees Fahrenheit (180 degrees Celsius).
- Using cooking spray, grease six 8-ounce (250-ml) soufflé plates.
- 1 tablespoon superfine sugar, poured onto each dish and generously coated, removing any excess. In a heatproof dish or the top half of a double boiler, combine the chocolate and cream.
- Set over a pot of boiling water or the bottom half of a double boiler and whisk until the chocolate is melted and properly blended (make sure the bottom of the bowl does not touch the water). Allow to cool slightly before serving.
- In a large mixing basin, beat the egg yolks with the remaining superfine sugar with a handheld electric mixer until pale, thick, and creamy.
- In a separate bowl, whisk together the cornstarch, brown sugar, and milk until smooth. Pour into a saucepan and simmer, stirring constantly, for 5 minutes over medium heat, or until thickened. Set everything to cool somewhat before stirring into the chocolate mixture.
- Clean the mixer beaters and whip the egg whites until firm peaks form in a large clean mixing dish.
- Fill the soufflé dishes to about 14 inch (5 mm) below the rim with the chocolate mixture, gently folding in with a big metal spoon. Place the dishes on a baking sheet and bake for 20 to 25 minutes, or until the soufflés have risen to their full potential. If preferred, dust with confectioners' sugar and serve right away, since they will sink if left to stand.

18. Amaretti Tiramisu

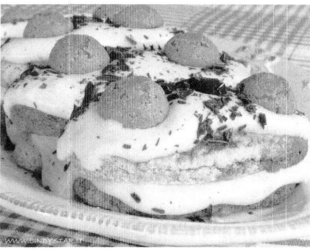

Prep time: 2hr-10 min | Serves: 6-8 | Difficulty: Moderate
Nutrition: Calories: 311 kcal | Fat: 7.1 g | Protein: 44 g | Carbohydrates: 16 g

Ingredients

- 4 large eggs, separated
- 1/2 cup superfine sugar, plus more for the coffee (optional)
- 12 ounces reduced-fat cream cheese, at room temperature
- 1 cup strong brewed coffee
- 1/4 cup Marsala or amaretto (optional)
- About 30 Amaretti

Chocolate Sauce

- 1/2 teaspoon instant coffee
- 2/3 cup confectioners' sugar
- 2 heaping tablespoons unsweetened cocoa powder, plus more for dusting

Instructions

- In a large mixing basin, beat the egg yolks and superfine sugar with a handheld electric mixer until thick, pale, and creamy.
- For 3 to 4 minutes, beat in the cream cheese until it is creamy and thoroughly blended. Clean the beaters in the mixer. In a large clean mixing basin, whisk the egg whites until stiff peaks form.
- Gently incorporate the egg whites into the cream cheese mixture using a big metal spoon. In a small bowl, combine the coffee, sugar to taste, and liqueur (if using). Each Amaretti cookie should be dipped in coffee.
- Fill each of the six glass dessert plates with 1 cookie and a few teaspoons of the cream cheese filling. Finish with a cream cheese layer and the remaining cookies and filling.
- Dissolve the instant coffee in 2 to 3 tablespoons boiling water to produce the chocolate sauce. In a small mixing bowl, sift the confectioners' sugar and cocoa together, then add the coffee mixture and stir until smooth.

- Drizzle the chocolate sauce on top of the tiramisu and finish with a dusting of cocoa powder. Before serving, cover and chill for at least 2 hours, ideally overnight.

19. Irish Cream Delights

Prep time: 3hr | Serves: 6 | Difficulty: Moderate
Nutrition: Calories: 321 kcal | Fat: 8 g | Protein: 6 g | Carbohydrates: 22 g

Ingredients
- 1/2 cup light cream
- 1/2 cup packed light brown sugar
- 2 cups milk, lactose-free milk, or suitable plant-based milk
- 1/2 cup Irish cream liqueur, such as Baileys
- 1/4 cup cornstarch
- Shaved chocolate, for serving

Instructions
- In a medium saucepan, combine the cream, brown sugar, and 13/4 cup (435 ml) of the milk and simmer over medium heat until almost boiling.
- Add the liquor and mix well. To make a smooth paste, combine the cornstarch and the remaining 14 cups (60 ml) of milk.
- Gradually add to the heated cream mixture, frequently stirring to avoid lumps, then simmer, constantly stirring, for about 5 minutes over medium heat, until thickened. (Do not allow it to boil.)
- Fill six 4-ounce (125-ml) ramekins with the pudding.
- Allow cooling completely before covering with plastic wrap and chilling for 3 to 4 hours, or until set.
- Just before serving, garnish with shaved chocolate.

20. Berry and Chocolate Fudge Sundaes

Prep time: 20 min | Serves: 6-8 | Difficulty: Moderate
Nutrition: Calories: 302 kcal | Fat: 10 g | Protein:11 g | Carbohydrates:17 g

Ingredients
Chocolate Fudge Sauce
- 3 tablespoons unsalted butter
- 1/2 cup packed light brown sugar
- 1/2 cup light cream
- 2 heaping tablespoons unsweetened cocoa powder
- 1/4 cup good-quality dark chocolate buttons or chips
- 1-1/3 cups blueberries
- 1-2/3 cups raspberries
- 3-1/3 cups strawberries, hulled, halved if large
- 4 cups gluten-free, lactose-free vanilla ice cream

Instructions
- Melt the butter in a small saucepan over low heat to produce the chocolate fudge sauce.
- Stir in the dark chocolate, brown sugar, milk, cocoa, and cocoa powder until the chocolate has melted and the sauce is smooth.
- Allow cooling to room temperature after removing from the heat. In a mixing dish, combine the berries. Scoop the ice cream into serving cups or bowls, top with the berries, then drizzle generously with chocolate fudge sauce.

21. Warm Lemon Tapioca Pudding

Prep time: 35 min | Serves: 6 | Difficulty: Moderate
Nutrition: Calories: 179 kcal | Fat: 8 g | Protein: 7 g | Carbohydrates: 14 g

Ingredients
- 4 lemons
- 4 cups low-fat milk, lactose-free milk, or suitable plant-based milk
- 1/2 cup pearl tapioca or sago
- 1/3 cup superfine sugar

Instructions
- Slice the zest of all four lemons into 34-inch (2-cm) strips with a vegetable peeler. Make a 1/2 cup lemon juice by juicing the lemons.
- In a medium saucepan, combine the milk and lemon zest and bring to a boil over high heat. Reduce the heat to low and continue to cook for another 2 minutes.
- Remove the lemon zest and toss it out. Stir the tapioca into the milk until it is completely combined. Simmer for 20 to 25 minutes, often stirring, until the tapioca becomes transparent jelly-like balls.
- Turn off the heat. Pour the sugar and lemon juice into six glass dessert plates and mix well. Serve right away.

22. White Chocolate–Mint Pots

Prep time: 3hr | Serves: 4 | Difficulty: Moderate
Nutrition: Calories: 202 Kcal | Fat: 13 g | Protein: 16 g | Carbohydrates:13 g

Ingredients
- 2 cups milk, lactose-free milk, or suitable plant-based milk
- 1/4 cup light cream
- 1/2 cup superfine sugar
- 1/4 teaspoon peppermint extract (more to taste)
- 3 or 4 drops green food coloring
- 4 ounces white chocolate chips, plus more for decorating
- 1/4 cup cornstarch
- Mint leaves

Instructions
- In a small saucepan over medium heat, bring 13/4 cup (185 ml) milk, cream, sugar,

peppermint essence, and food coloring to just below a boil (do not let it boil).

- Stir in the white chocolate chips until they are all melted. To make a smooth paste, combine the cornstarch and the remaining 14 cups (60 ml) of milk.
- Gradually add the white chocolate mixture to the white chocolate mixture, frequently stirring to avoid lumps. Cook, constantly stirring, for 5 minutes, or until the sauce has thickened.
- Fill four 7-ounce (200-ml) ramekins with the mixture. Allow cooling completely at room temperature before refrigerating for 3 to 4 hours, or until firm.
- Just before serving, garnish with additional white chocolate chips and mint leaves.

---

23. Cappuccino and Vanilla Bean Mousse Duo

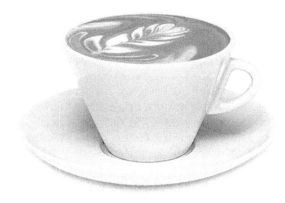

Prep time: 3hr-25 min | Serves: 6 | Difficulty: Moderate
Nutrition: Calories: 149 kcal | Fat: 9 g | Protein: 6 g | Carbohydrates:12 g
Ingredients
- Nonstick cooking spray
- 8 ounces good-quality white chocolate, broken into pieces
- 2/3 cup light cream
- 1 heaping tablespoon unflavored gelatin powder
- 4 large eggs, separated, at room temperature
- 1 cup light whipping cream
- 1/4 cup superfine sugar
- 1 teaspoon vanilla bean paste or 1 to 2 teaspoons vanilla extract
- 2 teaspoons instant coffee
- Edible organic flowers (optional)

Instructions
- Use nonstick cooking spray to coat six 5-ounce (150 ml) cups or ramekins.
- In a heatproof dish or the top half of a double boiler, combine the chocolate and light cream. Set over a pot of boiling water or the bottom

portion of a double boiler and whisk until melted and properly blended (make sure the bottom of the bowl does not touch the water).
- Allow 15 to 20 minutes for cooling. In a small heatproof basin, pour 12 cups (125 ml) of cold water and mix in the gelatin with a fork. Set the gelatin aside for 5 minutes or until it has softened.
- Fill a bigger bowl halfway with hot water, add the gelatin bowl, and whisk regularly until the gelatin is completely dissolved. Stir the gelatin into the cooled chocolate mixture, then one at a time, add the egg yolks.
- Half of the chocolate mixture should be transferred to another bowl. In a clean mixing basin, whisk the whipping cream and sugar with a handheld electric mixer until the mixture is thick and the sugar is dissolved. Half of the whipped cream should be placed in a smaller bowl. Clean the beaters in the mixer.
- In a large clean mixing basin, whisk the egg whites until stiff peaks form. To one of the chocolate mixture dishes, add the vanilla extract. Fold this into one of the whipped cream dishes with a big metal spoon until thoroughly blended.
- Finally, fold half of the beaten egg whites in gently. Pour the mixture into the glasses. Cover and chill for 1 hour, or until completely set. Allow the remaining bowls to come to room temperature.
- Dissolve the coffee in 2 tablespoons hot water and add it into the remaining chocolate mixture after an hour. Fold the remaining whipped cream into this, then fold in the remaining egg whites carefully.
- Pour over the vanilla layer in the glasses. Cover and chill for another 2 hours or until set. Garnish with flowers just before serving, if preferred.

---

24. Cinnamon Panna Cotta with Pureed Banana

Prep time: 3hr-35 min | Serves: 4 | Difficulty: Moderate
Nutrition: Calories: 370 kcal | Fat: 10 g | Protein: 5 g | Carbohydrates:15 g
Ingredients
- Nonstick cooking spray
- 12/3 cups light cream
- 1/2 cup milk, lactose-free milk, or suitable plant-based milk
- 1/2 cup superfine sugar
- 1 teaspoon ground cinnamon
- 1 teaspoon vanilla extract
- 21/4 teaspoons unflavored gelatin powder
- Ice cubes
- 2 ripe bananas, peeled
- 2 teaspoons light brown sugar

Instructions

- Cooking spray four 4-ounce (125 ml) dariole molds, custard cups, or tall ramekins. In a medium saucepan over low heat, combine the cream, milk, superfine sugar, cinnamon, and vanilla.
- Cook for 20 minutes, stirring occasionally and taking care not to let it boil, or until the mixture is thick enough to coat the back of a spoon.
- Take the pan from the heat and transfer the contents into a medium heatproof bowl. In a small heatproof dish, mix together 1 tablespoon cold water and the gelatin with a fork. Allow for 5 minutes or until the gelatin has started to gel.
- Fill a bigger bowl halfway with hot water, add the gelatin bowl, and whisk regularly until the gelatin is completely dissolved.
- Incorporate the cream mixture using a whisk. Fill a large mixing dish halfway with ice cubes. Place the bowl with the cream mixture on the ice for about 10 minutes, whisking every few minutes.
- As the mixture cools, it will thicken. Carefully pour it into the molds once it has thickened enough to coat the back of a spoon. Refrigerate for 2 to 3 hours, covered, until set. In a mixing bowl, mash the bananas and brown sugar with a fork until smooth and well blended.
- Dip each mold in hot water for a few seconds before turning it out onto plates to serve. Fill a piping bag with the pureed banana and use it to garnish the plates (or dollop directly onto the panna cotta, if preferred).

25. Orange-Scented Panna Cotta

Prep time: 2hr | Serves: 4 | Difficulty: Moderate
Nutrition: Calories: 269 kcal | Fat: 9 g | Protein: 7 g | Carbohydrates: 27 g
Ingredients
- Nonstick cooking spray

Orange Topping
- 2 tablespoons plus 2 teaspoons fresh orange juice, strained
- 2 tablespoons plus 2 teaspoons boiling water
- 2 tablespoons plus 2 teaspoons sugar
- 1 1/2 teaspoons unflavored gelatin powder
- 1-2/3 cups light cream
- 1/2 cup milk, lactose-free milk, or suitable plant-based milk
- 1/2 cup superfine sugar
- 3 to 4 heaping tablespoons finely grated orange zest
- 2 tablespoons plus 2 teaspoons fresh orange juice, strained
- 2 1/4 teaspoons unflavored gelatin powder
- Ice cubes
- Orange segments, for serving

Instructions

- Cooking spray four 4-ounce (125 ml) dariole molds, custard cups, or tall ramekins. In a small heatproof dish, mix all of the topping ingredients.
- Place the bowl over a bigger basin of boiling water and whisk until all of the gelatin is dissolved. Fill each cup with a quarter of the orange topping.
- Refrigerate for 1–2 hours, or until completely set. In a medium saucepan over low heat, combine the cream, milk, superfine sugar, orange zest, and orange juice. Cook for 20 minutes, stirring occasionally and taking care not to let it boil or until it has thickened enough to coat the back of a spoon.
- Take the pan from the heat and transfer the contents into a medium heatproof bowl. In a small heatproof bowl, pour 1 tablespoon cold water and mix in the gelatin with a fork.
- Allow for 5 minutes or until the gelatin has started to gel. Fill a bigger bowl halfway with hot water, add the gelatin bowl, and whisk regularly until the gelatin is completely dissolved.
- Incorporate the cream mixture using a whisk. Fill a second big basin halfway with ice cubes. Place the bowl with the cream mixture on the ice for about 10 minutes, whisking every few minutes. As the mixture cools, it will thicken.
- Carefully pour it over the orange topping in the molds once it has thickened enough to coat the back of a spoon. Refrigerate for 2 to 3 hours, covered, until set.
- Dip the mold in hot water for a few seconds before turning it out onto plates to serve. Serve with fresh orange segments on top.

26. Maple Syrup Bavarian Cream with Quick Pecan Brittle

Prep time: 4hr-20 min | Serves: 6 | Difficulty: Moderate
Nutrition: Calories: 318 kcal | Fat: 7 g | Protein: 11 g | Carbohydrates: 14 g
Ingredients
- Nonstick cooking spray
- 3 large egg yolks, at room temperature
- 1/2 cup superfine sugar
- 1/2 cup maple syrup
- 1/2 cup low-fat milk, lactose-free milk, or suitable plant-based milk
- 1 heaping tablespoon unflavored gelatin powder
- Ice cubes
- 1 cup light whipping cream

Quick Pecan Brittle
- 13/4 ounces gluten-free butterscotch candies
- 1/2 cup pecans, coarsely crushed

Instructions

- Grease six 4-ounce dariole molds, custard cups, or tall ramekins with cooking spray.
- Place the egg yolks and sugar in a medium bowl and beat with a handheld electric mixer for 2 to 3 minutes, until thick and pale.
- Combine the maple syrup and milk in a medium saucepan over low heat. Whisk in the egg mixture and stir with a wooden spoon over very low heat for 5 minutes, or until thick enough to coat the back of the spoon.
- Don't let it boil. Remove from the heat and pour into a medium heatproof bowl. Add 3 tablespoons of cold water to a small heatproof bowl and whisk in the gelatin with a fork. Set it aside for 5 minutes or until the gelatin has begun to gel.
- Fill a larger bowl with boiling water, set the bowl containing the gelatin in it, and constantly stir until the gelatin has completely dissolved. Whisk the gelatin into the maple mixture until smooth. Fill a large bowl with ice cubes.
- Place the bowl with the maple mixture on the ice and whisk every few minutes for about 10 minutes. The mixture will thicken as it cools. Beat the cream in a medium bowl with a handheld electric mixer until thick. Fold into the cooled maple mixture with a large metal spoon until well combined.
- Pour evenly into the molds, then place the molds on a baking sheet, cover with plastic wrap, and refrigerate for 4 to 5 hours. To make the pecan brittle, combine the butterscotch and pecans in a small food processor or blender and process until coarsely crushed (don't overdo it, or you will be left with crumbs).
- To serve, dip each mold into hot water for a few seconds, then turn it out onto plates. Sprinkle generously with the pecan brittle.

27. Lemon Tart

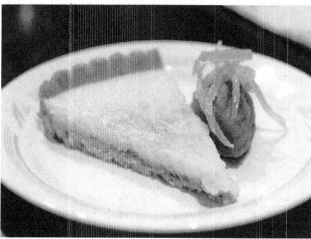

Prep time: 1hr-10 min | Serves: 8-10 | Difficulty: Moderate

Nutrition: Calories: 408 kcal | Fat: 12 g | Protein: 11 g | Carbohydrates: 25 g

Ingredients

- Nonstick cooking spray

Tart Crust

- 1 cup superfine white rice flour
- 1/2 cup cornstarch, plus more for kneading
- 1/2 cup soy flour
- 1 teaspoon xanthan gum or guar gum
- 1/4 cup superfine sugar
- 10 tablespoons cold unsalted butter, diced
- About 1/2 cup ice water
- 3/4 cup superfine sugar
- One 8-ounce package mascarpone
- 1 heaping tablespoon finely grated lemon zest
- 2/3 cup fresh lemon juice
- 4 large eggs
- Confectioners' sugar, for dusting

Instructions

- Preheat the oven to 350 degrees Fahrenheit (180 degrees Celsius). Using cooking spray, grease a 9-inch (23-cm) fluted tart pan.
- Sift the rice flour, cornstarch, soy flour, and xanthan gum into a bowl to form the crust.
- Add the superfine sugar and butter to a food processor and pulse until the mixture resembles fine bread crumbs.
- Add the cold water a spoonful at a time while the engine is running to produce a soft dough. Using cornstarch, lightly dust your work surface. Knead the dough on the work surface until it is smooth.
- Refrigerate for 30 minutes after wrapping in plastic wrap. Roll out the dough between two sheets of parchment paper to about an 18-inch thickness (2 to 3 mm). To neaten the edges, ease the crust into the pan and trim the edges.
- Bake for 10 minutes, or until gently brown, after lining the crust with parchment paper and filling it with pie weights or rice. Remove the

parchment and weights. Reduce the oven temperature to 325 degrees Fahrenheit (160 degrees Celsius).

- In a medium bowl, whisk the superfine sugar, mascarpone, lemon zest, and lemon juice with a handheld electric mixer to make the filling. One at a time, add the eggs, beating thoroughly after each addition.
- Fill the heated crust with the filling and bake for 30 to 35 minutes, or until set. In the pan, cool fully. Before serving, dust with confectioners' sugar.

28. Citrus Rice Tart with Raspberry Sauce

Prep time: 2hr-45 min| Serves: 8-10| Difficulty: Moderate
Nutrition: Calories: 256 kcal |Fat:9 g| Protein:5 g| Carbohydrates:17 g
Ingredients
- Nonstick cooking spray
- 1 cup medium-grain white rice
- 1/4 cup sugar
- 1/3 cup cornstarch
- 3 large eggs
- 1/2 cup light cream
- 1/2 teaspoon vanilla extract
- Grated zest of 1 orange
- 3/4 cup fresh orange juice
- Grated zest of 1 lemon
- RASPBERRY SAUCE
- One 15-ounce can raspberry in syrup, drained, reserving the juice.
- 1/4 cup raspberry juice (from the can)
- 1 heaping tablespoon confectioners' sugar
Instructions
- Preheat the oven to 325 degrees Fahrenheit (160 degrees Celsius). Using cooking spray, grease a 9-inch (23-cm) fluted tart or pie pan. In a large saucepan, bring 612 cups (1.5 liters) of water to a boil.
- Cook, stirring periodically, for 12 minutes, or until the rice is soft, adding the rice and sugar as needed.
- To cool, drain and rinse under cold water. In a medium mixing bowl, whisk together the cornstarch, eggs, cream, vanilla, orange zest and juice, and lemon zest.
- Mix in the rice well. Bake for 35 to 40 minutes, or until just set, in the tart pan.
- Refrigerate for 2 to 3 hours after removing from the oven and let it cool to room temperature. Remove 30 minutes before serving from the refrigerator.
- Remove the outside rim of your pan if it has a detachable bottom. In a blender or food processor, combine all of the ingredients to make the raspberry sauce.
- Serve drizzled over the tart.

29. Lemon Tartlets

Prep time: 45 min | Serves: 12 | Difficulty: Moderate
Nutrition: Calories: 294 kcal |Fat:9 g| Protein:12 g| Carbohydrates:19 g
Ingredients
- Nonstick cooking spray
Lemon Filling
- 1/2 cup cornstarch
- 1 1/4 cups water
- Grated zest of 2 lemons
- 3/4 cup fresh lemon juice
- 4 tablespoons unsalted butter, cut into cubes, at room temperature
- 2/3 cup sugar
- 2 large egg yolks
- 1 batch Tart Crust dough, chilled
- Gluten-free, lactose-free ice cream, for serving
Instructions
- Preheat the oven to 325 degrees Fahrenheit (170 degrees Celsius). Using cooking spray, grease twelve tartlet pans or a 12-cup muffin pan.
- To create the filling, whisk together the cornstarch and 1 tablespoon of water in a small saucepan until smooth.
- Stir in the remaining water to ensure there are no lumps, then add the lemon zest, lemon juice, butter, and sugar and cook, constantly stirring, for 3 to 5 minutes, until the sauce has thickened.
- Allow cooling for 10 minutes after removing from the heat. In a separate bowl, whisk together the egg yolks. Pour into a bowl, cover, and chill until completely chilled.
- In the meantime, layout the cold dough between two pieces of parchment paper to an 18-inch thickness (2 to 3 mm). To fit the pan or cups, cut out 12 circles using a pastry cutter.
- Trim the sides of the pan or cups to make them tidy. Preheat oven to 350°F and bake for 12 to 15 minutes, or until golden brown.
- Allow cooling completely on a wire rack. Fill the tartlet crusts with the cold lemon filling and serve with ice cream.

30. Cinnamon and Chestnut Flan

Prep time: 1hr| Serves: 10-12| Difficulty: Moderate
Nutrition: Calories: 311 kcal |Fat: 7.1 g| Protein: 44 g| Carbohydrates: 16 g
Ingredients
- Nonstick cooking spray
- 1 batch Tart Crust dough chilled
- 3/4 cup superfine sugar
- 2 tablespoons ground cinnamon
- One 14-ounce can fat-free sweetened condensed milk
- One 8-ounce package mascarpone or reduced-fat cream cheese, at room temperature
- 1 1/2 cups chestnut meal

- 4 large eggs
- Confectioners' sugar, for dusting
- Gluten-free, lactose-free ice cream, for serving

Instructions

- Preheat the oven to 350 degrees Fahrenheit (170 degrees Celsius). Using cooking spray, grease a 9-inch (23-cm) fluted quiche pan.
- Roll out the cold dough between two pieces of parchment paper to about an 18-inch thickness (2 to 3 mm).
- Trim the edges of the crust and ease it into the flan dish. Bake for 10 minutes, or until gently brown, after lining the crust with parchment paper and filling it with pie weights or rice. Remove the baking sheet from the oven and lower the temperature to 325°F (160°C).
- Remove the parchment and weights. Meanwhile, to create the filling, in a food processor or blender, add the superfine sugar, cinnamon, condensed milk, mascarpone, chestnut meal, and eggs and pulse until smooth and thoroughly incorporated.
- Fill the heated crust with the filling. Preheat oven to 350°F and bake for 50–60 minutes, or until firm.
- Remove from the pan and set aside to cool fully before serving.
- Serve with ice cream and a dusting of confectioners' sugar.

31. Lemon Cheesecake

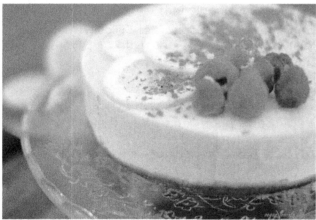

Prep time: 3hr-15 min| Serves: 10-12| Difficulty: Moderate

Nutrition: Calories: 308 kcal |Fat:11 g| Protein:12 g| Carbohydrates:17 g

Ingredients

- 9 ounces gluten-free vanilla cookies, crushed (about 2½ cups)
- 4 tablespoons unsalted butter, melted

Cheesecake Filling

- 1 heaping tablespoon unflavored gelatin powder
- One 8-ounce package of reduced-fat cream cheese, at room temperature

- ¾ cup superfine sugar
- 2 tablespoons plus 2 teaspoons fresh lemon juice
- 1 to 2 heaping tablespoons grated lemon zest
- 1⅓ cups light whipping cream

Lemon Topping

- 1½ teaspoons unflavored gelatin powder
- 3 tablespoons unsalted butter, cut into cubes, at room temperature
- ½ cup superfine sugar
- 1 large egg yolk, lightly beaten
- 1 teaspoon grated lemon zest
- 2 tablespoons plus 2 teaspoons fresh lemon juice

Instructions

- In a medium mixing dish, combine the crumbled cookies and melted butter.
- In the bottom of an 8-inch (20-cm) springform pan, press evenly. Refrigerate the filling and topping while you work on the filling.
- To create the filling, fill a small heatproof basin with 12 cups (125 ml) cold water and mix in the gelatin with a fork. Allow to sit for 5 minutes or until the gelatin begins to gel.
- Fill a bigger mixing bowl halfway with hot water, add the gelatin bowl, and whisk regularly until the gelatin is completely dissolved. In a food processor or blender, combine the cream cheese, sugar, lemon juice, lemon zest, and dissolved gelatin and process for 1 to 2 minutes, until smooth.
- In a medium mixing basin, whisk the cream with a handheld electric mixer until it thickens. Fold the whipped cream into the cream cheese mixture using a big metal spoon. Fill the cookie crust with the filling.
- Cover and chill for 3 hours, or until firm. To prepare the topping, fill a small heatproof basin with 1/2 cup (125 ml) cold water and mix in the gelatin with a fork. Allow to sit for 5 minutes or until the gelatin begins to gel. Fill a bigger bowl halfway with hot water, add the gelatin bowl, and whisk regularly until the gelatin is completely dissolved.
- In a small saucepan, combine the dissolved gelatin, butter, sugar, egg yolk, lemon zest, and juice.
- Stir for about 15 minutes over low heat or until the sauce is thick enough to coat the back of a spoon. Allow cooling to room temperature before serving.
- Return the cheesecake to the refrigerator for at least 3 hours, or until firm, to spread the topping evenly over the filling.

32. Baked Blueberry Cheesecakes

Prep time: 3hr-20min| Serves: 9| Difficulty: Moderate
Nutrition: Calories: 341 Kcal |Fat: 18 g| Protein: 6 g|
Carbohydrates: 24 g

Ingredients

- 7 ounces gluten-free vanilla cookies, crushed (about 2 cups)
- 4 tablespoons unsalted butter, melted
- 2 cups fresh or frozen blueberries
- Two 8-ounce packages of reduced-fat cream cheese at room temperature
- One 14-ounce can fat-free sweetened condensed milk
- 2 teaspoons vanilla extract
- 1/2 cup light whipping cream
- 2 large eggs
- 1/4 cup (35 g) cornstarch

Instructions

- Preheat the oven to 325°F (160°C). Mix together the crushed cookies and melted butter, then press into the bottom of nine 4-inch (10 cm) springform pans.
- Divide the blueberries evenly over the cookie crusts.
- Combine the cream cheese, condensed milk, vanilla, cream, eggs, and cornstarch in a food processor or blender and process until smooth.
- Pour the batter over the crusts. Bake for 15 to 20 minutes, until lightly golden and firm to the touch. Allow to cool completely in the pans, then cover and refrigerate for 3 hours before serving.

33. Chocolate Tart

Prep time: 2hr| Serves: 10-12| Difficulty: Moderate
Nutrition: Calories: 374 Kcal |Fat: 18 g| Protein: 23 g |Carbohydrates: 16 g

Ingredients

- Nonstick cooking spray
- 7 ounces gluten-free chocolate cookies, crushed (about 2 cups)
- 5 tablespoons unsalted butter, melted

Chocolate Filling

- 8 ounces good-quality dark chocolate, broken into pieces
- 10 tablespoons unsalted butter, cut into cubes, at room temperature
- 3/4 cup superfine sugar
- 2 teaspoons vanilla extract
- 1/4 cup coffee liqueur (optional)
- 5 large eggs, at room temperature
- Unsweetened cocoa powder for dusting
- Gluten-free, lactose-free, ice cream, for serving

Instructions

- Preheat the oven to 300 degrees Fahrenheit (150 degrees Celsius). Using cooking spray, grease a 9-inch (23-cm) fluted tart pan. In a medium mixing dish, combine the crumbled cookies and melted butter.
- In the bottom of the tart pan, press evenly. While you're making the filling, keep it refrigerated. Place the chocolate in a small heatproof dish or the top half of a double boiler to prepare the filling.
- Set over a pot of boiling water or the bottom portion of a double boiler, occasionally stirring until melted (make sure the bottom of the bowl does not contact the water). Allow cooling slightly before serving.
- In a medium mixing bowl, whisk the butter, sugar, vanilla, coffee liqueur (if using), and 1 egg with a handheld electric mixer until pale and creamy.
- Mix in the melted chocolate until everything is nicely mixed. Remove from the equation. Clean the beaters in the mixer. In a large mixing basin, whisk the remaining eggs for 3 to 5 minutes or until they have doubled in volume.
- Pour the chocolate mixture into the eggs and beat on low speed for 1 to 2 minutes, or until they are completely blended. Fill the cookie crust equally with the filling and bake for 45 to 50 minutes, or until firm.
- Remove from the oven and set aside to cool to room temperature before refrigerating for 2 to 3 hours. Serve with ice cream and a heavy dusting of chocolate powder.

34. Pecan and Maple Tarts

Prep time: 45 min| Serves: 24| Difficulty: Moderate
Nutrition: Calories:234 kcal |Fat:12 g| Protein:14 g| Carbohydrates:27 g

Ingredients

- Nonstick cooking spray
- 2 batches Tart Dough, chilled Filling
- 1 tablespoon unsalted butter, at room temperature
- 1/4 cup packed light brown sugar
- 1/2 teaspoon vanilla extract
- 1 large egg
- 1/4 cup maple syrup
- 1/2 cup pecans, roughly chopped
- Confectioners' sugar, for dusting (optional)

Instructions

- Preheat the oven to 325 degrees Fahrenheit (170 degrees Celsius). Using cooking spray, grease two 12-cup mini tartlets or tiny muffin pans.
- Using parchment paper, line a baking sheet. Roll out the cold pastry dough between two pieces of parchment paper to about an 18-inch thickness (2 to 3 mm).
- To fit the small tartlet pans, use a scalloped 1- to 112-inch (3 to 4 cm) pastry cutter to cut out 24 round crusts.

- Place in the cups and tidy up the edges. Cut out 24 miniature stars with a star-shaped cookie cutter (or any preferred form).
- On the baking sheet, arrange the stars. Preheat the oven to 350°F and bake the crusts and stars until golden brown (the crusts will take about 10 minutes, but the stars will only need 7 to 8 minutes).
- Remove the pan from the oven and place it on a wire rack to cool. Preheat the oven to 350 degrees Fahrenheit (180 degrees Celsius). In a small mixing basin, cream together the butter, brown sugar, and vanilla with a handheld electric mixer until smooth.
- Stir in the chopped pecans after beating in the egg and maple syrup. Fill the crusts equally with the filling and bake for 5–10 minutes, or until the filling is set (it should remain firm when given a gentle shake).
- While the tarts are still warm, place a star on each one.
- Cool for 10 minutes in the pans before transferring to a wire rack to cool fully. If desired, dust with confectioners' sugar.

35. Carrot Cake with Cream Cheese Frosting

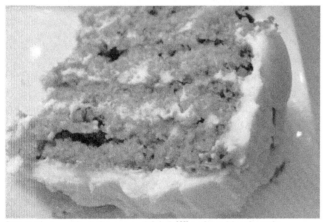

Prep time: 1hr| Serves: 10| Difficulty: Moderate
Nutrition: Calories:277 kcal |Fat:11 g| Protein:14 g| Carbohydrates: 31 g
Ingredients
- Nonstick cooking spray
- 1/3 cup superfine white rice flour
- 1/3 cup cornstarch
- 2 teaspoons gluten-free baking powder
- 1 teaspoon baking soda
- 1 teaspoon xanthan gum or guar gum
- 1 heaping tablespoon ground cinnamon
- 1 heaping tablespoon pumpkin pie spice
- 2 cups almond flour
- 1 cup packed light brown sugar
- 2 medium carrots, grated
- 1/3 cup walnuts, chopped
- 4 large eggs, separated

Cream Cheese Frosting
- One 8-ounce package reduced-fat cream cheese
- 1 tablespoon plus 1 teaspoon fresh lemon juice
- 1/2 cup confectioners' sugar
Instructions
- Preheat the oven to 325 degrees Fahrenheit (160 degrees Celsius). Cooking spray an 812 x 412 inch (22 x 11.5 cm) loaf pan and line it with parchment paper, allowing an overhang on the two long edges to assist pull the cake out afterward.
- In a large mixing bowl, sift together the rice flour, cornstarch, baking powder, baking soda, xanthan gum, cinnamon, and pumpkin pie spice three times (or whisk in the bowl until well combined).
- Combine the almond flour, brown sugar, carrots, walnuts, and egg yolks in a mixing bowl. In a medium mixing bowl, whisk the egg whites with a handheld electric mixer until firm peaks form.
- With a big metal spoon, gently incorporate the egg whites into the carrot batter. Fill the pan halfway with batter and bake for 45 to 50 minutes, or until firm to the touch (a toothpick inserted into the center should come out clean).
- Cool for 10 minutes in the pan before turning out onto a wire rack to cool fully. To create the cream cheese frosting, whisk together the cream cheese, lemon juice, and confectioners' sugar until smooth.
- After the cake has cooled, spread the icing on top and serve.

36. Layered Tahitian Lime Cheesecake
Prep time: 2hr-15 min| Serves: 10-12| Difficulty: Moderate
Nutrition: Calories: 269 kcal |Fat:11 g| Protein:12 g| Carbohydrates:15 g
Ingredients
- 9 ounces gluten-free vanilla cookies, crushed
- 4 tablespoons butter, melted
- 2 tablespoons unflavored gelatin powder
- Two 8-ounce packages of reduced-fat cream cheese at room temperature
- One 14-ounce can fat-free sweetened condensed milk
- 1/3 cup coconut liqueur
- 3 tablespoons plus 1 teaspoon fresh lime juice
- Finely grated zest of 1 lime
- 1 to 2 drops of green food coloring
Instructions
- Mix together the crushed cookies and melted butter in a medium bowl. Press evenly into the bottom of a 9-inch (23 cm) springform pan.
- Place in the refrigerator while you prepare the topping. Add 1/2 cup (125 ml) cold water to a

small heatproof bowl and whisk in the gelatin with a fork.

- Set aside for 5 minutes or until the gelatin has begun to gel. Fill a larger bowl with boiling water, set the bowl containing the gelatin in it, and constantly stir until the gelatin has completely dissolved.
- Combine the dissolved gelatin, cream cheese, and condensed milk in a food processor or blender and process for 1 minute or until smooth. Pour half of the mixture into a clean bowl; there should be about 2 cups (500 ml). Add the coconut liqueur to the bowl and mix it in well. Pour over the cookie crust and freeze for 10 minutes.
- Add the lime juice, lime zest, and food coloring to the remaining batter in the food processor and process for 30 seconds or until well combined. Remove the cheesecake from the freezer—it should be just set.
- Pour the lime mixture over the coconut layer, then refrigerate for 2 to 3 hours to set completely before serving.

37. Orange and Poppy Seed Cake

Prep time: 1hr-45 min| Serves: 10| Difficulty: Moderate
Nutrition: Calories:266 kcal |Fat:8.7 g| Protein:12 g| Carbohydrates:14 g
Ingredients
- Nonstick cooking spray
- 2 oranges
- 1 1/4 cups almond flour
- 1 teaspoon gluten-free baking powder
- 1/2 cup (65 g) superfine white rice flour
- 2 tablespoons poppy seeds
- 5 large eggs
- 1 1/4 cups sugar
Instructions
- Preheat the oven to 325°F (170°C). Grease a 9-inch (23 cm) springform pan with cooking spray and line with a parchment paper circle.
- Boil the oranges in a medium pot of boiling water for 20 minutes, covered. Drain.
- In a food processor or blender, puree the softened oranges (seeds, pith, and all!) for 3 to 4 minutes to get a smooth paste.
- Allow cooling before serving. Sift the almond flour, baking powder, and rice flour into a mixing bowl three times (or whisk in the bowl until well combined).
- Add the poppy seeds and mix well. In a medium mixing basin, whisk together the eggs with a handheld electric mixer for 5 minutes, or until thick and creamy.
- Mix in the sugar until everything is completely blended. Stir the orange paste into the dry

ingredients, then use a big metal spoon to fold it into the egg mixture.

- Fill the pan halfway with batter and bake for 50 to 60 minutes, or until golden brown and firm to the touch (a toothpick inserted into the center should come out clean).
- Cool for 15 minutes in the pan, then remove the outer ring and cool fully on a wire rack.

38. Rich White Chocolate Cake

Prep time: 1hr-40 min| Serves: 12| Difficulty: Moderate
Nutrition: Calories:496 kcal |Fat:9 g| Protein:19 g| Carbohydrates:42 g
Ingredients
- Nonstick cooking spray
- 15 tablespoons unsalted butter, cut into cubes
- 7 ounces good-quality white chocolate, broken into pieces
- 2 1/4 cups packed light brown sugar
- 3/4 cup soy flour
- 3/4 cup tapioca flour
- 1 cup superfine white rice flour
- 1/2 cup cornstarch
- 2 teaspoons xanthan gum or guar gum
- 1 teaspoon baking soda
- 1 teaspoon gluten-free baking powder
- 2 teaspoons vanilla extract
- 2 large eggs
- Confectioners' sugar, for dusting
Instructions
- Preheat the oven to 300 degrees Fahrenheit (150 degrees Celsius). Using cooking spray, grease a 9-inch (23-cm) springform pan. In a medium heatproof dish or the top half of a double boiler, combine the butter, white chocolate, brown sugar, and 1 1/2 cups (375 ml) boiling water.
- Set over a pot of boiling water or the bottom half of a double boiler and whisk until the chocolate and butter are melted, and everything is properly blended (make sure the bottom of the bowl does not touch the water). Allow cooling to room temperature before serving.
- In a medium mixing bowl, sift the soy flour, tapioca flour, rice flour, cornstarch, xanthan gum, baking soda, and baking powder three times (or whisk in the bowl until well combined).
- With a handheld electric mixer, whip the cooled white chocolate mixture, vanilla, and eggs until smooth.
- Bake for 45 minutes after pouring the batter into the pan. Cover with foil and bake for another 15 to 30 minutes, or until firm (a toothpick inserted into the center should come out clean).
- Cool for 15 minutes in the pan, then remove the outer ring and cool fully on a wire rack.
- Before serving, dust with confectioners' sugar.

39. Flourless Chocolate Cake

Prep time: 1hr-25 min | Serves: 8-10 | Difficulty: Moderate

Nutrition: Calories:398 kcal | Fat:8 g | Protein:16 g | Carbohydrates:18 g

Ingredients

- Nonstick cooking spray
- 1/3 cup unsweetened cocoa powder, plus more for dusting
- 10 tablespoons unsalted butter, cut into cubes, at room temperature
- 5 ounces good-quality dark chocolate, broken into pieces
- 1 1/4 cups packed light brown sugar
- 1 1/4 cups almond flour
- 4 large eggs, separated
- Gluten-free, lactose-free ice cream, for serving (optional)

Instructions

- Preheat the oven to 300°F (150°C). Grease a 9-inch (23 cm) springform pan with cooking spray and line with a parchment paper circle.
- Combine the cocoa, butter, dark chocolate, and 1/3 cup (80 ml) water in a medium saucepan over low heat and stir until melted and smooth.
- Remove from the heat and stir in the brown sugar, almond flour, and egg yolks. Transfer to a large bowl and let cool to room temperature.
- Beat the egg whites in a clean bowl with a handheld electric mixer until soft peaks form.
- Gently fold the egg whites into the cooled chocolate mixture in two batches.
- Pour the batter into the prepared springform pan and bake for 55 to 65 minutes, until firm when pressed gently in the center.
- Cool in the pan for 20 minutes, then remove the outer ring and turn it out onto a wire rack to cool completely.
- Dust with additional cocoa and serve with ice cream, if desired.

40. Moist Chocolate Cake

Prep time: 1h-15 min | Serves: 10-12 | Difficulty: Moderate

Nutrition: Calories:369 kcal | Fat:11 g | Protein:14 g | Carbohydrates:21 g

Ingredients

- Nonstick cooking spray
- 1 cup plus 2 tablespoons superfine white rice flour
- 1/2 cup cornstarch
- 1/2 cup potato flour
- 2/3 cup unsweetened cocoa powder
- 2 teaspoons gluten-free baking powder
- 1 teaspoon baking soda
- 1 teaspoon xanthan gum or guar gum
- 2 large eggs

- 1 1/2 cups superfine sugar
- 3 tablespoons unsalted butter, melted
- 3/4 cup gluten-free, low-fat vanilla yogurt
- 2/3 cup low-fat milk, lactose-free milk, or suitable plant-based milk

Chocolate Frosting

- 1 1/2 cups confectioners' sugar
- 2 to 3 heaping tablespoons unsweetened cocoa powder
- 7 tablespoons unsalted butter, at room temperature
- 1/4 cup low-fat milk, lactose-free milk, or suitable plant-based milk

Instructions

- Preheat the oven to 325 degrees Fahrenheit (170 degrees Celsius). Cooking sprays a 9-inch (23-cm) springform pan and line it with a parchment paper circle.
- In a large mixing bowl, sift together the rice flour, cornstarch, potato flour, cocoa, baking powder, baking soda, and xanthan gum three times (or whisk in the bowl until well combined).
- In a medium mixing bowl, whisk together the eggs and superfine sugar until thick and frothy. Stir in the melted butter, yogurt, and milk until everything is thoroughly incorporated.
- Add to the dry ingredients and mix for 2 to 3 minutes with a wooden spoon until fully incorporated and no lumps remain.
- Fill the pan halfway with batter and bake for 45 to 55 minutes, or until firm to the touch (a toothpick inserted in the center should come out clean).
- Cool for 10 minutes in the pan before removing the outer ring and transferring to a wire rack to cool fully.
- Sift the confectioners' sugar and cocoa into a mixing dish to make the chocolate frosting.
- Mix in the butter and milk until everything is completely mixed. Using a spatula, spread evenly over the cooled cake.

41. Hazelnut–Sour Cream Cake with Blueberry Jam

Prep time: 1hr | Serves: 10-12 | Difficulty: Moderate

Nutrition: Calories:386 kcal | Fat:11 g | Protein:23 g | Carbohydrates:28 g

Ingredients

- Nonstick cooking spray
- 13 tablespoons unsalted butter, cut into cubes at room temperature
- 1 1/2 cups superfine sugar
- 2 teaspoons vanilla extract
- 3 large eggs
- 3/4 cup superfine white rice flour
- 1/3 cup soy flour
- 1/4 cup cornstarch
- 1 teaspoon ground cinnamon
- 1 teaspoon baking soda

- 2 teaspoons gluten-free baking powder
- 1 teaspoon xanthan gum or guar gum
- 1 cup hazelnut flour
- 1 cup light sour cream

Cream Cheese Filling
- 4 ounces reduced-fat cream cheese, at room temperature
- 1/2 cup hazelnut flour
- 1 teaspoon ground cinnamon
- 2/3 cup confectioners' sugar
- 1 tablespoon plus 1 teaspoon fresh lemon juice
- 1/2 cup blueberry jam, plus more for garnish

Instructions
- Preheat the oven to 350 degrees Fahrenheit (180 degrees Celsius). Cooking spray two 8-inch (22-cm) cake pans and line with parchment paper circles
- In a large mixing basin, beat the butter, superfine sugar, and vanilla with a handheld electric mixer until thick, pale, and creamy.
- One at a time, add the eggs, beating thoroughly after each addition. In a medium mixing bowl, sift together the rice flour, soy flour, cornstarch, cinnamon, baking soda, baking powder, and xanthan gum three times (or whisk in the bowl until well combined).
- Add the hazelnut flour and mix well. Gently combine the dry ingredients into the butter mixture in two parts, alternating with the sour cream, using a big metal spoon.
- Pour the batter into the pans in an equal layer. Bake for 35–40 minutes, or until a toothpick inserted in the middle comes out clean.
- Cool for 10 minutes in the pans before turning out onto a wire rack to cool fully. In a medium mixing bowl, combine all of the ingredients for the cream cheese filling and stir well.
- Over one of the cake layers, spread the jam, then slightly over half of the cream cheese filling. Spread the remaining cream cheese mixture on top of the second cake layer.
- Dollop blueberry jam on top as a garnish.

42. Brownie Batter Bowls
Prep time: 35 min | Serves: 6 | Difficulty: Easy
Nutrition: Calories:211 kcal | Fat:11 g | Protein:15 g | Carbohydrates:28 g
Ingredients
- 1/4 cup butter softened, plus more for greasing ramekins
- 1 tablespoon unsweetened cocoa powder
- 1/2 cup sugar
- 1 tablespoon cornstarch
- 6 ounces semi-sweet chocolate, chopped
- 1 teaspoon vanilla extract
- 2 large eggs, lightly beaten
- 6 tablespoons vanilla lactose-free ice cream
- 2 tablespoons pomegranate seeds

Instructions
- Preheat the oven to 300 degrees Fahrenheit. Using a dab of butter, grease the bottom and halfway up the sides of six 4- to 5-ounce ramekins, then sprinkle with cocoa powder. On a baking sheet, arrange the ramekins.
- Combine the sugar and cornstarch in a small bowl.
- In a medium microwave-safe dish, combine the chocolate and butter. Microwave for 1 minute on high, then stir. The rep at 20- to 30-second intervals until the chocolate and butter are completely melted. Toss the melted chocolate with the sugar mixture and the vanilla extract. Add the eggs one at a time, beating firmly with a wooden spoon after each addition.
- Place the baking sheet in the oven and divide the batter among the ramekins. Bake for 30 minutes, or until the brownie around the sides of each ramekin is puffy and cracked, but the inside is still soft. Allow it cool for 15 minutes on a cake rack before serving with a dollop of ice cream and a few pomegranate seeds.

43. Chocolate -Dipped Almond Biscotti

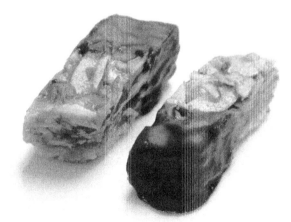

Prep time: 35 min | Serves: 24 | Difficulty: Easy
Nutrition: Calories:211 kcal | Fat:9 g | Protein:11 g | Carbohydrates: 19g
Ingredients
- 1/2 cup salted butter, softened
- 1 cup sugar
- 2 large eggs
- 2 tablespoons water
- 1 tablespoon almond extract
- 1 tablespoon vanilla extract
- 1/2 cup almond flour
- 3/4 cup/80 grams sorghum flour
- 1 3/4 cups/190 grams Authentic Foods Superfine Brown Rice Flour
- 6 tablespoons tapioca starch
- 3 tablespoons cornstarch
- 3 tablespoons arrowroot powder
- 2 tablespoons ground chia seeds

- 2 teaspoons baking powder
- ½ cup almond slices
- 1 cup semi-sweet chocolate chips
- 2 teaspoons coconut oil

Instructions

- Preheat the oven to 325 degrees Fahrenheit. Prepare two big baking sheets by lining them with foil.
- Using a wooden spoon, combine the butter and sugar in a large mixing basin. One at a time, add the eggs, pounding vigorously after each addition. Stir in the almond and vanilla extracts, as well as the water.
- Combine the flours, tapioca starch, cornstarch, and arrowroot powder in a medium mixing bowl, then toss in the chia seeds and baking powder until thoroughly combined. Add about a quarter of this mixture to the wet components at a time, mixing well after each addition. If necessary, add 1 tablespoon of rice flour at a time until the dough is firm and holds its shape. Add the almonds and mix well.
- On each baking sheet, cut the dough in half and make a 3-inch-wide loaf approximately 1 inch thick. With wet hands, smooth the tops of the loaves. Bake for 45 to 50 minutes, or until brown and firm to the touch, swapping oven positions of the baking pans after the first 20 minutes.
- Cool for 5 minutes on the baking pans, then wrap securely in foil and set aside to cool.
- Preheat the oven to 300 degrees Fahrenheit.
- 1 loaf should be unwrapped and placed on a cutting board. Using a large serrated knife and a gentle sawing motion cut the bread on the diagonal into 34-inch-thick pieces.
- Handle the bread with care and support. Then arrange the slices in a single layer on an oiled baking sheet (carefully so they don't fracture or break). Repeat with the other loaf and another baking sheet, reserving any crumbs that form. Bake for 40 to 50 minutes, or until golden brown all over. Allow the cookies to cool completely in the cooling oven after turning off the oven and cracking up the door.
- In a small glass cup or dish, combine the chocolate chips and coconut oil and microwave on high for 30 seconds, stirring after each interval, until smooth and melted.
- Place each biscotti on parchment or wax paper after dipping one end into the chocolate. Any residual crumbs should be sprinkled on top of the heated chocolate. Keep the biscotti in an airtight container until ready to serve once the chocolate has solidified.

44. Lemon -Pecan Bars

Prep time: 35 min | Serves: 8 | Difficulty: Easy
Nutrition: Calories: 141 Kcal | Fat: 18 g | Protein: 6 g | Carbohydrates: 14 g

Ingredients

- ⅓ cup salted butter
- ⅔ cup oat flour
- ⅔ cup finely ground pecan flour
- 4 large eggs
- 1⅓ cups granulated sugar
- 1 teaspoon vanilla extract
- 1 teaspoon almond extract
- ⅓ cup fresh lemon juice
- 1 tablespoon cornstarch
- 1½ teaspoons baking powder
- Pinch of salt
- Confectioners' sugar (optional)

Instructions

- Preheat the oven to 350 degrees Fahrenheit.
- Heat the butter in a microwave-safe medium bowl on high for 15 seconds to soften it slightly. With a wooden spoon, whisk together the flours, 1 egg, 13 cups granulated sugar, and the vanilla and almond extracts until a soft dough forms. In a 9-inch square baking dish, press the dough. Bake for 30 minutes, or until firm to the touch and golden brown around the edges, on a rack in the lower third of the oven. Preheat the oven to 350 degrees Fahrenheit.
- With an electric mixer on medium-high, beat the remaining 1 cup sugar, lemon juice, cornstarch, baking powder, remaining 3 eggs, and salt for 3 minutes in a medium bowl.
- Return the baking dish to the oven and pour the contents over the crust. Bake on the same rack for 20 minutes, then decrease to 300°F and bake for another 10 minutes, or until the custard is light golden brown and fluffy. When the dish is inverted, it should not seem runny under the surface.
- Before cutting the lemon bars into squares, let them cool fully in the pan.
- If desired, dust with confectioners' sugar right before serving. Refrigerate leftovers in an airtight container.

45. Raspberry-Lime Ice Pops

Prep time: 35 min | Serves: 10 | Difficulty: Easy
Nutrition: Calories: 274 Kcal | Fat: 18 g | Protein: 23 g | Carbohydrates: 6 g

Ingredients

- 1½ cups cold water
- 10 tablespoons sugar
- 4 tablespoons fresh lime juice (from 2 limes)
- 1½ cups mashed fresh (about 3 cups) or frozen-thawed (12 ounces)
- raspberries
- 10 wooden pop sticks

Instructions

- Bring the water and sugar to a boil in a medium saucepan over medium heat, constantly stirring until the sugar is dissolved. Remove from the heat and whisk in the raspberries and lime juice. Fill the molds with the mixture using a kitchen funnel. Dip a pop stick into each mold a couple of times to press any air bubbles to the top, then tap the molds on the counter several times to settle the mixture in the molds.
- For 1 hour, place the molds in the freezer.
- Soak one end of 10 wooden ice-pop sticks in about 2 inches of cold water in a water glass.
- Dry the sticks with a towel before inserting them into the ice pop molds. Freeze for another 4 hours at least. Depending on the temperature of your freezer, the freezing time may vary.
- Submerge the ice-pop molds in extremely warm water for about 30 seconds to unmold and serve, then unmold and serve right away. Leftover pops may be frozen for many weeks if wrapped in sandwich bags.

46. Five-Ingredient Peanut Butter Cookies

Prep time: 35 min| Serves: 28| Difficulty: Easy
Nutrition: Calories:264 kcal |Fat:7 g| Protein:13 g| Carbohydrates:19 g

Ingredients

- 1 large egg
- 1 cup peanut butter
- ¾ cup sugar, plus extra for forming cookies
- ¼ cup miniature semi-sweet chocolate chips
- ⅛ teaspoon sea salt or kosher salt flakes

Instructions

- Preheat the oven to 350 degrees Fahrenheit.
- Combine the egg, peanut butter, and 34 cup sugar in a medium mixing bowl until smooth, then toss in the chocolate chips. Form the dough into twenty-eight 1-inch balls using your hands or a tiny cookie scoop and place them on two ungreased cookie trays.
- To produce a crisscross pattern, press the back of the fork into the dough of the first biscuit. Dip the tines of the fork in some loose sugar before flattening the tops of the cookies with the fork to about a 14-inch thickness.
- Season the cookies with a pinch of salt.
- Preheat the oven to 350°F and bake the cookies for 12 to 14 minutes, or until puffy in the center and hard around the edges. Make sure they aren't over-baked. Allow the cookies to cool completely before storing them in an airtight container.

47. Vegan Khir Pudding

Prep time: 20 min | Serves: 4| Difficulty: Easy
Nutrition: Calories: 102 Kcal |Fat: 13 g| Protein: 16 g| Carbohydrates: 3 g

Ingredients

- 1 cup cashews, soaked in water for 4 hours, and drained
- 1 to 11/2 cups water
- 2 to 3 tablespoons maple syrup, or to taste
- Pinch of sea salt
- 1 to 2 teaspoons of cardamom, or to taste
- 1 /2 cup cooked brown rice or whole-grain noodles (such as rice or buckwheat noodles of your choice)
- Dash of saffron (optional)
- 1/4 cup slivered almonds (optional)

Instructions

- In a blender, combine the cashews, water, maple syrup, sea salt, and cardamom; season to taste.
- Toss cooked rice or noodles with cashew milk and a splash of saffron and almonds, as well as an extra drizzle of maple syrup if preferred.

48. Coconut Currant Cookies

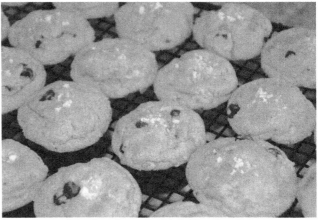

Prep time: 20 min | Serves: 6| Difficulty: Easy
Nutrition: Calories: 171 kcal |Fat:8g| Protein:12 g| Carbohydrates:18 g

Ingredients

- 1 egg
- 1 /2 cup honey
- 1 /4 teaspoon salt
- 1 /2 cup almond flour
- 1 1/2 cups shredded coconut
- 1 /2 cup chopped walnuts
- 1 /2 cup currants

Instructions

- Preheat oven to 350 degrees Fahrenheit.
- Combine the egg, honey, and salt in an electric mixer or blender. Mix in the almond flour until everything is nicely combined. Mix in the coconut, walnuts, and currants until everything is well blended.

- Preheat oven to 350°F and bake for 10 to 12 minutes.

49. Coconut Bread
Prep time: 20 min| Serves: 6| Difficulty: Easy
Nutrition: Calories: 198 kcal |Fat:9 g| Protein:12 g| Carbohydrates: 25 g
Ingredients
- 2⁄3 cups coconut flour
- 5 eggs
- 1 teaspoon organic vanilla
- 2 teaspoons cinnamon
- 1/2 teaspoon salt
- 1 tablespoon of gluten-free baking powder
- 1/4 cup plus 1 tablespoon honey

Instructions
- Preheat the oven to 330 degrees.
- In a mixing dish, combine 1 teaspoon cinnamon, salt, baking powder, and 14 cups honey.
- Fill a greased 9-x-5-inch loaf pan or an ungreased silicone bread pan halfway with batter.
- Sprinkle the remaining cinnamon and honey over the dough and bake for 45 to 50 minutes.

50. Date Syrup
Prep time: 10 min| Serves: 6| Difficulty: Easy
Nutrition: Calories: 60 Kcal |Fat: 0.3 g| Protein: 1 g| Carbohydrates: 14.1 g
Ingredients
- 20 to 25 honey or Medjool dates
- 1 cup filtered, spring, or alkaline water
Instructions
- Pit the dates and cover them with the water in a bowl. Soak for 3 to 4 hours.
- Blend the dates and the soaking water in a blender until smooth.

51. Angel's Decadent Whipped Cream
Prep time: 5 min| Serves: 6| Difficulty: Easy
Nutrition: Calories:287 kcal |Fat:14 g| Protein:9 g| Carbohydrates:23g
Ingredients
- 1 cup macadamia nuts, soaked in water for 4 hours, and drained
- 1/2 cup water
- 1/2 cup Date Syrup or agave, or more to taste
- 1 teaspoon organic vanilla
- 1 tablespoon cold-pressed coconut oil
Instructions
- Blend all the ingredients in a blender until smooth and creamy in texture.

52. Frozen Fruit Pops
Prep time: 30 min to 2 hours| Serves: 4| Difficulty: Easy
Nutrition: Calories: 191 kcal |Fat:8 g| Protein:12 g| Carbohydrates:14 g
Ingredients
- 2 cups fresh mango 1 teaspoon lemon juice
- 1 teaspoon brown sugar or agave (optional)
- 1/2 cup water
Instructions
- In a food processor, puree the fruit and lemon juice until the smooth; taste and adjust the sweetness with brown sugar or agave nectar if required. Place the mixture in tiny glasses or big ice cube trays and freeze until it becomes slushy (15 to 45 minutes, depending on cup size and the temperature of your freezer).
- Insert the Popsicle sticks when the mixture is slushy and freeze for up to 2 hours.

53. Banana Smoothie
Prep time: 5 min| Serves: 2| Difficulty: Easy
Nutrition: Calories: 102 Kcal |Fat: 13 g| Protein: 16 g| Carbohydrates: 3 g
Ingredients
- 3 bananas
- 1 1/2 cup lactose-free milk
- 1 teaspoon honey
- 1/3 cup ice cubes
Instructions
- Blend together all the ingredients until smooth.

54. Raspberry Smoothie
Prep time: 5 min| Serves: 2| Difficulty: Easy
Nutrition: Calories: 114 kcal |Fat: 10 g| Protein: 3 g| Carbohydrates:17 g
Ingredients
- 1 cup raspberries
- 1 1/2 cup lactose-free milk
- 1 teaspoon honey
- 1/3 cup ice cubes
Instructions
- Blend together all the ingredients until smooth.

55. Nutty Breakfast Smoothie
Prep time: 5min| Serves: 2| Difficulty: Moderate
Nutrition: Calories: 134 kcal |Fat:7 g| Protein:12 g| Carbohydrates:18 g
Ingredients:
- 2 bananas
- 2 cups spinach
- 1 cup water
- 1 tablespoon almond butter
Instructions:
- Cut up the bananas and spinach.

- Put all the ingredients in a blender. Blend until smooth and enjoy

56. Safe and Soothing Smoothie

Prep time: 5min | Serves: 1 | Difficulty: Moderate
Nutrition: Calories:201 kcal | Fat:13 g | Protein:11 g | Carbohydrates: 23 g
Ingredients:
- 1 small, ripe banana
- 1 cup strawberries, fresh or frozen
- 2 tablespoons hulled hemp seeds (no soaking required)
- 1 to 2 tablespoons pea powder protein (such as provided)
- 1 cup liquid (water, coconut juice, or half coconut juice and half coconut milk)
- Natural sweetener (such as agave, stevia, or Just Like Sugar) to taste (optional)

Instructions:
- In a high-powered blender or food processor, combine the banana, strawberries, hemp seeds, and pea powder. Blend in the liquid, making sure all of the components are covered.
- Taste the combined mixture and adjust the sweetness as needed (if desired). To incorporate any sweetener, give the mixture another short blend.

57. Banana and Greens Delight Smoothie

Prep time: 5min | Serves: 4 | Difficulty: Moderate
Nutrition: Calories: 69 Kcal | Fat: 0.3 g | Protein:5 g | Carbohydrates: 14.1 g
Ingredients:
- 1 banana, cut up
- 2 cups baby spinach, chopped
- 1 apple, cored, peeled, and cut up
- 1 pear, cored, peeled, and cut up
- 2 cups water

Instructions:
- Blend all of the ingredients together in a blender or with a powerful hand blender.
- Blend until smooth, then serve.

58. Lovely Bones Juice

Prep time: 5min | Serves: 2 | Difficulty: Moderate
Nutrition: Calories: 125 kcal | Fat:7 g | Protein:4 g | Carbohydrates:19 g
Ingredients:
- 2 apples, quartered
- 5 kale leaves
- 1 handful parsley (about 1/2 cup)
- Juice of 1/4 of a lemon (about 1/16 cup)
- 1-inch ginger
- 1 celery stalk

Instructions:
- Alternatively, you can chop the ingredients, combine them in a blender, and then filter the liquid through a nut milk bag (for more information on this procedure, see the nearby sidebar "Juicer or nut milk bag: That is the question").
- Fill glasses with the mixture and enjoy.

59. Ginger Love!

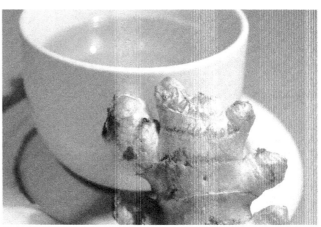

Prep time: 5min | Serves: 2 | Difficulty: Moderate
Nutrition: Calories: 102 Kcal | Fat: 13 g | Protein: 16 g | Carbohydrates: 3 g
Ingredients:
- 1/4 inch ginger
- 2 apples, quartered
- Juice of 1/2 a lemon (about 1/8 cup)

Instructions:
- Using a juicer, puree the ginger and then the quartered apples, or chop, combine, and filter through a nut milk bag.
- Serve with a squeeze of lemon juice.

60. Pick Me Up

Prep time: 5min | Serves: 3 | Difficulty: Moderate
Nutrition: Calories: 161 kcal | Fat: 2g | Protein: 9.5g | Carbohydrates: 25 g
Ingredients:
- 1 bunch cilantro (about 12 ounces)
- 3 apples, cored and quartered
- 1 medium cucumber, cut lengthwise 8 to 10 celery stalks
- Juice of 3 lemons (about 3/4 cup)

Instructions:
- Cilantro, apple, cucumber, and celery can be juiced or chopped, blended, and strained through a nut milk bag.
- Serve with a squeeze of lemon juice.

61. Soaking Nuts and Seeds

Prep time: 5min | Serves: 1 | Difficulty: Moderate
Nutrition: Calories: 165 kcal | Fat: 1.8 g | Protein:12 g | Carbohydrates:11 g
Ingredients:
- 1 cup nuts or seeds of your choice
- 1/4 teaspoon of sea salt Water (enough to cover nuts/seeds)

Instructions:
- Set aside after rinsing the nuts or seeds three times in a fine strainer.
- In a dish or other soaking container, combine the salt and water, then add the nuts/ seeds. Seeds should be soaked for at least 4 hours, while nuts should be soaked for at least 8 hours. Remove the nuts/seeds from the soaking liquid and thoroughly rinse them with fresh water.

62. Cashew Milk

Prep time: 5min | Serves: 3 | Difficulty: Moderate
Nutrition: Calories: 102 Kcal | Fat: 13 g | Protein: 16 g | Carbohydrates: 3 g
Ingredients:
- 1 cup raw cashews, soaked (see Soaking Nuts and Seeds earlier in this chapter)
- 10 honey dates, soaked for 1 hour 2 cups water

Instructions:
- Blend the cashews and honey dates with 1 cup of water in a high-powered blender until a thick cream forms. Blend on high for 2 minutes after slowly adding the balance of the water.
- Using a nut milk bag, strain the mixture and collect the milk in a bowl.

63. Essential Nut Milk

Prep time: 10min | Serves: 2 | Difficulty: Moderate
Nutrition: Calories: 60 Kcal | Fat: 0.3 g | Protein: 1 g | Carbohydrates: 14.1 g
Ingredients:
- 1/2 cup raw almonds, shelled and soaked
- 2 cup liquid
- 1 banana, ripe, or 1 teaspoon maple syrup or honey (optional)

Instructions
- One cup water, 1 banana, maple syrup, honey, or agave nectar (if desired). To make a smooth cream, blend for another 1 to 2 minutes. Blend for 2 minutes while gently adding the second cup of water to the blender.
- Line the strainer with a cheesecloth or a cloth coffee filter and place it over a large basin.
- Pour the milk slowly into the sieve and let it filter through, using a spatula if necessary to increase the flow. Pull the cheesecloth's edges together to make a ball, and then squeeze to extract another half cup of nut milk.

64. A Fine Pot of Tea

Prep time: 12min | Serves: 4 | Difficulty: Moderate
Nutrition: Calories:88 kcal | Fat:2 g | Protein: 3 g | Carbohydrates:13 g
Ingredients:
- 4 tablespoons peppermint (dry)
- 12 teaspoons peppermint (fresh) 4 c. boiling water
- 1 tsp. honey (or more to taste)

Instructions
- Fill a teapot halfway with boiling water and add your herbs.
- Fill the pot with water. Cover the hole immediately to prevent steam from escaping and carrying the flavor and healing with it.
- Steep the herbs for 10 minutes before straining the tea into a cup through a fine-mesh tea strainer. For taste, add the honey.

65. Silky Chai (Tea) Nut Milk

Prep time: 5min | Serves: 6 | Difficulty: Moderate
Nutrition: Calories: 60 Kcal | Fat: 0.3 g | Protein: 1 g | Carbohydrates: 14.1 g
Ingredients:
- 2 cups raw almonds, soaked (see Soaking Nuts and Seeds earlier in this chapter)
- 5 to 6 cups pure water
- 1 teaspoon vanilla extract
- 2 tablespoons raw honey or agave or 6 pitted dates (optional)
- 1 teaspoon nutmeg, or to taste
- 1 1/2 teaspoon cinnamon, or to taste
- 1/2 teaspoon cardamom, or to taste

Instructions:
- In a blender, combine the soaked almonds and water and blend until the mixture is liquefied.
- Strain the mixture through a nut milk bag over a large mixing basin.
- Return the milk to the blender, add the remaining ingredients, and blend briefly to combine everything.

66. Lemonade

Prep time: 15min | Serves: 6 | Difficulty: Moderate
Nutrition: Calories: 31 kcal | Fat: 0.4 g | Protein:0.6 g | Carbohydrates:9 g
Ingredients:
- 6 lemons' juice (about 112 cups)
- 6 quarts of cold water 12 to 1 teaspoon stevia, or
- 1 cup Just Like Sugar

Instructions
- Combine the lemon juice, water, and just like Sugar or stevia in a big pitcher.
- Serve the lemonade over ice, garnished with a lemon slice or two.

67. Rich and Moist Chocolate Cake

Prep time: 45min | Serves: 6 | Difficulty: Moderate
Nutrition: Calories: 211 kcal | Fat:16 g | Protein:7 g | Carbohydrates:43 g

Ingredients:
- 1/2 cup brown rice flour
- 1/4 cup millet or sorghum flour
- 1/4 cup potato starch
- 1/4 cup tapioca flour
- 1/2 cup plus
- 2 tablespoons unsweetened cocoa powder
- 1 teaspoon xanthan gum
- 1 1/4 teaspoons baking soda
- 1 cup maple crystals
- 3/4 teaspoon sea salt
- 1 tablespoon organic vanilla
- 1/2 cup almond or rice milk
- 1 /2 cup Earth Balance margarine, room temperature, plus more for pan greasing
- 1 egg, beaten
- 3/4 cup brewed coffee, room temperature

Instructions
- Preheat the oven to 350 degrees Fahrenheit. Using margarine or coconut oil, grease an 8-inch round cake pan, adding and greasing a round layer of parchment paper if your pan likes to cling.
- In a large mixing bowl, combine the flours, potato starch, cocoa powder, xanthan gum, baking soda, maple crystals, and salt.
- Mix the vanilla, milk, margarine, and egg in a separate large mixing bowl at low speed using a hand mixer. Continue to mix with the hand mixer after adding the dry ingredients. Blend in the coffee until well combined.
- Smooth out the top of the batter in the cake pan. Preheat the oven to 350°F and bake for 30–35 minutes, rotating the pan halfway through. When a toothpick inserted in the center comes out clean, remove it from the oven.

68. Pineapple Upside-Down Cake

Prep time: 45min | Serves: 6 | Difficulty: Moderate
Nutrition: Calories: 181 kcal | Fat:9.5 g | Protein:12 g | Carbohydrates:34 g

Ingredients:
- 2 cups almond flour, or more as needed for consistency
- 3 eggs
- 4 tablespoons butter, melted
- 1/2 cup honey
- 3/4 teaspoon organic vanilla extract
- 1/4 teaspoon cinnamon powder
- 1/2-pound fresh pineapple, thinly sliced (about 8 slices)

Instructions
- Preheat oven to 350 degrees Fahrenheit. Using butter, grease a 9-by-12-inch baking dish.

- By hand or with a hand mixer, combine the almond flour, eggs, butter, honey, vanilla, and cinnamon until smooth. If required, add extra almond flour to ensure the dough isn't too thin.
- In the bottom of the baking dish, layer the pineapple pieces. Pour the cake batter into the pan and smooth it out evenly. Bake for 30–40 minutes, or until a toothpick inserted in the middle comes out clean.

69. Cherry Cobbler

Prep time: 15min | Serves: 8 | Difficulty: Moderate
Nutrition: Calories: 274 Kcal | Fat: 18 g | Protein: 23 g | Carbohydrates: 6 g

Ingredients:
- 1 1/2 cups shredded coconut
- 1 1/2 cups walnuts
- 1/2 teaspoon salt
- 1/3 cup plus
- 1/2 cup pitted dates
- 3 cups frozen cherries, thawed and drained
- 2 teaspoons lemon juice
- 1/8 teaspoon cinnamon

Instructions
- In a food processor, combine the coconut, walnuts, and salt. 1 1/3 cup pitted dates, processed one at a time until coarse crumbs form; set aside.
- Combine 1 cup of the cherries, the rest of the dates, the lemon juice, and the cinnamon in a blender. Blend until the mixture is chunky. Combine the remaining 2 cups of cherries in a large mixing bowl.
- Fill a square glass baking dish halfway with the cherry mixture. Refrigerate until ready to serve, then top with crumble topping.

70. Vegan Lemon Meringue Pie

Prep time: 5min | Serves: 8 | Difficulty: Moderate
Nutrition: Calories: 278 kcal | Fat:13 g | Protein:8 g | Carbohydrates:13 g

Ingredients:
- 2 cups cashews, soaked
- Pinch of sea salt
- 4 tablespoons unsweetened coconut milk
- Juice of 1 lemon (about 1/4 cup)
- 2 to 4 tablespoons maple or agave syrup (optional)
- 4 to 8 tablespoons water
- Lemon Meringue Pie Crust (see the following recipe)
- 1/4 cup unsweetened shredded coconut

Instructions
- In a blender, combine the salt, coconut milk, cashews, lemon juice, syrup (if desired), and half of the water until a thick, creamy consistency is achieved; add the remaining water toward the

end to reach the desired consistency without causing the filling to separate.

- Drizzle the filling over the crust and top with shredded coconut. Refrigerate the pie for 30 minutes before cutting to allow it to firm up.

71. Lemon Meringue Pie Crust

Prep time: 5min | Serves: 8 | Difficulty: Moderate
Nutrition: Calories: 141 Kcal | Fat: 18 g | Protein: 6 g | Carbohydrates: 14 g
Ingredients:

- 4 tablespoons ground flaxseed
- 4 tablespoons brown rice protein powder
- 1/2 teaspoon stevia
- 1 to 2 teaspoons flaxseed oil
- 1 teaspoon cinnamon
- 1 teaspoon water

Instructions

- In a 9-inch pie pan, combine the ground flaxseed, brown rice protein powder, stevia, flax seed oil, cinnamon, and water.
- Cover the bottom of the pie plate with the mixture.

Unit Conversion Chart

Conversion Chart

Oven Temperatures

No Fan	Fan Forced	Fahrenheit
120°c	100°c	250°c
150°c	130°c	300°c
160°c	140°c	325°c
180°c	160°c	350°c
190°c	170°c	375°c
200°c	180°c	400°c
230°c	210°c	450°c
250°c	230°c	500°c

SR Flour = Self Raising

Cup and Spoons

Cup	Metric
¼ Cup	60ml
1/3 Cup	80ml
½ Cup	125ml
1 Cup	250ml
Spoon	**Metric**
¼ Teaspoon	1.25ml
½ Teaspoon	2.5ml
1 Teaspoon	5ml
2 Teaspoons	10ml
1 Tablespoon	20ml

Liquids

Cup	Metric	Imperial
	30ml	1 fl oz
¼ Cup	60ml	2 fl oz
1/3 Cup	80ml	3 ½ fl oz
	100ml	2 ¾ fl oz
½ Cup	125ml	4 fl oz
	150ml	5 fl oz
¾ Cup	180ml	6 fl oz
	200ml	7 fl oz
1 Cup	250ml	8 ¾ fl oz
1 ¼ Cups	310ml	10 ½ fl oz
1 ½ Cups	375ml	13 fl oz
1 ¾ Cups	430ml	15 fl oz
	475ml	16 fl oz
2 Cups	500ml	17 fl oz
2 ½ Cups	625ml	21 ½ fl oz
3 Cups	750ml	26 fl oz
4 Cups	1L	35 fl oz
5 Cups	1.25L	44 fl oz
6 Cups	1.5L	52 fl oz
8 Cups	2L	70 fl oz
10 Cups	2.5L	88 fl oz

Mass

Metric	Imperial
10g	¼ oz
15g	½ oz
30g	1 oz
60g	2 oz
90g	3 oz
125g	4 oz (¼ lb)
155g	5 oz
185g	6 oz
220g	7 oz
250g	8 oz (½ lb)
280g	9 oz
315g	10 oz
345g	11 oz
375g	12 oz (¾ lb)
410g	13 oz
440g	14 oz
470g	15 oz
500g	16 oz (1 lb)
750g	24 oz (1 ½ lb)
1kg	32 oz (2 lb)
1.5kg	48 oz (3 lb)

How to Read Food Labels Without Being Tricked

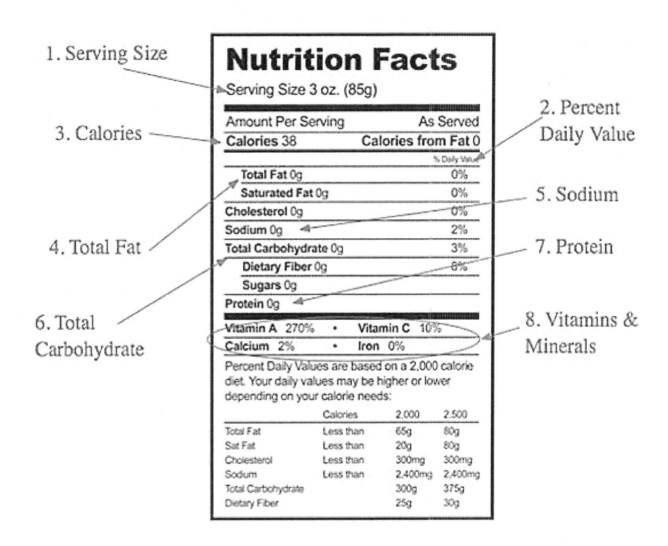

1. Serving Size

3. Calories

4. Total Fat

6. Total Carbohydrate

2. Percent Daily Value

5. Sodium

7. Protein

8. Vitamins & Minerals

30-Day Meal Plan

Day	Breakfast	Lunch	Dinner
1	Bacon and Zucchini Crustless Quiche	Baked Macaroni and Cheese	Smoked Tuna Risotto
2	Scrambled Eggs	Pesto -Baked Chicken	Lasagna
3	Omelet Wraps	Chana Masala	Beef Risotto with Whole Grain Mustard and Spinach
4	Light Omelet with Chicken and Spinach	Chicken Korma	Asian Duck and Pea Risotto
5	Roasted Sweet Potato and Bell Pepper Frittata	Asian-Style Chicken Noodle Soup	Lamb and Eggplant Risotto with Middle Eastern Spices
6	Cheese and Herb Scones	Company Roast Chicken	Grilled Snapper on Lemon and Spinach Risotto
7	Chocolate Scones	Easy Chicken Enchilada Casserole	Chicken Risotto with Roasted Squash and Sage
8	Blueberry Pancakes	Baked Eggplant Parmesan	Chicken Fried Rice
9	Pumpkin Muffins	Italian Wedding Soup	Pizza Crust
10	Banana–Chocolate Chip Muffins	Polenta Pizza Squares	Smoked Salmon
11	Vanilla-Rhubarb Muffins	Portuguese Fisherman's Stew	Autumn Veggie
12	Ginger and Pecan Muffins	Shrimp Fried Rice	Pesto Margherita
13	Cheesy Corn Muffins	Skillet Buffalo Chicken and Spinach Salad	Potato and Rosemary
14	Spinach and Tomato Muffins	Maple -Bourbon Baked Salmon	Grilled Fish with Coconut-Lime Rice
15	High-Fiber Muffins with Zucchini and Sunflower Seeds	Spaghetti and Meatballs	Baked Atlantic Salmon on Soft Blue Cheese Polenta
16	Chili-Cheese Muffins	Marinated Steak Kebabs	Chicken with Olives, Sun-Dried Tomato, and Basil with Mediterranean Vegetables
17	Smoothie Magic	Taco Salad Deluxe	Pan-Fried Chicken with Brown Butter–Sage Sauce

18	Golden French Toast	Traffic Light Chili	Chile Chicken Stir-Fry
19	Sweet Potato Hash	Veggie Burger of Your Dreams	Spanish Chicken with Creamy Herbed Rice
20	Breakfast Scones	West African Sweet Potato Soup	Chicken and Vegetable Curry
21	Hand-Milled Gluten-Free Breakfast Cereal	Pasta with Fresh Tomato, Olives, and Pecorino	Chicken Parmigiana
22	Caramelized Banana and Date "Porridge" (SCD)	Tuna Macaroni and Cheese Bake	Baked Chicken and Mozzarella Croquettes
23	Soaked Oats Porridge	Speedy Spaghetti Bolognese	Tarragon Chicken Terrine
24	Strawberries and Cream Oatmeal	Penne with Meatballs	Soy-Infused Roast Chicken
25	Cinnamon Pancakes with Ghee	Seafood Pasta with Salsa Verde	Swiss Chicken with Mustard Sauce
26	Gluten-Free Pumpkin Spice Bread	Smoked Chicken Pasta	Chicken Pockets
27	Shannon's Non-Dairy "Yogurt."	Vegetable Pasta Bake	Mild Lamb Curry
28	Cheese Omelet	Roasted Lamb Racks on Buttered Mashed Rutabaga	Pork and Vegetable Fricassee with Buttered Quinoa
29	Vanilla-Rhubarb Muffins	Chicken Korma	Lasagna
30	Smoothie Magic	Company Roast Chicken	Chicken Fried Rice

1. How is irritable bowel syndrome (IBS) diagnosed?

A skilled medical practitioner determines the diagnosis of IBS. When alternative medical explanations have been ruled out, the diagnosis is based on the Rome III criteria for recurring abdominal pain or discomfort for at least three days per month for the previous three months, linked with two or more of the following symptoms:

Defecation relieves pain; commencement of pain is linked to a change in bowel frequency (either diarrhea or constipation); onset of pain is linked to a change in stool appearance (loose, watery or pellet-like).

2. Hard cheese is suitable for Lactose intolerant or not?

Lactose content in aged cheeses is either negligible or inadequate to create difficulties for most people. The FODMAP Friendly laboratory testing criteria have been passed by hard cheeses.

3. Can I not consume any food containing almonds?

No, it depends on how many almonds are in a serving of the almond-containing food product. If a product carries the FODMAP Friendly designation, it signifies that the fructan content per serving is suitable for people on a low FODMAP diet.

4. Do FODMAP friendly and Fructose Friendly labelled foods are same?

No, FODMAP Friendly certified goods are the only ones that have met the requirements of the ACCC-approved certified trademark.

5. What happens when FODMAPs are consumed?

The bacteria that live in your intestines quickly ferment FODMAPs. They draw more water into your stomach, which might lead to an increase in gas production. This causes bloating and distension, as well as changes in the way your gut muscles contract. Irritable bowel syndrome (IBS) sufferers may have gastrointestinal pain as a result (such as diarrhea and constipation). FODMAPs are usually tolerated well by those who do not have IBS.

6. How true is that cooking changes FODMAPs so that they are easily digested?

Canning and preserving foods under acidic conditions (such as pickling) had the biggest influence on FODMAP levels in meals, according to our findings. Water-soluble FODMAPs (GOS) seep into the brine combination from canned legumes (lentils and chickpeas). If you're on a low-FODMAP diet, discard the brine and carefully wash your beans before eating.

The combination of acid (from the vinegar) and FODMAP leaching drastically lowered the fructan content of pickled artichokes (a poorly absorbed carbohydrate that comes within the FODMAP umbrella).

While extremely high temperatures can also break down FODMAPs, we've found that the degree to which this happens varies greatly.

7. Can I make food tasty without adding onion or garlic?

Because garlic and onions are high in FODMAP fructan, they are not permitted on the Low FODMAP Diet. On the other hand, onions and garlic may be employed to flavour your cuisine.

Because FODMAPs aren't soluble in oil, utilising garlic-infused oil to reintroduce Flavor to your meals is a great way to do so. This may be done by sautéing whole garlic cloves (not crushed or finely minced) in oil for 1-2 minutes to let the oil flavour emerge. Remove and discard the garlic clove after that because it will still be high in FODMAPs.

8. What makes dried fruits high FODMAP but fresh fruit low FODMAP?

To create dried fruit, you must first remove the water from the fresh fruit. During this process, all sugars (and hence FODMAPs) contained in the raw fruit are concentrated. Fructans, which aren't found in fresh fruit, have also been detected in dried fruits.

When compared to its original size, dried fruit shrinks dramatically. As a result, it's easy to consume too much fruit without recognizing it! That is why portion sizes are so important.

Some dried fruits, such as cranberries, are high in FODMAPs only if consumed in large amounts. Dried cranberries are low in FODMAPs and should be tolerated in modest doses by most people with IBS.

9. Can you list meat in FODMAPs?

Because animal protein sources such as meat, poultry, fish, and eggs contain very little or no carbohydrate, FODMAPs are comparatively low. However, high FODMAP ingredients such as bread crumbs, onions, garlic, marinades, sauces, and gravies should be avoided while making these recipes. Because animal protein sources such as meat, poultry, fish, and eggs contain very little or no carbohydrate, FODMAPs are comparatively low. However, high FODMAP ingredients such as breadcrumbs, onions, garlic, marinades, and sauces/gravies should be avoided while making these recipes.

Conclusion

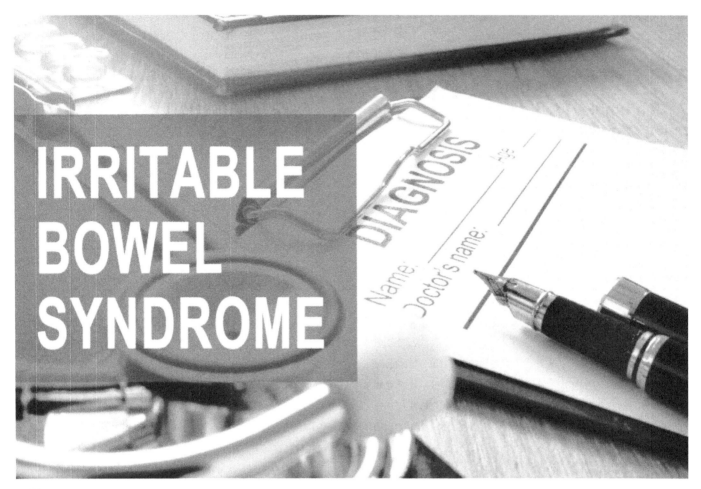

For years, IBS has been a difficult condition for individuals and their doctors. We've seen a lot of medications, and food fads come and go. So it's good that Sue Shepherd and Peter Gibson have created a diet based on strong scientific and physiological processes for many IBS patients. The low-FODMAP diet may be customized and adapted to each patient when combined with proper medical care, which includes testing for small intestine bacterial overgrowth and fructose and lactose intolerance. This book also has a wide range of mouth-watering recipes that can surely guide about how to properly enjoy in the diet.

Made in the USA
Coppell, TX
10 October 2022

83687754R00098